FREE Study Skills Videos/DVD Offer

Dear Customer,

Thank you for your purchase from Mometrix! We consider it an honor and a privilege that you have purchased our product and we want to ensure your satisfaction.

As part of our ongoing effort to meet the needs of test takers, we have developed a set of Study Skills Videos that we would like to give you for FREE. These videos cover our *best practices* for getting ready for your exam, from how to use our study materials to how to best prepare for the day of the test.

All that we ask is that you email us with feedback that would describe your experience so far with our product. Good, bad, or indifferent, we want to know what you think!

To get your FREE Study Skills Videos, you can use the **QR code** below, or send us an **email** at studyvideos@mometrix.com with *FREE VIDEOS* in the subject line and the following information in the body of the email:

- The name of the product you purchased.
- Your product rating on a scale of 1-5, with 5 being the highest rating.
- Your feedback. It can be long, short, or anything in between. We just want to know your impressions and experience so far with our product. (Good feedback might include how our study material met your needs and ways we might be able to make it even better. You could highlight features that you found helpful or features that you think we should add.)

If you have any questions or concerns, please don't hesitate to contact me directly.

Thanks again!

Sincerely,

Jay Willis
Vice President
jay.willis@mometrix.com
1-800-673-8175

SCAN HERE

Mometrix
TEST PREPARATION

Mometrix

TEST PREPARATION

Maternal Newborn Nursing Exam Secrets Study Guide

Exam Review and Practice Test for the Maternal Newborn Nurse Test

Written and edited by Mometrix Test Prep

Mometrix offers volume discount pricing to institutions. For more information or a price quote, please contact our sales department at sales@mometrix.com or 888-248-1219.

Hardback
ISBN 13: 9781516718764
ISBN 10: 1516718763

Dear Future Exam Success Story

First of all, **THANK YOU** for purchasing Mometrix study materials!

Second, congratulations! You are one of the few determined test-takers who are committed to doing whatever it takes to excel on your exam. **You have come to the right place.** We developed these study materials with one goal in mind: to deliver you the information you need in a format that's concise and easy to use.

In addition to optimizing your guide for the content of the test, we've outlined our recommended steps for breaking down the preparation process into small, attainable goals so you can make sure you stay on track.

We've also analyzed the entire test-taking process, identifying the most common pitfalls and showing how you can overcome them and be ready for any curveball the test throws you.

Standardized testing is one of the biggest obstacles on your road to success, which only increases the importance of doing well in the high-pressure, high-stakes environment of test day. Your results on this test could have a significant impact on your future, and this guide provides the information and practical advice to help you achieve your full potential on test day.

Your success is our success

We would love to hear from you! If you would like to share the story of your exam success or if you have any questions or comments in regard to our products, please contact us at **800-673-8175** or **support@mometrix.com**.

Thanks again for your business and we wish you continued success!

Sincerely,
The Mometrix Test Preparation Team

TABLE OF CONTENTS

Introduction

Thank you for purchasing this resource! You have made the choice to prepare yourself for a test that could have a huge impact on your future, and this guide is designed to help you be fully ready for test day. Obviously, it's important to have a solid understanding of the test material, but you also need to be prepared for the unique environment and stressors of the test, so that you can perform to the best of your abilities.

For this purpose, the first section that appears in this guide is the **Secret Keys**. We've devoted countless hours to meticulously researching what works and what doesn't, and we've boiled down our findings to the five most impactful steps you can take to improve your performance on the test. We start at the beginning with study planning and move through the preparation process, all the way to the testing strategies that will help you get the most out of what you know when you're finally sitting in front of the test.

We recommend that you start preparing for your test as far in advance as possible. However, if you've bought this guide as a last-minute study resource and only have a few days before your test, we recommend that you skip over the first two Secret Keys since they address a long-term study plan.

If you struggle with **test anxiety**, we strongly encourage you to check out our recommendations for how you can overcome it. Test anxiety is a formidable foe, but it can be beaten, and we want to make sure you have the tools you need to defeat it.

Secret Key #1 – Plan Big, Study Small

There's a lot riding on your performance. If you want to ace this test, you're going to need to keep your skills sharp and the material fresh in your mind. You need a plan that lets you review everything you need to know while still fitting in your schedule. We'll break this strategy down into three categories.

Information Organization

Start with the information you already have: the official test outline. From this, you can make a complete list of all the concepts you need to cover before the test. Organize these concepts into groups that can be studied together, and create a list of any related vocabulary you need to learn so you can brush up on any difficult terms. You'll want to keep this vocabulary list handy once you actually start studying since you may need to add to it along the way.

Time Management

Once you have your set of study concepts, decide how to spread them out over the time you have left before the test. Break your study plan into small, clear goals so you have a manageable task for each day and know exactly what you're doing. Then just focus on one small step at a time. When you manage your time this way, you don't need to spend hours at a time studying. Studying a small block of content for a short period each day helps you retain information better and avoid stressing over how much you have left to do. You can relax knowing that you have a plan to cover everything in time. In order for this strategy to be effective though, you have to start studying early and stick to your schedule. Avoid the exhaustion and futility that comes from last-minute cramming!

Study Environment

The environment you study in has a big impact on your learning. Studying in a coffee shop, while probably more enjoyable, is not likely to be as fruitful as studying in a quiet room. It's important to keep distractions to a minimum. You're only planning to study for a short block of time, so make the most of it. Don't pause to check your phone or get up to find a snack. It's also important to **avoid multitasking**. Research has consistently shown that multitasking will make your studying dramatically less effective. Your study area should also be comfortable and well-lit so you don't have the distraction of straining your eyes or sitting on an uncomfortable chair.

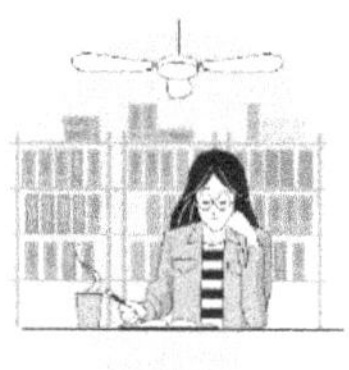

The time of day you study is also important. You want to be rested and alert. Don't wait until just before bedtime. Study when you'll be most likely to comprehend and remember. Even better, if you know what time of day your test will be, set that time aside for study. That way your brain will be used to working on that subject at that specific time and you'll have a better chance of recalling information.

Finally, it can be helpful to team up with others who are studying for the same test. Your actual studying should be done in as isolated an environment as possible, but the work of organizing the information and setting up the study plan can be divided up. In between study sessions, you can discuss with your teammates the concepts that you're all studying and quiz each other on the details. Just be sure that your teammates are as serious about the test as you are. If you find that your study time is being replaced with social time, you might need to find a new team.

Secret Key #2 – Make Your Studying Count

You're devoting a lot of time and effort to preparing for this test, so you want to be absolutely certain it will pay off. This means doing more than just reading the content and hoping you can remember it on test day. It's important to make every minute of study count. There are two main areas you can focus on to make your studying count.

Retention

It doesn't matter how much time you study if you can't remember the material. You need to make sure you are retaining the concepts. To check your retention of the information you're learning, try recalling it at later times with minimal prompting. Try carrying around flashcards and glance at one or two from time to time or ask a friend who's also studying for the test to quiz you.

To enhance your retention, look for ways to put the information into practice so that you can apply it rather than simply recalling it. If you're using the information in practical ways, it will be much easier to remember. Similarly, it helps to solidify a concept in your mind if you're not only reading it to yourself but also explaining it to someone else. Ask a friend to let you teach them about a concept you're a little shaky on (or speak aloud to an imaginary audience if necessary). As you try to summarize, define, give examples, and answer your friend's questions, you'll understand the concepts better and they will stay with you longer. Finally, step back for a big picture view and ask yourself how each piece of information fits with the whole subject. When you link the different concepts together and see them working together as a whole, it's easier to remember the individual components.

Finally, practice showing your work on any multi-step problems, even if you're just studying. Writing out each step you take to solve a problem will help solidify the process in your mind, and you'll be more likely to remember it during the test.

Modality

Modality simply refers to the means or method by which you study. Choosing a study modality that fits your own individual learning style is crucial. No two people learn best in exactly the same way, so it's important to know your strengths and use them to your advantage.

For example, if you learn best by visualization, focus on visualizing a concept in your mind and draw an image or a diagram. Try color-coding your notes, illustrating them, or creating symbols that will trigger your mind to recall a learned concept. If you learn best by hearing or discussing information, find a study partner who learns the same way or read aloud to yourself. Think about how to put the information in your own words. Imagine that you are giving a lecture on the topic and record yourself so you can listen to it later.

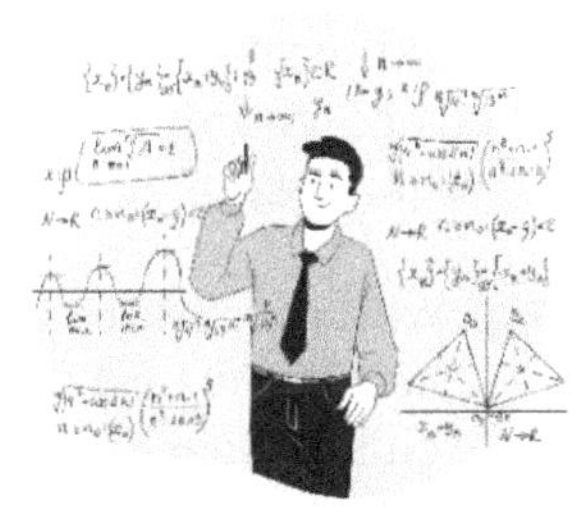

For any learning style, flashcards can be helpful. Organize the information so you can take advantage of spare moments to review. Underline key words or phrases. Use different colors for different categories. Mnemonic devices (such as creating a short list in which every item starts with the same letter) can also help with retention. Find what works best for you and use it to store the information in your mind most effectively and easily.

Secret Key #3 – Practice the Right Way

Your success on test day depends not only on how many hours you put into preparing, but also on whether you prepared the right way. It's good to check along the way to see if your studying is paying off. One of the most effective ways to do this is by taking practice tests to evaluate your progress. Practice tests are useful because they show exactly where you need to improve. Every time you take a practice test, pay special attention to these three groups of questions:

- The questions you got wrong
- The questions you had to guess on, even if you guessed right
- The questions you found difficult or slow to work through

This will show you exactly what your weak areas are, and where you need to devote more study time. Ask yourself why each of these questions gave you trouble. Was it because you didn't understand the material? Was it because you didn't remember the vocabulary? Do you need more repetitions on this type of question to build speed and confidence? Dig into those questions and figure out how you can strengthen your weak areas as you go back to review the material.

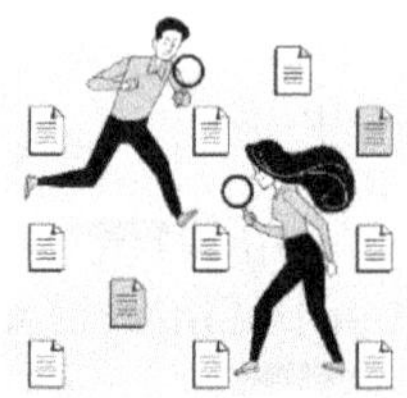

Additionally, many practice tests have a section explaining the answer choices. It can be tempting to read the explanation and think that you now have a good understanding of the concept. However, an explanation likely only covers part of the question's broader context. Even if the explanation makes perfect sense, **go back and investigate** every concept related to the question until you're positive you have a thorough understanding.

As you go along, keep in mind that the practice test is just that: practice. Memorizing these questions and answers will not be very helpful on the actual test because it is unlikely to have any of the same exact questions. If you only know the right answers to the sample questions, you won't be prepared for the real thing. **Study the concepts** until you understand them fully, and then you'll be able to answer any question that shows up on the test.

It's important to wait on the practice tests until you're ready. If you take a test on your first day of study, you may be overwhelmed by the amount of material covered and how much you need to learn. Work up to it gradually.

On test day, you'll need to be prepared for answering questions, managing your time, and using the test-taking strategies you've learned. It's a lot to balance, like a mental marathon that will have a big impact on your future. Like training for a marathon, you'll need to start slowly and work your way up. When test day arrives, you'll be ready.

Start with the strategies you've read in the first two Secret Keys—plan your course and study in the way that works best for you. If you have time, consider using multiple study resources to get different approaches to the same concepts. It can be helpful to see difficult concepts from more than one angle. Then find a good source for practice tests. Many times, the test website will suggest potential study resources or provide sample tests.

Practice Test Strategy

If you're able to find at least three practice tests, we recommend this strategy:

Untimed and Open-Book Practice

Take the first test with no time constraints and with your notes and study guide handy. Take your time and focus on applying the strategies you've learned.

Timed and Open-Book Practice

Take the second practice test open-book as well, but set a timer and practice pacing yourself to finish in time.

Timed and Closed-Book Practice

Take any other practice tests as if it were test day. Set a timer and put away your study materials. Sit at a table or desk in a quiet room, imagine yourself at the testing center, and answer questions as quickly and accurately as possible.

Keep repeating timed and closed-book tests on a regular basis until you run out of practice tests or it's time for the actual test. Your mind will be ready for the schedule and stress of test day, and you'll be able to focus on recalling the material you've learned.

Secret Key #4 – Pace Yourself

Once you're fully prepared for the material on the test, your biggest challenge on test day will be managing your time. Just knowing that the clock is ticking can make you panic even if you have plenty of time left. Work on pacing yourself so you can build confidence against the time constraints of the exam. Pacing is a difficult skill to master, especially in a high-pressure environment, so **practice is vital**.

Set time expectations for your pace based on how much time is available. For example, if a section has 60 questions and the time limit is 30 minutes, you know you have to average 30 seconds or less per question in order to answer them all. Although 30 seconds is the hard limit, set 25 seconds per question as your goal, so you reserve extra time to spend on harder questions. When you budget extra time for the harder questions, you no longer have any reason to stress when those questions take longer to answer.

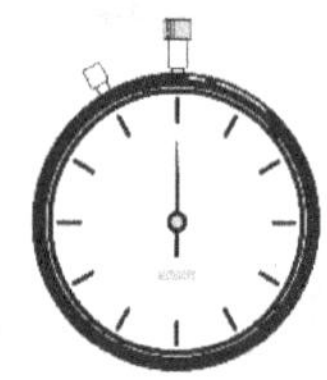

Don't let this time expectation distract you from working through the test at a calm, steady pace, but keep it in mind so you don't spend too much time on any one question. Recognize that taking extra time on one question you don't understand may keep you from answering two that you do understand later in the test. If your time limit for a question is up and you're still not sure of the answer, mark it and move on, and come back to it later if the time and the test format allow. If the testing format doesn't allow you to return to earlier questions, just make an educated guess; then put it out of your mind and move on.

On the easier questions, be careful not to rush. It may seem wise to hurry through them so you have more time for the challenging ones, but it's not worth missing one if you know the concept and just didn't take the time to read the question fully. Work efficiently but make sure you understand the question and have looked at all of the answer choices, since more than one may seem right at first.

Even if you're paying attention to the time, you may find yourself a little behind at some point. You should speed up to get back on track, but do so wisely. Don't panic; just take a few seconds less on each question until you're caught up. Don't guess without thinking, but do look through the answer choices and eliminate any you know are wrong. If you can get down to two choices, it is often worthwhile to guess from those. Once you've chosen an answer, move on and don't dwell on any that you skipped or had to hurry through. If a question was taking too long, chances are it was one of the harder ones, so you weren't as likely to get it right anyway.

On the other hand, if you find yourself getting ahead of schedule, it may be beneficial to slow down a little. The more quickly you work, the more likely you are to make a careless mistake that will affect your score. You've budgeted time for each question, so don't be afraid to spend that time. Practice an efficient but careful pace to get the most out of the time you have.

Secret Key #5 – Have a Plan for Guessing

When you're taking the test, you may find yourself stuck on a question. Some of the answer choices seem better than others, but you don't see the one answer choice that is obviously correct. What do you do?

The scenario described above is very common, yet most test takers have not effectively prepared for it. Developing and practicing a plan for guessing may be one of the single most effective uses of your time as you get ready for the exam.

In developing your plan for guessing, there are three questions to address:

- When should you start the guessing process?
- How should you narrow down the choices?
- Which answer should you choose?

When to Start the Guessing Process

Unless your plan for guessing is to select C every time (which, despite its merits, is not what we recommend), you need to leave yourself enough time to apply your answer elimination strategies. Since you have a limited amount of time for each question, that means that if you're going to give yourself the best shot at guessing correctly, you have to decide quickly whether or not you will guess.

Of course, the best-case scenario is that you don't have to guess at all, so first, see if you can answer the question based on your knowledge of the subject and basic reasoning skills. Focus on the key words in the question and try to jog your memory of related topics. Give yourself a chance to bring the knowledge to mind, but once you realize that you don't have (or you can't access) the knowledge you need to answer the question, it's time to start the guessing process.

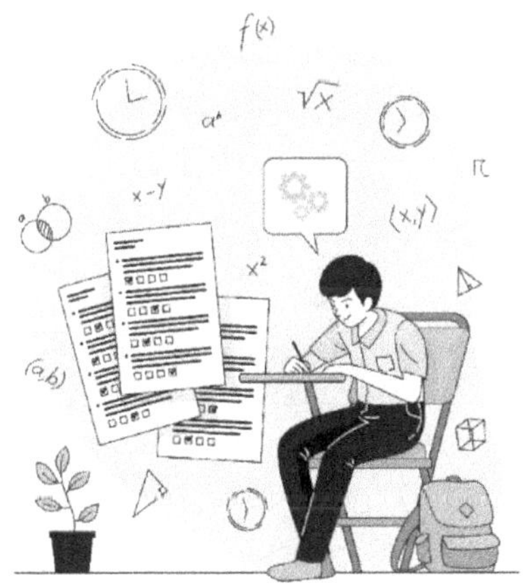

It's almost always better to start the guessing process too early than too late. It only takes a few seconds to remember something and answer the question from knowledge. Carefully eliminating wrong answer choices takes longer. Plus, going through the process of eliminating answer choices can actually help jog your memory.

Summary: Start the guessing process as soon as you decide that you can't answer the question based on your knowledge.

How to Narrow Down the Choices

The next chapter in this book (**Test-Taking Strategies**) includes a wide range of strategies for how to approach questions and how to look for answer choices to eliminate. You will definitely want to read those carefully, practice them, and figure out which ones work best for you. Here though, we're going to address a mindset rather than a particular strategy.

Your odds of guessing an answer correctly depend on how many options you are choosing from.

Number of options left	5	4	3	2	1
Odds of guessing correctly	20%	25%	33%	50%	100%

You can see from this chart just how valuable it is to be able to eliminate incorrect answers and make an educated guess, but there are two things that many test takers do that cause them to miss out on the benefits of guessing:

- Accidentally eliminating the correct answer
- Selecting an answer based on an impression

We'll look at the first one here, and the second one in the next section.

To avoid accidentally eliminating the correct answer, we recommend a thought exercise called **the $5 challenge**. In this challenge, you only eliminate an answer choice from contention if you are willing to bet $5 on it being wrong. Why $5? Five dollars is a small but not insignificant amount of money. It's an amount you could afford to lose but wouldn't want to throw away. And while losing $5 once might not hurt too much, doing it twenty times will set you back $100. In the same way, each small decision you make—eliminating a choice here, guessing on a question there—won't by itself impact your score very much, but when you put them all together, they can make a big difference. By holding each answer choice elimination decision to a higher standard, you can reduce the risk of accidentally eliminating the correct answer.

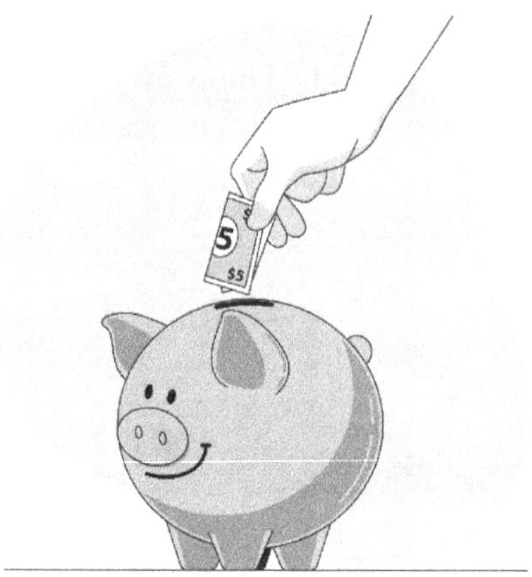

The $5 challenge can also be applied in a positive sense: If you are willing to bet $5 that an answer choice *is* correct, go ahead and mark it as correct.

Summary: Only eliminate an answer choice if you are willing to bet $5 that it is wrong.

Which Answer to Choose

You're taking the test. You've run into a hard question and decided you'll have to guess. You've eliminated all the answer choices you're willing to bet $5 on. Now you have to pick an answer. Why do we even need to talk about this? Why can't you just pick whichever one you feel like when the time comes?

The answer to these questions is that if you don't come into the test with a plan, you'll rely on your impression to select an answer choice, and if you do that, you risk falling into a trap. The test writers know that everyone who takes their test will be guessing on some of the questions, so they intentionally write wrong answer choices to seem plausible. You still have to pick an answer though, and if the wrong answer choices are designed to look right, how can you ever be sure that you're not falling for their trap? The best solution we've found to this dilemma is to take the decision out of your hands entirely. Here is the process we recommend:

Once you've eliminated any choices that you are confident (willing to bet $5) are wrong, select the first remaining choice as your answer.

Whether you choose to select the first remaining choice, the second, or the last, the important thing is that you use some preselected standard. Using this approach guarantees that you will not be enticed into selecting an answer choice that looks right, because you are not basing your decision on how the answer choices look.

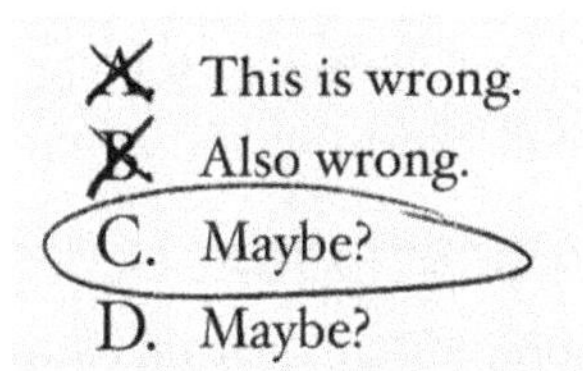

This is not meant to make you question your knowledge. Instead, it is to help you recognize the difference between your knowledge and your impressions. There's a huge difference between thinking an answer is right because of what you know, and thinking an answer is right because it looks or sounds like it should be right.

Summary: To ensure that your selection is appropriately random, make a predetermined selection from among all answer choices you have not eliminated.

Test-Taking Strategies

This section contains a list of test-taking strategies that you may find helpful as you work through the test. By taking what you know and applying logical thought, you can maximize your chances of answering any question correctly!

It is very important to realize that every question is different and every person is different: no single strategy will work on every question, and no single strategy will work for every person. That's why we've included all of them here, so you can try them out and determine which ones work best for different types of questions and which ones work best for you.

Question Strategies

✓ Read Carefully

Read the question and the answer choices carefully. Don't miss the question because you misread the terms. You have plenty of time to read each question thoroughly and make sure you understand what is being asked. Yet a happy medium must be attained, so don't waste too much time. You must read carefully and efficiently.

✓ Contextual Clues

Look for contextual clues. If the question includes a word you are not familiar with, look at the immediate context for some indication of what the word might mean. Contextual clues can often give you all the information you need to decipher the meaning of an unfamiliar word. Even if you can't determine the meaning, you may be able to narrow down the possibilities enough to make a solid guess at the answer to the question.

✓ Prefixes

If you're having trouble with a word in the question or answer choices, try dissecting it. Take advantage of every clue that the word might include. Prefixes can be a huge help. Usually, they allow you to determine a basic meaning. *Pre-* means before, *post-* means after, *pro-* is positive, *de-* is negative. From prefixes, you can get an idea of the general meaning of the word and try to put it into context.

✓ Hedge Words

Watch out for critical hedge words, such as *likely, may, can, sometimes, often, almost, mostly, usually, generally, rarely,* and *sometimes.* Question writers insert these hedge phrases to cover every possibility. Often an answer choice will be wrong simply because it leaves no room for exception. Be on guard for answer choices that have definitive words such as *exactly* and *always.*

✓ Switchback Words

Stay alert for *switchbacks.* These are the words and phrases frequently used to alert you to shifts in thought. The most common switchback words are *but, although,* and *however.* Others include *nevertheless, on the other hand, even though, while, in spite of, despite,* and *regardless of.* Switchback words are important to catch because they can change the direction of the question or an answer choice.

⊘ Face Value

When in doubt, use common sense. Accept the situation in the problem at face value. Don't read too much into it. These problems will not require you to make wild assumptions. If you have to go beyond creativity and warp time or space in order to have an answer choice fit the question, then you should move on and consider the other answer choices. These are normal problems rooted in reality. The applicable relationship or explanation may not be readily apparent, but it is there for you to figure out. Use your common sense to interpret anything that isn't clear.

Answer Choice Strategies

⊘ Answer Selection

The most thorough way to pick an answer choice is to identify and eliminate wrong answers until only one is left, then confirm it is the correct answer. Sometimes an answer choice may immediately seem right, but be careful. The test writers will usually put more than one reasonable answer choice on each question, so take a second to read all of them and make sure that the other choices are not equally obvious. As long as you have time left, it is better to read every answer choice than to pick the first one that looks right without checking the others.

⊘ Answer Choice Families

An answer choice family consists of two (in rare cases, three) answer choices that are very similar in construction and cannot all be true at the same time. If you see two answer choices that are direct opposites or parallels, one of them is usually the correct answer. For instance, if one answer choice says that quantity x increases and another either says that quantity x decreases (opposite) or says that quantity y increases (parallel), then those answer choices would fall into the same family. An answer choice that doesn't match the construction of the answer choice family is more likely to be incorrect. Most questions will not have answer choice families, but when they do appear, you should be prepared to recognize them.

⊘ Eliminate Answers

Eliminate answer choices as soon as you realize they are wrong, but make sure you consider all possibilities. If you are eliminating answer choices and realize that the last one you are left with is also wrong, don't panic. Start over and consider each choice again. There may be something you missed the first time that you will realize on the second pass.

⊘ Avoid Fact Traps

Don't be distracted by an answer choice that is factually true but doesn't answer the question. You are looking for the choice that answers the question. Stay focused on what the question is asking for so you don't accidentally pick an answer that is true but incorrect. Always go back to the question and make sure the answer choice you've selected actually answers the question and is not merely a true statement.

⊘ Extreme Statements

In general, you should avoid answers that put forth extreme actions as standard practice or proclaim controversial ideas as established fact. An answer choice that states the "process should be used in certain situations, if…" is much more likely to be correct than one that states the "process should be discontinued completely." The first is a calm rational statement and doesn't even make a definitive, uncompromising stance, using a hedge word *if* to provide wiggle room, whereas the second choice is far more extreme.

⊘ Benchmark

As you read through the answer choices and you come across one that seems to answer the question well, mentally select that answer choice. This is not your final answer, but it's the one that will help you evaluate the other answer choices. The one that you selected is your benchmark or standard for judging each of the other answer choices. Every other answer choice must be compared to your benchmark. That choice is correct until proven otherwise by another answer choice beating it. If you find a better answer, then that one becomes your new benchmark. Once you've decided that no other choice answers the question as well as your benchmark, you have your final answer.

⊘ Predict the Answer

Before you even start looking at the answer choices, it is often best to try to predict the answer. When you come up with the answer on your own, it is easier to avoid distractions and traps because you will know exactly what to look for. The right answer choice is unlikely to be word-for-word what you came up with, but it should be a close match. Even if you are confident that you have the right answer, you should still take the time to read each option before moving on.

General Strategies

⊘ Tough Questions

If you are stumped on a problem or it appears too hard or too difficult, don't waste time. Move on! Remember though, if you can quickly check for obviously incorrect answer choices, your chances of guessing correctly are greatly improved. Before you completely give up, at least try to knock out a couple of possible answers. Eliminate what you can and then guess at the remaining answer choices before moving on.

⊘ Check Your Work

Since you will probably not know every term listed and the answer to every question, it is important that you get credit for the ones that you do know. Don't miss any questions through careless mistakes. If at all possible, try to take a second to look back over your answer selection and make sure you've selected the correct answer choice and haven't made a costly careless mistake (such as marking an answer choice that you didn't mean to mark). This quick double check should more than pay for itself in caught mistakes for the time it costs.

⊘ Pace Yourself

It's easy to be overwhelmed when you're looking at a page full of questions; your mind is confused and full of random thoughts, and the clock is ticking down faster than you would like. Calm down and maintain the pace that you have set for yourself. Especially as you get down to the last few minutes of the test, don't let the small numbers on the clock make you panic. As long as you are on track by monitoring your pace, you are guaranteed to have time for each question.

⊘ Don't Rush

It is very easy to make errors when you are in a hurry. Maintaining a fast pace in answering questions is pointless if it makes you miss questions that you would have gotten right otherwise. Test writers like to include distracting information and wrong answers that seem right. Taking a little extra time to avoid careless mistakes can make all the difference in your test score. Find a pace that allows you to be confident in the answers that you select.

⊘ KEEP MOVING

Panicking will not help you pass the test, so do your best to stay calm and keep moving. Taking deep breaths and going through the answer elimination steps you practiced can help to break through a stress barrier and keep your pace.

Final Notes

The combination of a solid foundation of content knowledge and the confidence that comes from practicing your plan for applying that knowledge is the key to maximizing your performance on test day. As your foundation of content knowledge is built up and strengthened, you'll find that the strategies included in this chapter become more and more effective in helping you quickly sift through the distractions and traps of the test to isolate the correct answer.

Now that you're preparing to move forward into the test content chapters of this book, be sure to keep your goal in mind. As you read, think about how you will be able to apply this information on the test. If you've already seen sample questions for the test and you have an idea of the question format and style, try to come up with questions of your own that you can answer based on what you're reading. This will give you valuable practice applying your knowledge in the same ways you can expect to on test day.

Good luck and good studying!

Pregnancy, Birth Risk Factors and Complications

Antenatal Factors

Maternal Age

Adolescent

Adolescent mothers age 15 and older are not at higher risk than those over 20 if they have **adequate prenatal care** and follow guidelines and recommendations, but this is often not the case. Teenage mothers are more likely to smoke and to gain inadequate weight, increasing the likelihood of premature delivery, low-birth-weight infants, iron deficiency anemia, and preeclampsia/eclampsia. Additionally, there is increased risk of cephalopelvic disproportion, because the mother may not be fully mature physically. Teenagers 15-19 also have increased risk of sexually transmitted infections, such as gonorrhea, herpes, chlamydia, and syphilis. Many also drink alcohol and take illicit drugs, increasing the incidence of fetal abnormalities. In many cases, the male partner has little education, lacks employment, and may not be able to provide emotional or financial support. Adolescent partners are often of similar social and educational background to the mothers, may not have completed development, and may not be prepared for fatherhood. The nurse should remain non-judgmental and supportive, educating the adolescent and encouraging good prenatal care.

Mature, Over 35

Many women have chosen to delay pregnancy, resulting in a marked increase in pregnancy among **women over 35**. These mothers tend to be better educated and more financially secure than younger mothers. If the mother is in good health, pregnancy poses little increased risk; however, the risk of **death associated with pregnancy** does increase with age. Those over 40 have about 5 times the risk of those under 25. Additionally, those over 35 are more likely to have **preexisting health problems**, such as diabetes or hypertension, which increases risk. They are more likely to have a C-section, placenta previa, abruptio placentae, and spontaneous abortion. There may also be increased risk to the fetus. The incidence of Down syndrome increases with mothers over 35, and markedly increases in those over 40, so these mothers are more likely to want genetic testing. Macrosomia and congenital malformations are also more common. Older mothers with unplanned pregnancies may be concerned about their age, long-term care of the child, retirement plans, and lifestyle changes.

Multiple Gestations

In vitro fertilization and ovulation-inducing drugs have increased the incidence of high order **multiple gestations** over the past 30 years. The trend of delayed childbearing has led to an increase in twin/multiple gestations. Infants born from multiple gestations are more likely to be born prematurely and with low birth weights. The incidence of premature birth and low birth weight is proportional to the number of fetuses. There may be growth restriction/growth discordance, oligohydramnios, and restriction of movement of one or more of the fetuses. Approximately 50% of twins and 90% of triplets are born premature, compared to 10% of singletons. With this increase in prematurity and the proportion of infants born with low birth weight, there are increased morbidities, such as cerebral palsy and intellectual disability. The risk for genetic disorders, such as neural tube defects, gastrointestinal defects, and cardiac abnormalities is twice that of single gestations.

Multiparity

Grand multiparity is ≥5 deliveries of live or stillborn infants at ≥20 weeks, although some studies suggest risks increase after 4 deliveries. **Great grand multiparity** is usually considered ≥10 deliveries.

Risks associated with multiparity include increased incidence of placenta previa, abruptio placentae, preeclampsia, and hemorrhage. Rates of C-sections are increased significantly. Grand multiparas often have **poor prenatal care** and tend to have increased rates of disease, such as diabetes mellitus and hypertension, but studies show that with proper prenatal care, those without health problems have risks comparable to those with lower parity. Younger multiparous women have fewer complications than older multiparous women, so some of the increased risks may be primarily age-related. Fetal complications include macrosomia, SGA, and malpresentation (breech).

Lifestyle Factors Impacting the Fetus and Neonate

Many **maternal factors** have an impact on the fetus and newborn:

- **Stress**: Stress effects the neurodevelopment of the fetus, resulting in behavioral and neurological impairments as the child grows. The fetus exposed to maternal stress has less variability in fetal heart rate. If the mother is depressed, the fetus tends to be more active; and if anxious, less active.
- **Health habits**: Smoking can result in low birth rate, spontaneous abortion, placental abruption, preterm birth and developmental problems in the infant. Alcohol is a teratogen and can lead to fetal alcohol syndrome with cognitive and physical impairment and skeletal and organ malformations.
- **Exercise**: Can improve circulation, improve sleep, elevate mood, decrease duration of labor, and prevent excess weight gain. However, it can also impair oxygenation to the fetus and increase risk of maternal falls.

Maternal Nutrition

The nutrition of the mother has a profound effect on the developing embryo/fetus. Caloric needs vary widely depending on the mother's age, size, weight, metabolism, and general health. Energy needs of the mother usually remain stable during the first trimester, but an additional **300 calories** a day are needed during the second and third trimesters for a singleton, and **600 calories** a day are needed for twins. Recommended nutrient intake for pregnant women is shown below:

Vit. A (µg/d)	Vit. C (mg/d)	Vit. D (µg/d)	Vit. E (mg/d)	Vit. K (µg/d)	Ca (mg/d)	Phos. (mg/d)
750-770	80-85	≥5	15	75-90	1000-1300	700-1250

Generally, a pregnant woman requires about 71 g of **protein** daily (3 meat servings or equivalent) and 4-5 cups of milk (or equivalent). Diet should include 2-4 servings of fruit and 3-5 servings of vegetables. **Simple carbohydrates** (sugar, flour) should be limited and replaced by whole grains, which are high in B vitamins. **Fat** should constitute about 30% of total caloric intake. Iron intake should be about 27 mg per day.

Maternal Malnutrition

Maternal malnutrition can have a profound effect on the developing fetus. If malnutrition occurs during the stages of cell division, then cells may not divide properly, causing permanent damage. If malnutrition occurs when cells are enlarging, then correcting the nutritional deficit can reverse damage. Maternal weight gain must be adequate:

- Underweight: 28-40 lb
- Normal weight: 25-35 lb
- Overweight: 15-25 lb
- Obese: 15 lb

Mothers who are malnourished or underweight have increased perinatal losses and preterm births. Neonates often have lower Apgar score and low birth weight (<2500 g). Women with eating disorders are more likely to have infants that are small for gestational age. Vitamin and mineral deficiencies can result in a number of problems for the developing fetus:

- Thiamine: congestive heart failure, stillbirths
- Folic acid: megaloblastic anemia, neural tube defects
- Vitamin D and calcium: skeletal defects

Infants of obese and morbidly obese women are often macrosomic (large) and may suffer fetal distress, early neonatal death, meconium aspiration, shoulder dystocia, and/or complications from Cesarean birth.

Impact of Maternal Obesity and Age on Pregnancy

The numbers of mothers who are **obese** or **older than 35 years of age** are increasing. Both conditions increase the risk of **morbidity and mortality** for the mother and fetus. Complications of pregnancy are more numerous in these two groups and include a higher risk of ischemic events, preeclampsia, gestational diabetes, stillbirth, and premature births. Labor and delivery can be complicated by macrosomia, failure to progress, Cesarean section deliveries, problems with anesthetics, and postpartum hemorrhages. Infection and wound dehiscence are more common. Fetal anomalies such as spina bifida and ventral wall defects are more common, as well as disrupted growth patterns and an increased risk of fetal demise.

Effects of Obesity on Labor, Fetus, and Newborn

A pregnant woman is considered **obese** with weight 50% greater than ideal weight, weight greater than 200 lb (91 kg), or BMI greater than 29. The woman is at an increased risk of developing gestational diabetes mellitus and hypertension. The second stage of labor is often prolonged because the myometrium is overstretched. Additionally, labor is difficult and associated with macrosomia and shoulder dystocia, which can cause permanent brachial plexus injury in the newborn. Because of excessive fatty tissue in the abdomen, monitoring of fetal heart rate and contractions may be difficult. During labor and delivery, the woman is at increased risk of uterine rupture and lacerations. The obese pregnant woman is more likely to require Cesarean but is at risk for excessive blood loss during surgery (>1000 mL), difficulty with intubation, and prolonged operative time as well as the need for hysterectomy. Postoperatively, the woman is at greater risk of complications (DVT and infection).

Issues of Pregnancy Post-Bariatric Surgery

Patients are usually advised to avoid pregnancy for at least 12 months (sometimes as long as 24 months) following **bariatric surgery** to give the patient time to stabilize weight loss. Pregnancy soon after surgery may result in small-for-gestational-age neonates. The primary concern with pregnancy post-bariatric surgery is the **maternal nutritional status** because many patients have deficiencies of protein, iron, and calcium as well as vitamin deficiencies (especially vitamins B12 and D), and their caloric intake may be 500-1000 kcal/day, which is not sufficient to support pregnancy. Thus, the patient's nutritional status should be monitored at least every trimester. The patient may need to eat several small nutritious meals daily. Additionally, absorption of medications may be impaired, and symptoms of pregnancy (nausea, vomiting, discomfort) may mimic those of post-bariatric complications, so careful evaluation is necessary. Patients still overweight are at increased risk of hypertension and gestational diabetes. Labor and delivery should progress normally in post-bariatric patients. Bariatric surgery is not an indication for Cesarean although rates tend to be high.

Anxiety and Depressive Disorders

Pregnancy-specific anxiety is high in pregnant women, especially in the first and third trimesters, but the rates of **anxiety and depressive disorders** are similar to those of non-pregnant women. Approximately 10-13% of pregnant women suffer from depression. Rates of OCD and generalized anxiety disorder show a slight increase during pregnancy, and panic attacks may start or worsen. Anxiety increases perceptions of pain by triggering release of catecholamines, which increase pelvic pain stimuli transmitted to the CNS and may be a major factor in labor pain. Additionally, anxiety increases muscle tension, decreasing the effectiveness of uterine contractions and prolonging labor. The increased pain further increases anxiety. Treatment to reduce anxiety includes providing analgesia to reduce pain, keeping the woman informed with accurate information about her progress, and ensuring comfort measures, such as relaxation exercises, massages, breathing techniques, and a quiet, calm environment.

Effects of Anti-Anxiety and Antidepressant Medications

Commonly used medications to treat anxiety and depression may pose risks to the fetus and newborn, so risks and benefits should be discussed with the physician. Typical medications include:

- **Benzodiazepines** (alprazolam, lorazepam, diazepam, clonazepam): Study results have been inconsistent in regards to whether benzodiazepines cause birth defects or developmental or behavioral problems, but the neonate may have withdrawal symptoms, such as dyspnea, tremors, jitters, excessive crying, and difficulty sleeping. Combining benzodiazepines with diphenhydramine may result in increased rate of stillbirths.
- **Buspirone**: Little data regarding pregnancy is available for this drug, but it is classified as a Class B drug.
- **SSRIs** (fluoxetine, sertraline, citalopram, paroxetine, escitalopram): May cause persistent pulmonary hypertension of the newborn if taken during the last half of the pregnancy. Paroxetine (Paxil) may result in congenital heart disease. Withdrawal symptoms in neonate may occur within 2 days of delivery and may be similar to those of benzodiazepines.
- **SNRIs** (venlafaxine, duloxetine): Similar to SSRIs, but withdrawal symptoms are less pronounced.

Alternate Treatments for Anxiety and Depression

Many pregnant women choose to avoid medications for anxiety and depression out of concern for possible adverse effects on the fetus, but these untreated disorders pose risks as well, so **alternate treatments** should be provided:

- **Bright light therapy**: the patient sits in front of a light box (10,000 lux) for 30 minutes in AM to treat depression.
- **Cognitive behavioral therapy**: helps the patient to control thought patterns and control depression and anxiety disorders.
- **Group therapy**: talking with others with similar anxiety provides emotional support.
- **Relaxation exercises/visualization**: helps the patient to control emotional response and to reduce anxiety.
- **Support/reassurance**: anticipating questions and providing clear and honest information about what to expect during pregnancy and the patient's progress can help to allay fears and reduce anxiety.
- **Exercise**: physical exercise, such as daily walks, can help to increase release of endorphins and increase feeling of wellbeing.

Antepartum Risk Factors and Complications

Preeclampsia and Eclampsia

Preeclampsia is a disorder that develops in approximately 5% of all pregnancies. It is defined as a new onset of elevated blood pressure of at least 140/90 on two occasions at least 4 hours apart. In addition to elevated BP, diagnosis requires one or more of the following complications after the 20th week of pregnancy: proteinuria, new-onset headaches or visual disturbances, thrombocytopenia, impaired liver or kidney function, or pulmonary edema. Proteinuria is a common feature of preeclampsia, but diagnostically, it is possible to have preeclampsia without proteinuria when there is evidence of significant end-organ dysfunction. Preeclampsia is more commonly seen after 34 weeks gestation. Delivery is the only cure for preeclampsia. If it is not severe, patients are often induced after 37 weeks gestation. In patients with severe features, induction should be considered after 34 weeks gestation. Antihypertensive treatment, such as thiazide, hydralazine, propranolol, labetalol, nifedipine, and methyldopa, is recommended for severe hypertension, as well as anticonvulsants if seizures occur. Magnesium sulfate is given prophylactically for severe preeclampsia and for treatment of seizures. **Eclampsia** is a complication of severe preeclampsia in which seizures occur. The main detrimental effect on the fetus occurs when longstanding hypertension leads to uteroplacental vascular insufficiency, which impairs the transfer of nutrients and oxygen to the fetus, resulting in intrauterine growth restriction (IUGR). Placental abruption also occurs more frequently. The IUGR is usually asymmetric (fetal head size is normal for gestational age). Infants who are born with IUGR and/or prematurity have increased morbidity and mortality.

HELLP Syndrome

HELLP syndrome occurs in 4-12% of those with preeclampsia, most often during weeks 27-37, but it may develop within 24 hours postpartum. It is characterized by the following:

- **H**—hemolysis
- **EL**—elevated liver enzymes
- **LP**—low platelet count

HELLP syndrome is most common in older multiparous mothers. Hypertension may be less pronounced than in others with preeclampsia. Pain in the right upper quadrant related to liver dysfunction may be misdiagnosed as gastrointestinal upset or gall bladder disease. Mothers often present with flu-like nonspecific symptoms, including headache, nausea and vomiting, and visual disturbances. Prompt diagnosis and treatment are necessary because of high mortality. Platelet transfusions are given if platelet counts are $<20,000/mm^3$ before vaginal delivery or $<50,000/mm^3$ before Cesarean section. The primary treatment is immediate delivery of the fetus as the mother may develop hepatic hemorrhage or permanent liver damage. Both the mother and the fetus are at risk. Neonates are at increased risk and may require mechanical ventilation. Complications include abruptio placentae, DIC, and postpartum hemorrhage.

Classes I to IV Cardiac Disease in Pregnancy

Maternal heart disease complicates approximately one percent of all pregnancies, with congenital heart disease accounting for more than half of the cases. Pre-pregnancy cardiac function is an excellent predictor of cardiac complications in pregnancy and is based on the New York Heart Association classification:

I. No cardiac insufficiency or activity limitations
II. Slight activity limitations: symptoms present with ordinary physical activity
III. Marked activity limitations: mild activity causes symptoms
IV. Inability to carry out physical activities without severe symptoms

The **maternal classification** affects the fetus. There is minimal danger to the fetus for mothers in Class I or Class II, but increased risk to both the mother and the fetus for Classes III and IV. Most medications cross the placenta, and the degree of safety during pregnancy has not been established for all of these. The most common drugs—heparin, digitalis glycosides, antiarrhythmics, thiazide, and loop diuretics—are not **teratogenic**. For Classes III and IV, delivery may be facilitated by low forceps or vacuum assistance, and Cesarean may be done if the mother or the fetus is in danger. Labor and delivery are particularly dangerous to the fetus because of inadequate oxygen and blood supply, so continuous fetal monitoring is essential.

Pregnancy with Congenital Heart Defects

With improved surgical repair techniques for **congenital heart defects,** many women survive to childbearing age. These are common **maternal defects**:

- Tetralogy of Fallot
- Ventricular and atrial septal defects
- Patent ductus arteriosus
- Coarctation of the aorta

If surgical correction was successful, there is no added **fetal risk**, but if the condition has not been completely repaired or involves cyanosis, pregnancy can put the fetus at risk because of inadequate oxygen supply. Mothers with cardiac disease have a 5-10% increased risk of having a baby with cardiac anomalies. Fetal echocardiography is recommended in pregnancy to evaluate the structure and function of the fetus' heart.

Marfan syndrome poses severe risks to the mother, with mortality rates of 25-50% because of possible rupture of the aorta, which also puts the fetus at risk. Additionally, because this is an autosomal dominant disorder, there is a 50% chance that an infant will inherit the syndrome.

Mitral valve prolapse usually does not pose a risk to the fetus.

Severe maternal cardiopulmonary disorders can result in death of the mother and/or fetus. However, the most common fetal complications are premature labor/birth and a fetus that is small for gestational age.

Infants of a Diabetic Mother (IDM)

Infants of a diabetic mother (IDM) suffer from increased morbidity and mortality. Glucose crosses the placenta, so when the mother has elevated blood glucose, the infant also has elevated blood glucose. Insulin does not cross the placenta. The pancreas of the fetus begins to produce insulin at about 20 weeks of gestation. Prior to the fetus producing insulin, the infant is exposed to elevated levels of glucose that restrict fetal growth. After week 20, the fetus responds to hyperglycemia with elevated production of insulin. The combination of elevated blood glucose and elevated insulin triggers rapid fetal growth, with increased fat and glycogen stores, hepatosplenomegaly, cardiomegaly, and increased head size. Sudden withdrawal from the consistent maternal source of glucose after birth, combined with the continued production of insulin by the newborn, result in hypoglycemia shortly after birth.

Maternal Sickle Cell Anemia

Sickle cell disease is a recessive genetic disorder of chromosome 11, causing hemoglobin to be defective so that red blood cells (RBCs) are sickle-shaped and inflexible, resulting in their accumulating in small vessels and causing painful blockage. There are 5 variations of sickle cell disease, with **sickle cell anemia** the most severe. Pregnant women with sickle cell anemia are at risk for urinary and pulmonary infections, congestive heart failure, and acute renal failure, all of which can trigger a vaso-occlusive crises that puts the fetus at risk. Perinatal mortality rates are about 18%, caused by sickling in the placenta. Neonates are at increased risk for prematurity and intrauterine growth restriction. Maternal infections must be treated promptly to avoid dehydration and/or fever that can trigger sickling. Steps to shorten the second stage of labor (oxytocin, forceps, episiotomy) may be necessary to protect the fetus if sickling occurs during labor.

Review Video: Sickle Cell Disease
Visit mometrix.com/academy and enter code: 603869

Pregnancy and Iron-Deficiency Anemia

Iron is necessary for the development of red blood cells. During pregnancy, the mother's plasma volume increases by about 50% but red cell mass increases less, so the **hematocrit** drops from a normal of 38-47% to as low as 30% (physiologic/iron deficiency anemia of pregnancy). Because the fetus takes iron from the mother, the mother's iron intake must compensate for this loss. When **hemoglobin** falls <10 g/dL, the mother is at increased risk of infection, preeclampsia, and postpartal hemorrhage, with associated dangers to the fetus. If hemoglobin falls <6 g/dL, the mother may suffer cardiac failure, and the fetus is at high risk, with increased rates of miscarriage, stillbirth, low birth weight, and neonatal death. Initial symptoms of iron deficiency include pallor, glossitis, headache, and pica, progressing to weakness, lethargy, confusion, ataxia, and cardiovascular abnormalities. Recommended treatment for iron-deficiency anemia is 60-120 mg daily of elemental iron. To promote absorption, it is best to avoid caffeine and dairy products within an hour of taking the iron supplement and to take some source of vitamin C with the iron.
Pregnancy and Folate/Folic Acid Deficiency Anemia

Folate/folic acid deficiency can result in **megaloblastic anemia**. Folate is the naturally occurring form of vitamin B9 and is necessary for DNA synthesis and the formation and maturation of red blood cells. Folic acid is the synthetic form of vitamin B9, used in supplements and added to processed foods. Causes of folate deficiency include inadequate diet, malabsorption syndromes (especially of the small intestine), medications that interfere with absorption (oral contraceptives, methotrexate, phenobarbital, and diphenylhydantoin), anorexia, alcoholism, and dialysis. Diagnostic findings include decreased hemoglobin, hematocrit, and folate (normal value is 3-25 mg/mL), as well as increased MCV and MCHV. Cobalamin level is normal and gastric analysis is positive for hydrochloric acid. Other blood studies are usually within normal range. RBCs are macrocytic and normochromic. Folate deficiency is associated with **neural tube defects**, such as myelomeningocele, spina bifida, and anencephaly in the fetus.

Signs and symptoms include:

- Asymptomatic (initially)
- GI disturbances, such as indigestion, anorexia, and weight loss
- Red, beefy-appearing tongue
- Pallor
- Weakness, fatigue
- Forgetfulness, impaired concentration

Treatment:

- Diet high in folate: green leafy vegetables, liver, citrus fruits, legumes, nuts, and grains
- Oral supplementation: L-Methylfolate 600-1000 mcg daily or folic acid 1-5 mg per day

Maternal Acidosis

Maternal pH directly impacts the pH of the fetus, particularly in the case of **metabolic acidosis**. Because the fetus is extremely vulnerable to even minor changes in pH, this can be a very threatening condition. Maternal acidosis is linked with decreased fetal pH (fetal acidosis), resulting in lower Apgar scores for these neonates. Maternal causes of acidosis include uncontrolled diabetes (leading to diabetic ketoacidosis), renal dysfunction, and severe diarrhea. Fetal acid-base balance should be closely monitored in mothers with these conditions. Should the fetus show signs of distress (FHR abnormalities, decreased fetal movement, etc.) and acidosis in the fetus be suspected, the mother should immediately be tested in the case that fetal acidosis is secondary to maternal acidosis.

Acute Fatty Liver Pregnancy (AFLP)

Acute fatty liver of pregnancy (AFLP) (the most common cause of liver failure during pregnancy) is characterized by micro-vesicular fat deposits throughout the liver that crowd out hepatocytes and interfere with liver function. AFLP, which is associated with genetic mutations, occurs in the third trimester or postpartal period. Women may exhibit nausea and vomiting, upper GI hemorrhage, coagulopathy, pancreatitis, hypoglycemia, hepatic encephalopathy (with confusion and altered mental status), hypertension, jaundice, general malaise, and renal and hepatic failure. Neonates may exhibit fatty acid oxidation defects that affect multiple body systems: cardiomyopathy, liver failure, myopathy, neuropathy, and hypoglycemia (nonketotic). Some may die *in utero* and 15% die after birth. The key to treatment of AFLP is immediate delivery of the fetus through labor induction or Cesarean (although coagulopathy may pose risks). Supportive care may include IV fluids, blood products, coagulation factors, and/or plasma exchange or plasmapheresis with continuous renal replacement therapy. Some women may require liver transplantation.

Maternal Systemic Lupus Erythematosus (SLE)

Systemic lupus erythematosus (SLE), a systemic reaction to collagen or connective tissue in the body, is believed to be triggered by an antibody-antigen immune response to an environmental agent, resulting in widespread damage of vessels and organs, primarily in females. Symptoms may include: malar and discoid rash; photosensitivity; oral ulcers; arthritis; serositis; and renal (proteinuria/nephritis), neurological (seizures, psychosis), and immunological disorders. Pregnant women with SLE have high rates of hypertension (up to 30%) and preeclampsia, especially with lupus nephritis, so they may need to continue immunosuppressive drugs during pregnancy. Women must be monitored carefully during pregnancy for flare-ups of SLE. Impaired circulation to the fetus may result from maternal decidual vasculopathy with placental infarction. Fetal risks include preterm delivery, fetal growth restriction, spontaneous abortion, and stillbirths. The newborn may inherit neonatal lupus, with symptoms appearing up to 4 weeks after birth. Indications include congenital heart block, autoimmune hemolysis, thrombocytopenia, and lupus dermatitis.

Review Video: Systemic Lupus Erythematosus
Visit mometrix.com/academy and enter code: 657082

Cholelithiasis and Cholecystitis

Pregnancy increases the risk of a woman developing **cholelithiasis** and **cholecystitis** because of increased levels of estrogen and increased biliary sludge (forerunner to gallstones). Symptoms occur when stones block the bile duct and may include RUQ pain, nausea, vomiting, low-grade fever, and mildly elevated white blood cell count. Some may have clay-colored stools and jaundice. Medical management has been most common in the first and third trimesters and surgical repair in the second trimester (when it is safest). However, early cholecystitis often recurs later in the pregnancy, increasing the risk of pre-term delivery and making surgery more difficult because of the size of the uterus, so some authorities advise against conservative treatment. Surgical procedures include laparoscopic cholecystectomy and endoscopic retrograde cholangiopancreatography for stones in the common bile duct. The fetus is usually unimpaired if the blockage is resolved.

Maternal Hypothyroidism and Hyperthyroidism

Maternal hypothyroidism threatens the development of the fetal brain and spinal cord. T4 is needed for proper development, and the fetus is not capable of T4 production during the critical period of growth. Decreased mental capacity or fetal death can occur.

Hyperthyroidism is difficult to detect since symptoms mimic normal pregnancy problems. The pregnant woman may have temporary hyperthyroidism in early pregnancy but levels should return to normal by the beginning of the second trimester. Continued high levels can cause thyroid crisis and result in fetal death or premature birth.

Review Video: What is Hyperthyroidism?
Visit mometrix.com/academy and enter code: 923159

Maternal Trauma

Maternal trauma can occur at any time during the pregnancy. Motor vehicle accidents are the leading cause of trauma to the pregnant woman. Maternal falls and trauma to the abdomen from domestic abuse are other common causes. Trauma to the abdomen by blunt force can result in abruptio placentae, placental injury, injury to the fetus, or uterine rupture causing fetal death by hemorrhage and hypoxia. Maternal hemorrhage and shock from traumatic injuries can result in both fetal and maternal death from hypoxia. Any trauma that compromises respiration will also cause hypoxia to the mother-fetal unit. Neurological trauma that results in shock, hemorrhage, or damage to the brain will also compromise the fetus when maternal vital functions deteriorate.

CHEAP TORCHES

CHEAP TORCHES is the acronym used to recall common causes of congenital and neonatal infections. Many congenital infections are present for at least a month prior to birth and remain present at birth:

C	Chickenpox (varicella)
H	Hepatitis (B, C, & E)
E	Enterovirus (RNA viruses, including coxsackievirus, echovirus, and poliovirus)
A	AIDS (HIV)
P	Parvovirus (B 19)
T	Toxoplasmosis
O	Other (Group B streptococcus, *Candida, Listeria*, TB, lymphocytic choriomeningitis)
R	Rubella (measles)
C	Cytomegalovirus
H	Herpes simplex virus
E	Every other STI (*Chlamydia*, gonorrhea, *Ureaplasma*, papillomavirus
S	Syphilis

Exposure to these pathogens *in utero* may cause a miscarriage or congenital defect, especially if the exposure was during the first trimester.

Review Video: Infant TORCH Syndrome
Visit mometrix.com/academy and enter code: 502502

CONGENITAL VARICELLA SYNDROME

Varicella infection (chickenpox) in the mother can affect the fetus in different ways, depending upon the time of exposure. **Congenital varicella syndrome** is characterized by many abnormalities, including eye abnormalities (cataracts, microphthalmia, pendular nystagmus, and retinal scarring), skin abnormalities (hypertrophy and cicatrix scarring), malformation of limbs, hypoplasia of digits, restricted growth, microcephalus, abnormalities of the brain and autonomic nervous system, developmental delay, and intellectual disability. Mortality rates are high (≥50%) for those with severe defects:

- First trimester: 1% risk of congenital varicella syndrome.
- Weeks 23-20: 2% risk of congenital varicella syndrome.
- 5 days before delivery to 2 days after delivery: Neonate may develop congenital varicella (20-25%).
- 6-12 days after delivery: Neonate may contract congenital varicella but, if breast-feeding, the child may receive the mother's antibodies, so the disease will be milder.

Fetal Exposure to Hepatitis

Routine screening of all pregnant women and all newborns helps to identify those infected with the **hepatitis B virus**. Infants are routinely immunized at discharge from hospital, at 2 months, and at 6 months of age. In the case of a premature infant, the immunization schedule is started when the infant weighs 2 kg or is 2 months old. If the mother is HVB-positive, surface antigen treatment of that infant should include careful bathing (wearing gloves) to remove all maternal blood and body fluids. The infant should also receive an IM injection of the hepatitis B immunoglobulin within 12 hours of birth. This immunoglobulin treatment is up to 95% effective in preventing the development of the disease in the infant.

Hepatitis C is rarely transmitted to the fetus, and of those infected, about 75% clear the infection by 2 years.

Hepatitis E poses the greatest risk to the mother, with a mortality of about 20% during pregnancy and an increased risk of fetal complications and death.

Fetal Exposure to Tuberculosis

Tuberculosis (TB), infection with *Mycobacterium tuberculosis,* does not appear to worsen with pregnancy and responds to treatment. The risk of transmission to the fetus is low. However, the fetus may acquire the infection directly from the mother's blood or from swallowing amniotic fluid, although most transmission occurs postpartum through maternal contact, so mothers with active disease should not have contact with a neonate until they are noninfectious. Fetal infection may cause death of the fetus, increased risk of miscarriage, or neonatal infection. If the mother's TB is untreated, the fetal death rate is 30-40%, so treating the mother during pregnancy is very important. Isoniazid (INH), rifampin, and ethambutol cross the placenta but do not appear to be teratogenic, and the need for treatment outweighs risks. Streptomycin should be avoided as it may result in sensorineural deafness in the neonate. Mothers with inactive disease taking medications may breastfeed.

Fetal Exposure to AIDS/HIV

Most children infected with AIDS/HIV acquire the infection from their mothers (vertical transmission). The perinatal transmission rate is 30% in untreated HIV positive mothers, usually acquired during delivery. Neonates are usually asymptomatic but are at risk for prematurity, low birth weight, and small for gestational age (SGA). Infants may show failure to thrive, hepatomegaly, interstitial lymphocytic pneumonia, recurrent infections, and CNS abnormalities. Optimal treatment reduces the perinatal transmission rate to as low as 1-2%:

- **Antiviral therapy during the pregnancy**: A reduced viral load in the mother lessens the likelihood of prenatal transmission.
- **Elective Cesarean**: Elective C-section before the amniotic membranes rupture is especially recommended for women with a viral load >1000 copies/mL and is associated with reduced rates of vertical transmission. Emergency Cesarean, rupture of membranes longer than 4 hours, and the need for an episiotomy all increase the likelihood of infection during delivery.
- **Antiviral medications for the neonate for the first 6 weeks of life**: The first dose should be given within 12 hours of delivery.
- **Avoiding breastfeeding**: The risk of HIV transmission with breastfeeding is 0.7% per month of breastfeeding.

Fetal Exposure to Parvovirus B19

Parvovirus B19 is a DNA virus that is very common and causes fever, malaise, and depression of progenitor cells in the bone marrow with a drop in reticulocyte count that can lead to anemia in those with preexisting low blood count. Most people are asymptomatic, although they can develop generalized rash and arthralgia/arthritis. Most mothers (≥50%) are seropositive with parvovirus before pregnancy and can become reinfected during pregnancy. Most infections do not adversely affect the fetus, but about 1-2% of maternal infections may cause spontaneous abortion or nonimmune hydrops fetalis. Hydrops fetalis is characterized by marked anemia, cardiac failure, and extramedullary hematopoiesis. A Parvovirus congenital infection syndrome may also occur with rash, anemia, and enlargement of the heart and liver.

Fetal Exposure to Toxoplasmosis

Toxoplasmosis, caused by a protozoal infection with *Toxoplasma gondii,* is a common disease. About 38% of pregnant women have antibodies from a previous infection, but about 1 in 1000 pregnant women become infected during pregnancy, primarily from eating undercooked meat, drinking unpasteurized goat's milk, or contacting infected cat feces, putting the fetus at risk. Risk to the fetus is greatest if the disease occurs during the first trimester, often causing severe fetal abnormalities, such as microcephaly and hydrocephalus, or miscarriage. However, risk of fetal transmission is greatest during the 3rd trimester, although 70% are born without indications of infection. Mild infection may manifest as retinochoroiditis at birth (with other symptoms delayed). Severe infection may result in convulsions and coma from CNS abnormalities, and the child may die in the neonatal period. Children who survive with severe infection may suffer blindness, deafness, and marked intellectual disability. If a diagnosis of fetal infection is made during pregnancy, the mother should be treated aggressively.

Fetal Exposure to GBS

Group B *Streptococcus* (GBS) is the most common neonatal bacterial infection. Many women are asymptomatic carriers. Screening of all pregnant women occurs between 37+0 and 37+6 weeks of gestation followed by antibiotic treatment of the mother during labor to prevent neonatal infection. A mother needs at least 4 hours' worth of antibiotic treatment for the infant to benefit. If an infant is born and the mother has not received the recommended treatment, the infant will often be treated with IV ampicillin and gentamicin for 10-14 days. If treatment is ineffective or impossible, the infant with a GBS infection that manifests in the first 24 hours after birth may develop pneumonia and/or meningitis, respiratory distress, floppiness, poor feeding, tachycardia, shock, and seizures. An infant may be asymptomatic at birth but have late-onset infection occurring at around 7 to 10 days old. Late-onset infections (usually meningitis) are generally more serious than earlier onset, and survivors often have serious damage, such as intellectual disability, quadriplegia, blindness, deafness, uncontrollable seizures, and hydrocephalus.

Fetal Exposure to Rubella

Women should always be vaccinated for rubella before becoming pregnant, as exposure to the virus has devastating effects on the newborn. The mother may not experience any symptoms of the disease or only mild symptoms like mild respiratory problems or rash. If the rubella exposure is during the first 4-5 months of pregnancy, the consequences for the infant are greater. Infants exposed to this virus *in utero* can develop a set of symptoms known as congenital rubella syndrome. This syndrome includes all or some of the following signs and symptoms:

- Intrauterine growth restriction (IUGR)
- Deafness
- Cataracts
- Jaundice
- Purpura
- Hepatosplenomegaly
- Microcephaly
- Chronic encephalitis
- Cardiac defects

Fetal Exposure to Cytomegalovirus

Cytomegalovirus, a member of the herpes simplex virus group, can cause asymptomatic infection in women. Over 50% of women are seropositive and may have chronic infections that persist for years. Cytomegalovirus is the most common intrauterine viral infection. Cytomegalovirus can be transmitted placentally or cervically during delivery (infecting ≤2.5% of neonates) and can put the fetus at high risk with death rates of 20-30% among infants born with symptoms. About 90% of survivors have neurological disorders, such as microcephaly, hydrocephalus, cerebral palsy, and/or intellectual disability. In less severe infections, symptoms (intellectual disability, hearing deficits, learning disabilities) may be delayed. Commonly, the neonate is small for gestational age (SGA). The brain and liver are commonly affected, but all organs can be infected. Multiple blood abnormalities can occur: anemia, hyperbilirubinemia, thrombocytopenia, and hepatosplenomegaly.

Fetal Exposure to Herpes Simplex Virus

Most pregnant women infected with herpes simplex virus (HSV) are asymptomatic and unaware of the infection. Most vertical transmissions occur when the neonate travels through a colonized birth canal. The risk of transmitting HSV during the birth process varies greatly, depending on if the infection is a new infection (primary) or a secondary outbreak. The transmission rate from women with a primary HSV infection is approximately 50%, while the transmission rate is 1-2% if the infection is a recurrence of HSV. Signs of a neonatal infection with HSV include:

- Skin, eye, and mucous membrane blistering at 10-12 days of life.
- Disseminated disease may spread to multiple organs, leading to pneumonitis, hepatitis, and intravascular coagulation.
- Encephalitis may be the only presentation, with signs of lethargy, irritability, poor feeding, and seizures.

A mother with active herpes should deliver by Cesarean section within 4-6 hours after membranes rupture. An infant that is inadvertently exposed to an active lesion should be treated with acyclovir.

Fetal Exposure to Chlamydia

Chlamydia is the most common sexually transmitted infection in the United States and can be passed on at the time of birth if the infant is delivered vaginally and comes into contact with contaminated vaginal secretions. The organism responsible for this infection is *Chlamydia trachomatis.* Because the mother infected with this organism is usually asymptomatic, preventive care for the newborn is essential. The usual infection site for the newborn is the eye, in the form of conjunctivitis. States now require all newborns to be given a prophylactic dose of either erythromycin or tetracycline ointment in the eyes at birth to prevent this infection. While the antibiotic ointment stops the eye infection, a few infants exposed to the pathogen will develop pneumonitis and/or ear infection.

Fetal Exposure to Syphilis

An infant can be exposed to the syphilis organism, *Treponema pallidum,* during gestation and become infected *in utero* starting with the 10th-15th week of gestation. Many infected fetuses abort spontaneously or are stillborn. An infant born infected with syphilis can be asymptomatic at birth or can have a full multi-system infection. An infant who is symptomatic may have non-viral hepatitis with jaundice, hepatosplenomegaly, pseudoparalysis, pneumonitis, bone marrow failure, myocarditis, meningitis, anemia, edema associated with nephritic syndrome, and a rash on the palms of the hands and soles of the feet. Other symptoms, such as interstitial keratitis and dental and facial abnormalities, may occur as the child develops. Treatment involves an aggressive regimen of penicillin administration with frequent follow-up until blood tests are negative.

Fetal Alcohol Syndrome

Fetal alcohol syndrome (FAS) is a syndrome of birth defects that develop as the result of maternal ingestion of alcohol. Fetal alcohol spectrum disorders (FASD) is an umbrella diagnosis that includes FAS along with infants impacted by alcohol in utero that do not meet the full FAS criteria. Despite campaigns to inform the public, women continue to drink during pregnancy, but no safe amount of alcohol ingestion has been determined. FAS includes:

- **Facial abnormalities**: Hypoplastic (underdeveloped) maxilla, micrognathia (undersized jaw), hypoplastic philtrum (groove beneath the nose), short palpebral fissures (eye slits between upper and lower lids).
- **Neurological deficits**: May include microcephaly, intellectual disability, motor delay, and hearing deficits. Learning disorders may include problems with visual-spatial and verbal learning, attention disorders, delayed reaction times.
- **Growth restriction**: Prenatal growth deficit persists with slow growth after birth.
- **Behavioral problems**: Irritability and hyperactivity. Poor judgment in behavior may relate to deficit in executive functions.

Indication of brain damage without the associated physical abnormalities is referred to as alcohol-related neurodevelopmental disorder (ARND).

Fetal Exposure to Tobacco/Nicotine

Tobacco smoke contains many substances known to be detrimental to a person's health. When a pregnant woman smokes, her fetus is exposed to carbon monoxide, nicotine, and hydrogen cyanide that all cross the placenta. Carbon monoxide displaces oxygen from hemoglobin, resulting in decreased oxygen delivery to the fetus. Exposure increases risk of miscarriage and perinatal death. Infants exposed *in utero* to tobacco may have the following problems:

- Decreased length, weight, and head circumference
- Increased rates of congenital birth defects, such as cleft palate or lip, limb reduction defects, and urinary tract anomalies
- Increased incidence of placenta previa, placental abruption, and preterm birth

If smoking continues after delivery, these further detrimental effects may occur:

- Sudden infant death syndrome
- Increased infant respiratory tract infections and childhood asthma
- Behavioral problems in later childhood

Fetal Exposure to Marijuana, PCP, and MDMA

Marijuana, phencyclidine (PCP), and methylenedioxymethamphetamine (MDMA or ecstasy) are popular club drugs that may be used by some women during pregnancy:

- **Marijuana**: This is often used along with alcohol and tobacco, so effects are difficult to assess, but there do not appear to be teratogenic effects; however, some studies report exposure can result in fine tremors, irritability, and prolonged startle response for the first 12 months after birth.
- **PCP**: One of the biggest problems with PCP is that mothers may have an overdose or psychotic response that can result in hypertension, hyperthermia, and coma, compromising the fetus.
- **MDMA**: Ecstasy is frequently used by teenagers and young adults. There is no clear evidence regarding effects on the fetus although some research suggests it may cause long-term impairments in learning.

Fetal Exposure to Amphetamines

Amphetamines are a class of drugs that cause CNS stimulation. The most commonly abused amphetamine is methamphetamine. Maternal use of these substances causes hypertension and tachycardia, which can cause miscarriage, abruptio placentae, and premature delivery. Vasoconstriction affects placental vessels, decreasing circulation, nutrition, and oxygen to the fetus. Methamphetamines can cross the placental barrier and cause fetal hypertension and prenatal strokes and damage to the heart and other organs. The neonate is commonly small for gestational age, often ≤5 pounds, full term but ≤10 percentile for weight, with shortened length and smaller head circumference. The neonate in withdrawal from maternal amphetamine use will suffer abnormal sleep patterns, often characterized by lethargy and excessive sleeping during the first few weeks, poor feeding, tremors, diaphoresis, miosis, frantic fist sucking, high-pitched crying, fever, excessive yawning, and hyperreflexia.

Fetal Exposure to Heroin

Heroin is a highly addictive, opioid narcotic that is a common drug of abuse. Heroin users are at increased risk of poor nutrition, iron deficiency anemia, and preeclampsia-eclampsia, all negatively affecting the fetus. Infants with prenatal heroin exposure display symmetric intrauterine growth restriction (IUGR) and are often born prematurely. About 60-80% of these infants will undergo neonatal abstinence syndrome (NAS). Heroin has a relatively short half-life and symptoms of NAR typically begin 48-72 hours after delivery. Several different body systems are affected by NAS and include:

- **CNS Dysfunction**
  - High-pitched cry
  - Hyperactive reflexes
  - Irritability
  - Tremors
- **GI Dysfunction**
  - Poor feeding
  - Periods of frantic sucking or rooting
  - Vomiting
  - Loose or watery stools
- **Miscellaneous Signs**
  - Frequent yawning
  - Sneezing multiple times
  - Sweating
  - Fever
  - Tachypnea

Fetal Exposure to Methadone

Methadone is commonly used to treat women who are addicted to opioids, such as heroin or prescriptive narcotics, as it blocks withdrawal symptoms and drug craving. An associated risk is that methadone crosses the placental barrier and exposes the fetus to the drug. Many female heroin users are of reproductive age, and methadone is often administered to pregnant women to decrease dangers associated with heroin, such as fluctuating levels of drug and exposure to hepatitis and HIV from sharing of needles. Exposure to methadone may result in miscarriage, stillbirth, intrauterine growth restriction, fetal distress, and low birth weight, although symptoms are usually less severe than with heroin. However, if the mother takes methadone and other drugs, this can compound the adverse effects. Additionally, sudden withdrawal from methadone may cause preterm labor or death of the fetus, so methadone should be monitored carefully.

Fetal Exposure to Cocaine

Cocaine/crack (freebase cocaine) is a nonopioid substance that readily crosses the placenta through simple diffusion. One of the most potent properties of cocaine is its ability to act as a vasoconstrictor. When a mother uses cocaine, the blood supply to the placenta is severely compromised when the vessels constrict, compromising blood flow and resulting in growth restriction and hypoxia. Cocaine also causes a programmed cell death (known as apoptosis) in the heart muscle cells of the fetus, resulting in cardiac dysfunction for the fetus. Maternal cocaine use increases the risk of premature birth and causes serious consequences for the neonate after birth. Maternal cocaine use can cause cerebral infarctions, non-duodenal intestinal atresia, anal atresia, NEC, defects of the limbs, and genitourinary defects. Cocaine stimulates the central nervous system by limiting the uptake of certain neurotransmitters, such as norepinephrine, serotonin, and dopamine. Cocaine has a direct toxic effect on the nervous system, so the infant will exhibit extreme irritability and tremors followed by sluggish, lethargic behavior.

Fetal Exposure to Prescription/OTC Drugs

Many OTC and prescription drugs have teratogenic effects on the developing fetus and can result in congenital abnormalities, growth restriction, intellectual disability, carcinogenesis, mutagenesis, and miscarriage. The degree of damage relates to multiple factors, such as the amount of drug reaching the fetus, the developmental period during which the drug is taken, and the duration for which the drug was taken. There are some recognizable syndromes:

- **Fetal warfarin (Coumadin) syndrome** (exposure 7-12 weeks): Nasal hypoplasia, laryngomalacia, atrial septal defects, patent ductus arteriosis, eye, ear, and skull abnormalities, intellectual disabilities and growth restriction, brachydactyly, and scoliosis. Exposure during 2nd and 3rd trimester may result in eye abnormalities (cataracts, optic atrophy), microphthalmia (eyes stop developing resulting in abnormally small eyes), fetal/maternal hemorrhage, and microcephaly.
- **Fetal hydantoin (Dilantin) syndrome** (exposure 1st trimester): Facial dysmorphism, microcephaly, underdeveloped nails (hands and feet), cleft left/palate, and developmental delays ranging from mild to severe.
- **Fetal valproate (Depakote) syndrome** (exposure 1st trimester): Facial dysmorphism, spina bifida, CNS and cardiac abnormalities, and delay in development.

Some drugs are classified as high risk (FDA classification D), but use is acceptable if the mother has a life-threatening illness or other drugs are not available, so neonates may exhibit adverse effects.

Drugs with high risk include and their adverse effects on the fetus/infant include:

- **ACE inhibitors** (2nd and 3rd trimesters): skull and pulmonary hypoplasia, renal tubular dysplasia, and oligohydramnios
- **Carbamazepine** (1st trimester): craniofacial defects, neural tube defects, restriction of growth, and hypoplasia of fingernails
- **Antineoplastic alkylating drugs** (1st to 3rd trimesters): eye disorders, including microphthalmia and cataracts, cardiac defects, renal agenesis, and cardiac abnormalities
- **Iodides** (3rd trimester): thyroid disorders, including goiter, and fetal hypothyroidism
- **Methimazole** (1st trimester): aplasia cutis
- **Lithium** (1st trimester): Ebstein anomaly, various cardiac abnormalities
- **Tetracycline** (2nd and 3rd trimesters): yellow discoloration of teeth, weakening of fetal bones, and dysplasia of tooth enamel

Some drugs are classified as extremely high risk (FDA classification X), and these drugs should not be used with women who are pregnant or might become pregnant because fetal risk outweighs benefits to mother:

- **Androgens** (1st trimester): Female fetus will become masculinized.
- **Retinoids**, such as isotretinoin, acitretin, tretinoin, and etretinate (1st trimester): Multiple deformities of heart, ears, face, limbs, & liver, cognitive impairment, thymic hypoplasia, microcephalus, hydrocephalus, microtia, and miscarriage.
- **Thalidomide** (days 34-60): Multiple facial, intestinal, cardiac, limb abnormalities, including lack of limbs and limb reductions, and deafness.
- **Vitamin A** (>18,000 IU/day): Multiple craniofacial deformities, microtia, cardiac abnormalities, atresia of bowel, limb reductions, and defects of urinary tract.

Fetal Assessment

Ultrasound

Ultrasound is an imaging technique that uses high-frequency sound waves to create computer images of vessels, tissues, and organs. Newer scans include two-dimensional Doppler readings. Fetal ultrasound can be done at about the fifth week of gestation and is commonly done at 20 weeks for all pregnant women. Ultrasound is typically done **transabdominally** (though it may also be done **transvaginally**) to evaluate the gestational sac and embryo/fetus, providing the most accurate measurement of gestational age.

Trimester	Purpose
First	Estimate gestational age (accuracy ±5-7 days) Assess vaginal bleeding Determine if multiple fetuses are present Examine for indications of birth defects of the brain/spine
Second	Estimate gestational age (accuracy ±7-10 days) Determine size and position of placenta, fetus, and umbilical cord Examine for indications of major birth defects (cardiovascular/neural tube)
Third	Estimate gestational age (accuracy ±21-30 days) Assess fetal viability Determine size and position of placenta, fetus, and umbilical cord Estimate volume of amniotic fluid

CVS

Chorionic villus sampling (CVS) is performed by inserting a catheter into the uterus to obtain placental villi for testing. The tissue may also be obtained through the abdominal wall if needed to safely reach the placenta. Chromosomal, DNA, and enzymatic analysis is done on the tissue. This test is best performed at 10-13 weeks of gestation. This test provides results during early pregnancy to either reassure parents or to provide information needed to decide whether to continue the pregnancy. There is a small risk of fetal injury resulting in death during the procedure.

Amniocentesis

Amniocentesis is done at 15-20 weeks to evaluate for genetic disease and at 30-35 weeks to determine fetal lung maturity. Ultrasound locates the placenta and fetus and identifies an area with adequate amniotic fluid. The needle is then inserted carefully to avoid major structures, the fetus, and arteries. A local anesthetic may be administered before insertion of a 22-gauge spinal needle into the uterine cavity. The first drops of fluid are discarded and a syringe attached. About 15-20 mL of amniotic fluid are withdrawn and placed in tubes, brown-tinted to shield the fluid from light that might break down bilirubin or other pigments. Ultrasound is again used to monitor removal of the needle, and the insertion point is checked for streaming (leakage of fluid). If the mother is Rh-negative, she is given Rh immune globulin immediately, unless already sensitized. The fetal heart rate is monitored. Miscarriage occurs in about 1 in 1600 amniocenteses. If the procedure is performed at 11-14 weeks, there is increased risk to the fetus. Infection of the placenta (chorioamnionitis) is a rare complication.

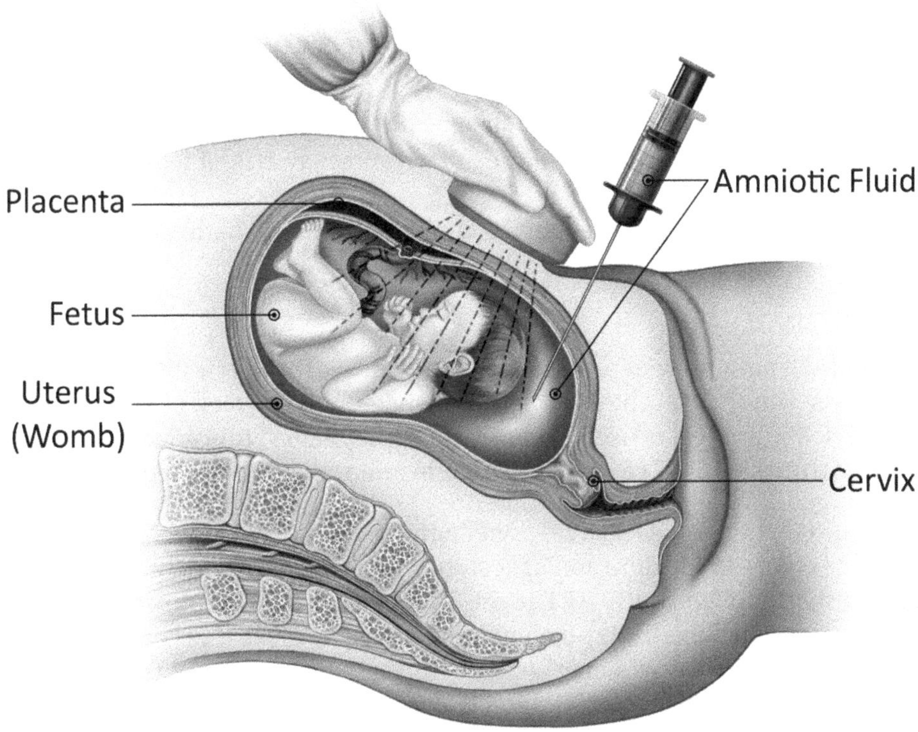

Biophysical Profile (BPP)

The fetal biophysical profile is a noninvasive antepartum test that uses ultrasound to evaluate four biophysical parameters: fetal respirations, fetal movement, fetal tone, and amniotic fluid volume. A separate nonstress test (NST) can also be performed to assess the fetal heart rate.

Measure	Discussion	Normal (2)	Abnormal (0)
Fetal Heart Rate	Measures fetal heart rate and acceleration with movement as measured by the NST	≥2 FHR accelerations of 15 bmp above baseline for ≥15 seconds in a 20-40-minute period (Reactive)	0-1 FHR accelerations in 40 minutes (Nonreactive)
Fetal Respirations	Assessed by ultrasound	≥1 episode of rhythmic breathing for ≥30 seconds in a 30-minute period	≤30 seconds of rhythmic breathing in 30 minutes
Fetal Movement	Assessed by ultrasound and tocodynamometer	≥3 separate movements in 30 minutes	≤2 movements in 30 minutes
Fetal Tone	Assessed by ultrasound	≥2 episodes of extension and flexion of arm/leg (or opening/closing of a hand)	No extension/flexion
Amniotic Fluid Volume	Assessed by ultrasound and amniotic fluid index	At least one single vertical pocket >2 cm	Largest single vertical pocket is ≤2 cm

Scoring:

- 10/10, 8/8 (NST omitted), or 8/10 (-2 points for either fetal movement, tone, or breathing but not amniotic fluid): Normal test result.
- 6/10 (-4 points for two of movement, tone, or breathing, but +2 points for amniotic fluid): Equivocal result—a significant possibility of developing fetal asphyxia cannot be excluded; test needs to be repeated or fetus needs to be delivered.
- 6/10 or 8/10 with 0 points for amniotic fluid: Abnormal; risk of fetal asphyxia within 1 week is high.
- 0-4/10: Abnormal; risk of fetal asphyxia within one week is high; delivery is usually indicated.

Alpha-Fetoprotein

Alpha-fetoprotein (AFT) is a protein produced by the yolk sac for the first 6 weeks of gestation and then by the fetal liver. Cutoff levels have been established for each week of gestation, with peak levels at about week 15. The test is used primarily to detect neural tube defects (NTDs), which develop in the first trimester. AFT can be measured in amniotic fluid or maternal serum.

Triple screening includes **serum AFT level** done in the second trimester. A positive result (which may be the result of errors in the duration of gestation) is followed by **ultrasound** and **amniocentesis** to check the **amniotic AFT level**. There is increased production of AFT with NTDs as well as abdominal wall defects and congenital nephrosis, so these levels can be used for assessment. (High quality ultrasound may also provide evidence of neural tube defects). The accuracy of tests varies depending upon the week of gestation. The most accurate results are acquired with testing during weeks 15-16. In addition to the serum AFT level, the Triple Screening also includes an examination of serum hCG (produced by the placenta) and estriol (produced by the placenta and the fetus).

Quad Screen

The Quad Screen is done between gestation weeks 16 and 20 to assess for risk of genetic abnormalities and is usually offered to all pregnant women but is especially important for those with the following risk factors: history of birth defects in family, age ≥35, use of teratogenic medications during pregnancy, diabetes mellitus with insulin use, exposure to high-dose radiation, and history of viral infection during pregnancy. The **Quad Screen** includes: (1) Alpha-fetoprotein (AFP), (2) Human chorionic gonadotropin (hCG), (3) Estriol (uE^3), and (4) Inhibin A (INH-A).

Disorder	AFP	hCG	uE^3	INH-A
Neural Tube Defects	High	Normal	Normal	Normal
Trisomy 21	Low	High	Low	High
Trisomy 18	Low	Low	Low	Low
Multiple Gestation	High	High	Normal	Normal

The fourth marker, inhibin A, improves the accuracy of screening for trisomy 21, especially in patients <35 years of age. With abnormal findings, an ultrasound may be used to verify weeks of gestation and an amniocentesis to confirm trisomy 21 or neural tube defects because of possible false positives.

Fetal Fibronectin Test

Fetal fibronectin (fFN) is a fetal extracellular glycoprotein that can be found in maternal cervical and vaginal secretions for the first 16-20 weeks of gestation, but then it is not found until near term.

The fetal fibronectin test is one that is carried out to assess the risk of preterm birth. If an increase in fFN is noted, this may be an indication that preterm labor may start, although this is not always the case. False positives may occur with fetal or maternal infection, cervical manipulation before collection of the specimen, sexual intercourse within 24 hours, lubricating gels, and vaginal bleeding. However, the absence of increased fFN almost always indicates that labor will not begin within the next 7 days. **Contraindications** include cervical dilation of ≥3 cm, suspected placental abruption or previa, vaginal bleeding, membrane rupture, or gestational age <22 weeks or >35 weeks. Special fFN kits are available for sample collection, which is taken with a speculum exam by rotating a swab across the vaginal fornix for 10 seconds and then inserting the swab into the collection tube.

PUBS

Percutaneous umbilical cord blood sampling (PUBS; also called cordocentesis) obtains fetal blood cells. A 22-gauge spinal needle is inserted into the umbilical vein at or very near the place where it joins the placenta while using ultrasound to guide placement. Fetal blood is collected and used to assess red cell and platelet status. Fetal blood cells are also used for genetic analysis with karyotyping available within 24-48 hours. Immunological, hematological, and metabolic studies can be done. The fetal acid-base balance can also be determined. Complications of the procedure include fetal injury or death, fetal bradycardia, amniotic fluid loss, vaginal bleeding, infections, or bleeding into the cord or from the fetus into the mother's circulation. The procedure may be done to verify results from other tests.

IUT

Indications for **intrauterine transfusion** (IUT) include various types of fetal anemia:

- **Erythrocyte alloimmunization**: CDE or other red cell antigens result in hemolytic anemia and lead to fetalis hydrops; antibodies build up with a first pregnancy and alloimmunization occurs with subsequent pregnancies.
- **Platelet alloimmunization**: Mother is alloimmunized against fetal paternal platelet antigens. This may occur with a first pregnancy. IUTs may be given to prevent cerebral hemorrhage but are required weekly and associated with significant morbidity.
- **Fetal-to-maternal hemorrhage**: IUT may be indicated if the hemorrhage is not ongoing, although cerebral hypoperfusion may result in irreversible neurological damage.
- **Infection**: Parvovirus B19 infection results in red cell hypoplasia and severe anemia. The fetus may develop viral myocarditis and, therefore, not respond well to the IUT.
- **Genetic disorders**: Alpha thalassemia major may be treated with IUT to correct the anemia and prevent fetal loss.

Risks associated with intrauterine transfusions include preterm rupture of membranes resulting in preterm delivery, fetal infection, maternal infection, fetal distress leading to cesarean, fetal fluid overload, and fetal/neonatal death.

Umbilical Artery Doppler Flow Study

Umbilical artery Doppler flow studies measure the blood flow waveform from the uterine arteries through the umbilical cord and help to calculate the systolic/diastolic (S/D) ratio. Umbilical artery Doppler flow studies are used during the third trimester for high-risk pregnancies to assess fetal wellbeing, signs of placental insufficiency, and intrauterine growth restriction or preeclampsia. The peak of the systolic waveform shows the maximum velocity of the blood flow when the fetal heart is contracting and the end-diastolic waveform shows the continuing flow of blood in the umbilical artery when the heart is relaxed. As the placenta matures and gestation advances in a normal pregnancy, there is increased flow during diastole and the S/D ratio decreases. However, with growth restriction, end-diastolic flow may be absent or even reversed (indicating the need for immediate delivery). If the absent or reverse end-diastolic flow is associated with maternal preeclampsia, then the fetus is at increased risk of hypoglycemia and polycythemia.

Tests for Fetal Lung Maturity

Tests for fetal lung maturity are important for monitoring a fetus if there is an indication for early termination of pregnancy. Pulmonary maturity is often an important factor in neonatal survival, as immaturity can result in respiratory distress syndrome (RDS). Commonly, two tests are used to confirm lung maturity. Tests of amniotic fluid include:

- **Lecithin/sphingomyelin (L/S) ratio:** The ratio of the surfactants lecithin and sphingomyelin changes during pregnancy, with L/S ratio at 0.5:1 early in pregnancy, 1:1 at 30-32 weeks, and 2:1 at 35 weeks. At 2:1, RDS is unlikely, although this finding is not always accurate for infants of diabetic mothers (IDM), as they may show an adequate ratio but still develop RDS. These neonates must be monitored carefully. This test is not accurate if the amniotic fluid contains blood or meconium.
- **Phosphatidylglycerol (PG):** This phospholipid first appears in surfactant at about week 35 in IDM with complications and week 36 in other pregnancies. Its presence is a sign of lung maturity.

Fetomaternal Hemorrhage and Kleihauer-Betke Test

Fetomaternal hemorrhage (FMH) occurs in many pregnancies without any signs or symptoms. A small amount of fetal blood in the maternal circulation (1-2 mL) has no clinical significance. Massive FMH (blood loss greater than 30 mL) occurs in about 3 of every 1,000 pregnancies, and is a major cause of stillbirths. Neonates' blood volume ranges from 85-100 mL/kg, so 30 mL of blood loss represents 10-12% of the blood volume in a 3 kg neonate. Risk factors for FMH include maternal trauma, placental abruption, placental tumors, third trimester amniocentesis, fetal hydrops, and twinning. One test used to diagnose the presence of FMH is the **Kleihauer-Betke (KB) test**, in which a sample of the mother's blood is examined for the presence of fetal hemoglobin. The KB test estimates the amount of hemorrhage that has taken place.

Fetal Scalp Blood Sampling

Fetal scalp blood sampling (FBS) can be obtained to check blood gases of the fetus during labor when membranes have already ruptured and there is access to the scalp. The most important parameters used are those of pH and base excess. These results can be affected by many factors, including length of time drawing the sample, exposure to air, improper handling or technique, drawing a sample during a contraction, maternal position, fever, hypertension, and the presence of caput succedaneum. A pH below 7 and base excess below -7 combined with signs of distress on electronic fetal heart monitor tracings will prompt an emergency birth. Fetal blood sampling requires skill and because of many false-positives, it is used infrequently. Scalp stimulation is used more often to determine FHR reactivity as a sign of fetal status.

Obtaining Umbilical Cord Blood Gases

Cord blood gases give a picture of the acid base status in the newborn's tissues at the time of birth. After birth, a segment of the umbilical cord is clamped on each end and placed on the delivery table until newborn status is determined. An accurate **pH and blood gas analysis** can be performed on this cord blood for up to 60 minutes after birth. ACOG recommends obtaining arterial and venous cord blood samples after cesarean sections for fetal distress, abnormalities during FHR evaluation in labor, low Apgar scores, growth restriction, maternal hypothyroidism, maternal fever, or multiple fetuses. When done rapidly after birth, the blood gas results can guide the treatment of the compromised neonate.

Fetal Heart Rate Monitoring During Labor

Continuous Fetal Heart Rate Monitoring

Fetal heart rate (FHR) monitoring is usually done by **electronic fetal monitoring** (EFM), as it provides a continuous tracing. FHR can be assessed by auscultation or ultrasound with an abdominal transducer, but tracings can be poor with an active fetus, maternal movement, and hydramnios. Intermittent monitoring is usually every 15 minutes in the first stage of labor and every 5 minutes in the second. Internal monitoring requires cervical dilation of ≥2 cm so an electrode can be applied to the fetal presenting part (head or buttocks). Internal scalp electrodes should not be used if the mother has a communicable disease, such as HIV, or with preterm infants. Telemetry with ultrasound or fetal ECG transducers and external uterine pressure transducers can also be used to monitor FHR. This type of battery-operated monitoring can be used while the mother ambulates, as it is less invasive. FHR patterns are evaluated against a baseline rate (rate for 10 minutes between contractions), usually 110-160 bpm.

NICHD Category I, II, and III Fetal Heart Rate Tracings

NICHD Category fetal heart tracings assess acid-base status at the time of observation only, as fetal status may change over time and the fetus's category may change:

- **I (Normal)**: Tracings indicate baseline FHR of 110-160 bpm with only moderate variability. There may be early decelerations but no late or variable decelerations. This category predicts normal acid-base status.
- **II (Indeterminate)**: May include numerous findings inconsistent with category I or III. Variability may be minimal or marked. Variability without recurrent decelerations may be absent. Accelerations after fetal stimulation may be absent. Deceleration may be prolonged, variable, or recurrent late with only moderate variability. Data is insufficient to categorize as normal or to assume abnormal acid-base status.
- **III (Abnormal)**: There is no variability in FHR with recurrent late decelerations, recurrent variable decelerations, or bradycardia. A sinusoidal pattern may be noted. This category predicts abnormal acid-base status.

External FHR Monitoring

External FHR monitoring may be used prior to the rupture of membranes and dilatation of the cervix because it is noninvasive; however, it is not as accurate as internal monitoring. A **transducer** is strapped to the abdomen to pick up the sounds of the fetal heart valves and blood ejection during systole. The resultant FHR is then displayed on the monitor. A gel is used to obtain proper conduction of sound from the fetal heart to the transducer. Leopold maneuvers determine fetal lie; the transducer is then applied over the back or chest of the fetus. A tocodynamometer is used to monitor uterine activity to allow correlation between fetal heart activity and uterine contractions. This method is problematic in the obese patient. It is also affected by maternal position and movement and fetal movement. Fetal heart tones may not be reliably obtained during a contraction.

Internal Fetal Heart Monitor

An internal fetal heart monitor may be used when the membranes are ruptured and the cervix is dilated to 2-3 cm. A **spiral electrode** is screwed into the fetal scalp. This allows the FHR to be more accurately distinguished from the maternal heartbeat. If fetal death has occurred, the maternal heart beat will be detected by the electrode. A reference electrode is attached to the maternal thigh. An intrauterine pressure monitoring catheter is inserted into the uterus next to the fetus to monitor contractions, allowing direct correlation between fetal heart activity and uterine contractions. Internal monitoring is the most accurate method of monitoring contractions and the FHR.

Fetal Heart Rate Abnormalities

Fetal heart rate usually varies with accelerations and decelerations. Fetal reactivity (accelerated fetal heart rate with fetal activity) begins at about 32 weeks. Heart rate often increases for periods of 20-40 minutes. These are causes for accelerated or decelerated fetal heart rate.

- **Tachycardia:** HR >160 for ≥10 minutes (severe, HR >180). Transient tachycardia occurs <10 minutes and is usually not significant. Tachycardia may result from early fetal hypoxia, prematurity, medications (such as terbutaline), fetal infection, maternal fever, or anxiety.
- **Bradycardia:** HR <120 for ≥10 minutes (severe, HR <80). Bradycardia at 100-119 is usually not significant, but bradycardia may indicate heart block or placentae abruptio. Uterine contractions slow the fetal heart rate because of compression of the head affecting cerebral blood flow, compression of the myometrial vessels of the uterus, and/or occlusion of the umbilical cord causing fetal hypertension or hypoxemia. Epidural anesthesia and medications such as narcotics and oxytocin can also cause decreased heart rate.

Review Video: Fetal Heart Rate
Visit mometrix.com/academy and enter code: 980576

Fetal Heart Rate Variability and Accelerations

Fetal heart rate **variability** shows sensitivity to oxygenation and acid-base status. Good variability indicates adequate oxygenation of the fetus's central nervous system (CNS). Decreased variability corresponds to fetal hypoxia and acidemia. Fetal heart rate variability is fluctuation in the fetal heart rate of two cycles or more, graded according to the range of amplitude:

- Absent: range not detectable
- Minimal: ≤5 bpm
- Moderate: 6-25 bpm
- Marked: >25 bpm

Short-term variability is a variation in amplitude of 3-8 bpm on a beat-to-beat basis. Long-term variability is an irregular pattern of variability of 3-5 cycles per minute with an amplitude of 5-15 bpm.

FHR **accelerations** are transient increases in fetal heart rate. Non-periodic accelerations relate to fetal movement. Periodic accelerations accompany contractions and/or compression of the umbilical cord and may indicate low amniotic fluid or dangerous cord compression.

Fetal Heart Rate Decelerations

Decelerations are transient decreases in FHR. They are categorized according to contraction cycle and waveform.

- **Early**: Caused by head compression as it descends the birth canal. Waveform is uniform, with onset just before or at the onset of contraction and the lowest level at the midpoint of contraction, inversely mirroring contraction. Range is usually 120-160 bpm. Deceleration may occur once or may repeat.
- **Late**: Caused by compression of vessels and uteroplacental insufficiency. Waveform is uniform, with shape reflecting contraction. Onset is late in the contraction and the lowest point is after the midpoint of the contraction. Range is 120-130 bpm. Deceleration may be occasional, consistent, or repetitive.
- **Variable**: Caused by umbilical cord compression. Waveform is variable with sharp drops and increases. Onset may be abrupt with fetal insult and not related to contraction. The lowest point is around the midpoint. The range is usually outside normal. Deceleration may be variable and occur once or repetitively. Repetitive deceleration may indicate fetal distress.

Artifacts on Fetal Heart Rate Tracing

Various **artifacts** (misleading fetal heart tracings) can occur when monitoring fetal heart rate, usually related to the maternal heart rate, which results in **signal ambiguity** (maternal heart rate displayed on FHR monitor). Artifacts can result from:

- **Maternal pacemaker interference**: Fetal electrode may record pacemaker firing.
- **Deceased fetus**: The maternal heartbeat may continue to register on the fetal electrode.
- **Superimposition**: The maternal heart rate or QRS complex may be superimposed on the fetal heart tracing.
- **Maternal heart rate tracing** displayed instead of fetal.

Artifacts and signal ambiguity should be suspected when the fetal heart rate continues at a low normal rate, at least 50% of contractions result in accelerations of FHR, and the FHR appears to decelerate to the maternal heart rate and does not return to baseline. If signal ambiguity is expected, the maternal pulse rate should be counted and traced and fetal and maternal tracings compared. To correct this, the FHR should be assessed with ultrasound, the Doppler sensor relocated, or a scalp electrode placed.

Uterine Contraction Assessment

Uterine contraction assessment is correlated with the FHR to determine if labor is progressing normally. Contractions can be palpated with the hands. They can also be externally monitored by using a tocodynamometer or internally monitored by inserting an intrauterine pressure catheter after the membranes are ruptured and the cervix is dilated to 2-3 cm. Contractions should be **assessed** for frequency (amount of time from the beginning of one contraction to the beginning of the next), duration (amount of time in seconds from the beginning to the end of the contraction), and intensity (mild, medium, or strong in strength). **Uterine resting tone** between contractions should also be determined. All four characteristics can be determined by palpation but it is a somewhat subjective method. External monitoring can determine the duration and frequency but not the intensity or resting tone. Internal monitoring is most accurate because the amniotic pressure is measured. It can be used to determine all four characteristics.

Abnormal Patterns of Uterine Activity

The desirable **pattern of uterine activity** during active labor is the presence of contractions every 2-3 minutes. Inadequate or abnormal patterns may develop, especially during oxytocin augmentation.

A pattern of **hyperstimulation** is the persistence of more than 5 contractions in a 10-minute period or contractions that occur within 1 minute of each other. They may be caused by maternal hormones or agents used to ripen the cervix or augment labor. They can cause fetal distress by interfering with uteroplacental blood flow.

Coupling or tripling occurs when contractions occur in groups of 2 or 3 with very little interval between, followed by a rest period of 2-5 minutes. This may occur as a result of incoordination of the uterine pacemakers or a decrease in sensitivity of oxytocin receptor sites in the uterine muscle.

Hypertonus and Uterine Tachysystole

Uterine hypertonus, a state in which the uterine muscle does not relax between contractions, may result from hormonal imbalance, immature genitals, infections, cervical failure, and fibroid tumors. Ineffectual contractions in the latent phase of labor become more frequent but do not result in dilation or effacement. The resting tone of the myometrium increases. The contractions may interfere with uteroplacental exchange, resulting in fetal distress. The pressure on the fetal head may result in cephalhematoma, caput succedaneum, or excessive molding. Oxytocin infusion or amniotomy may be used for treatment after assessment for cephalo-pelvic disproportion (CPD).

Uterine tachysystole is 6 or more contractions in a 10-minute period (averaged over 30 minutes) or a series of 2-minute or greater single contractions. Common causes include infection, dehydration, placental abruption, and induction. While associated with fetal heart decelerations, the fetus does not generally suffer adverse effects unless the uterine tachysystole is associated with hypertonus.

Intrauterine Resuscitation

In the case of NICDH Category III FHR patterns (indicating fetal acidosis) that demonstrate a sinusoidal pattern and are not responding to scalp stimulation, **in utero resuscitation** is indicated. The following actions should be taken for effective intrauterine resuscitation:

- **Reposition** the mother laterally (on the right or left side) to relieve any pressure that may be compressing the cord or causing insufficient perfusion of the placenta. Knees to the chest may be effective if the lateral position is not. Apply oxygen to the mother as a precaution (generally 8-10 L/min via nonrebreather mask).
- **Fluid resuscitation** with a bolus of 500-1000 mL Lactated Ringer's or normal saline. This improves placental perfusion and restores volume in the mother in the case of hypovolemia.
- If **uterotonic drugs** are being administered, stop them immediately. Blood flow to the placenta is decreased during contractions. **Tocolytics** (such as terbutaline) may also be administered to enhance uterine relaxation.
- If hypotension is potentially secondary to the epidural dosing, **consult anesthesia** to make changes or compensate for epidural associated hypotension.

Medications Used in Labor

ORIGIN OF PAIN DURING LABOR

The acute **pain of labor** is affected by variations in the individual patient, past experience and perception of pain, and past and present obstetrical procedures. Pain is affected by the rate of dilatation, intensity and length of contractions, fetal position, and fetal size. The lack of sleep and exhaustion reduces pain tolerance as the labor progresses. The mother's age and past pregnancy and delivery experiences also influence her perception of labor pain.

Physiologically, labor pain has its origin in uterine muscle hypoxia and the accumulation of lactic acid from uterine contractions. Pain also occurs with the stretching of the tissues in the lower uterine segment, cervix, ovaries, fallopian tubes, and uterine ligaments, followed by pain from the stretching of the pelvic floor, vagina, vulva, and perineum. Bone pain from pressure on the bony pelvis or lower spine contributes to discomfort. Pressure on the bladder, urethra, and rectum causes pain during the second stage as well.

PHARMACOLOGIC CONTROL OF LABOR PAIN

SYSTEMIC ANALGESICS DURING LABOR

Analgesics may be given during labor as needed, but because they cross the placenta and may depress the neonate's breathing, only the minimum amount required for maternal comfort should be given. The neonate's metabolic and excretory processes are immature, so drugs are cleared much more slowly by liver metabolism or urinary excretion once the umbilical cord is cut.

Opioids and sedatives may be given to decrease labor pain, allowing the woman to rest and decrease anxiety. They are usually given only when labor is well established, because they decrease labor contraction frequency and duration and FHR variability. If given too close to birth, CNS depression is increased in the fetus. This depression can persist after delivery, especially in premature infants, affecting Apgar scores. These drugs can also cause maternal respiratory depression and resultant fetal distress. Some drugs, such as morphine and benzodiazepines, are avoided because they can cause excessive fetal depression.

- **Fentanyl** (25-100 µg/hr IV) has a shorter onset (3-10 minutes) with one-hour duration and causes less fetal depression.
- **Butorphanol** (1-2 mg IV or IM every 4 hr) and **nalbuphine** (10-20 mg IV or IM every 3 hr) cause little respiratory effect and provide adequate relief of pain but may result in excessive sedation if given repeatedly.
- **Promethazine** (25-50 mg IM) **or propiomazine hydrochloride** (20-40mg IV or IM) may be given along with narcotics to decrease nausea and vomiting, provide relief of anxiety, and to reduce the dose of opioids.

Nitrous oxide is a weak anesthetic in high concentrations, but in low doses, it is an anxiolytic and an analgesic. While common in countries such as Australia, New Zealand, Canada and Great Britain, the use of **inhaled nitrous oxide** for pain management has only recently become more common in the United States. Nitrous oxide is self-administered by the patient by inhaling the gas through a mask 30-60 seconds prior to an expected contraction (due to its delayed effect). This may be difficult for the mother in later stages of labor. Because nitrous oxide does not accumulate in the lungs, it is safe for both the mother and fetus. It can cause nausea and vomiting or excessive sleepiness, so the mother should be assessed for these side effects.

> **Review Video: Calculating IV Drip Rates**
> Visit mometrix.com/academy and enter code: 396112

Regional Analgesia Used During Labor

Neuraxial Analgesia

Neuraxial analgesia techniques, including **epidurals, spinals, and combined epidural-spinal**, have grown in popularity. This is because they have a flexibility and effectiveness that make them ideal for this purpose. They cause less depression of the maternal and fetal CNS. These methods of providing regional anesthesia require skill to provide effective analgesia while retaining as much motor control as possible. A catheter placed in the epidural space delivers an infusion that is intermittent, continuous, or patient-controlled. Local anesthetics used include bupivacaine, lidocaine, and ropivacaine. Narcotics such as fentanyl, sufentanil, alfentanil, and remifentanil are often added to the infusion to lessen the amount of anesthetic used and therefore decrease the amount of motor blockage. The duration and quality of pain relief is also improved. Neuraxial analgesia provides better pain relief than systemic methods.

Lumbar Epidural

The most common form of regional anesthesia/analgesia for labor and delivery is the **lumbar epidural**. Dilute mixtures of local anesthetic and opioids are combined. The catheter is usually placed early so that it is available when pain relief is needed. At one time, epidurals were delayed until labor was well established, but the current trend is to administer it earlier if the fetus is in no distress, contractions are 3-4 minutes apart and persist for at least 60 seconds, and the fetal head is engaged with 3-4 cm of cervical dilation. The catheter is usually placed with the mother in a sitting position to ensure sacral spread. Placement is usually at L3 to L4 or L4 to L5. If inadvertent spinal placement occurs, spinal anesthesia/analgesia may be given or the catheter removed and replaced at a higher level. Most commonly, bupivacaine or ropivacaine (0.0625-0.125%) is given in combination with fentanyl (2-3 μg/mL) or sufentanil (0.3-0.5 μg/mL). If dilute anesthetic agents are used, the mother may be able to ambulate while receiving the epidural.

Intrathecal Analgesia with Opioids

Intrathecal (spinal) analgesia, injected into the subarachnoid space with only **opioids**, is sometimes used during the **first stage of labor**. Commonly used agents include morphine (0.25-0.5 mg), fentanyl (12.5-15 μg), and sufentanil (10-15 μg, mixed with 10 mL of low dose bupivacaine). Meperidine is the only agent that has local anesthetic characteristics. Higher doses are needed if spinal opioids are used alone, administered as a single dose, or given intermittently per catheter. This can result in higher risk of complications, maternal respiratory depression, and fetal depression. However, if given alone, opioids (except for meperidine) do not provide motor blockade or maternal hypotension, so the mother is able to push. However, the analgesic effect may not be adequate, and side effects (pruritis, nausea, and vomiting) related to the agent may occur. Morphine alone has a slow onset (45-60 minutes), although it provides 4 to 6 hours of analgesia with spinal administration. However, low doses may not provide adequate relief, and high doses increase side effects. Morphine is frequently combined with fentanyl for more rapid onset. Commonly, opioids are combined with local anesthetics.

Spinal Anesthesia (Saddle Block)

A saddle block, or spinal anesthesia, is usually given just before vaginal delivery to provide rapid **perineal anesthesia**. Spinal blocks are avoided during labor because they interfere with motor function. Because of this, other agents may be used during labor. Prior to receiving the spinal anesthesia, the patient is given a bolus of 500-1000 mL fluid. With the patient in a sitting position, a very small spinal needle (to prevent CSF leakage and post-spinal headache) is inserted into the subarachnoid space. Local anesthetics used include hyperbaric tetracaine, bupivacaine, or lidocaine, often with the addition of fentanyl or sufentanil to potentiate the effect. The agents are administered between contractions over about 30 seconds. The patient remains sitting for 3 minutes and then is placed in lithotomy position with left uterine displacement to prepare for delivery.

Pudendal Nerve Block

Visceral pain occurs in the first stage of labor from contractions and cervical dilation with afferent impulses entering the spinal cord at T10 and T11. However, during the second stage of labor, the stretching of the vagina and perineum caused by the descent of the fetus causes **somatic pain** with impulses carried by the pudendal nerves to the spinal cord at S2 to S4. **Pudendal nerve block** is used during the second stage (sometimes along with perineal infiltration) to reduce **somatic pain** when neuraxial blocks are contraindicated and for episiotomy and relaxation of the pelvic floor for forceps delivery. With the patient in lithotomy position, a transvaginal or transperineal approach is used to block the nerve. For the transvaginal approach (the most common), a Kobak needle or special guide (Iowa trumpet) is used to prevent inadvertent injection into the fetal head. Anesthetic agents include 10 mL of 1% lidocaine or 2% chloroprocaine. The transperineal approach may be used if the head is engaged.

General Anesthesia in Birth Process

General anesthesia is rarely used for vaginal birth but may be used for emergency procedures and Cesarean births if the mother is not a good candidate for epidural or subarachnoid block. Maternal complications can include aspiration of stomach contents, especially if the woman has not been NPO, and this can result in postoperative chemical pneumonitis. Therefore, an oral antacid is sometimes administered prior to anesthesia. A wedge should be placed under the woman's right hip to displace the uterus to the left prior to administration of anesthesia. The woman may experience respiratory depression, and this can affect the oxygenation of the fetus. General anesthesia can also result in relaxation of the uterine muscles, and if this persists in the postoperative period, it increases the risk of postpartum hemorrhage. General anesthesia is contraindicated with a high risk or preterm fetus because of fetal depression. Anesthesia usually affects the fetus within 2 minutes, so rapid delivery reduces risks to the fetus.

Tocolytics

Tocolysis suppresses preterm labor and premature birth, sometimes allowing time to administer betamethasone to accelerate maturity of fetal lungs. Tocolytics (some off-label) include the following:

- **Indomethacin,** an NSAID that inhibits prostaglandin production, can be used up to 32 weeks of gestation. It crosses the placenta and can cause reduction in amniotic fluid, leading to fetal distress, especially >32 weeks. Indomethacin can also cause premature closure of the ductus arteriosus. This medication is the first-line therapy for women 24-32 weeks gestation.
- **Nifedipine**, a calcium channel blocker that reduces muscle contractility, is most commonly used, as it is more effective and safer than many other drugs. It may increase fetal heart rate (FHR). This is second-line therapy for women 24-32 weeks gestation and first-line therapy for women 32-34 weeks gestation.
- **Terbutaline** is a beta-adrenergic asthma drug that also relaxes the uterine muscle. It may increase FHR. It can be used as second-line therapy at 32-34 weeks gestation when nifedipine is used in the 24-32 weeks gestational period.
- **Magnesium sulfate** is similar in action to terbutaline, but it requires close monitoring for maternal adverse effects. It crosses the placenta, and the neonate may suffer respiratory and motor depression.

Concurrent use of tocolytics is discouraged.

Complications of Labor

Complications Regarding Rupture of Membranes

There are various complications in regards to the rupture of membranes:

- **Premature rupture of membranes (PROM):** The chorioamniotic membrane breaks, ideally at term (40 weeks), prior to onset of labor. Rupture of membranes is premature if labor fails to begin within an hour. About 80% of women go into labor within 24 hours. If labor doesn't begin in 12-24 hours, the patient must be frequently monitored to ensure that adequate amniotic fluid remains, or labor may be induced or augmented to prevent infection if the child is at term.
- **Spontaneous rupture (SROM)** usually occurs in the early stage of labor during an intense contraction, causing the fluid to gush out of the vagina.
- **Preterm premature rupture of membranes (PPROM)** occurs in a woman <37 weeks of gestation and prior to the onset of labor. The patient is monitored, as with premature rupture. It is one of the leading causes of premature birth.
- **Prolonged rupture of membranes**: Prolonged PROM persists for greater than 18-24 hours prior to the onset of labor. It is associated with increased risk of infection in the neonate.

Preterm Premature Rupture of Membranes Causes and Fetal Viability

There are numerous **causes for PPROM**, including infections and digital pelvic exams. When a woman presents in labor, the estimated date of delivery should be obtained by determining the date of the last menstrual period (LMP) and using a gestation calculator wheel or estimating with Naegele's rule: first day LMP minus 3 months plus 7 days equals estimated date of delivery.

Fetal viability is very low before 23 weeks of gestation; by 25 weeks, delaying delivery for 2 days can increase survival rates by 10%. Tocolytic drugs, which have many negative side effects, may be used to delay delivery in order to administer glucocorticoids, such as betamethasone or dexamethasone, to improve fetal lung maturity between weeks 24 and 36.

Precipitous Labor/Birth

Precipitous labor and birth occurs when onset of labor to birth takes 3 hours or less, often because of strong uterine contractions and low muscle resistance in maternal tissue that promotes rapid dilatation of the cervix (or lacerations) and descent of the fetus. A primigravida may dilate 5 cm per hour; and a multigravida as quickly as 10 cm per hour. The neonate may have a low Apgar score and is at increased risk for aspiration of meconium and intracranial injury, such as subdural/dural tears. The strong uterine contractions may interfere with uterine blood flow and oxygenation of the fetus. Precipitous birth alone, by contrast, is usually an unexpected and sudden birth that takes place outside of the hospital or is unattended by a physician because there is no time to travel or get help. In these cases, the neonate is sometimes expelled into a toilet or onto the floor, causing injury.

Prolonged Labor

Prolonged labor results from dysfunctional uterine contractions, accounting for 50% of Cesareans in nulliparous women, but only 5% of Cesareans in multiparous women. Dysfunctional contractions are often irregular, exhibit low amplitude, and result in <1 cm cervical dilatation/hr. In some cases, contractions continue but cervical dilatation is arrested. The **labor patterns** below are associated with prolonged labor:

- **Hypertonic:** Ineffectual contractions in the latent phase of labor become more frequent but do not result in dilatation or effacement. The resting tone of the myometrium increases. The contractions may interfere with uteroplacental exchange, resulting in fetal distress. The pressure on the fetal head may result in cephalohematoma, caput succedaneum, or excessive molding. Oxytocin infusion or amniotomy may be used after assessment for cephalopelvic disproportion (CPD).
- **Hypotonic**: Fewer than 3 contractions occur in 10 minutes during active phase, with less than 1 cm dilatation per hour or arrest of dilatation. Treatment is the same as for hypertonic patterns.

Post-Term Pregnancy

Post-term pregnancy (>294 days or 42 weeks past 1st day of last menstrual period) occurs in 3-7% of pregnancies, and is often the result of errors in calculating due date, but true post-term pregnancies, while posing little risk to the mother, can increase the risk to the fetus, and vaginal birth may be facilitated by forceps or vacuum extractor. Increased fetal risks include:

- **Large for gestational age** (LGA), >4500g (about 10 pounds), which may result in prolonged labor, birth trauma with fractures or neurological injury, or Cesarean section.
- **Aspiration of meconium** occurs more frequently because a large fetus is more likely to expel meconium.
- **Post-maturity syndrome** related to restriction of growth in the uterus, often because of restricted blood flow, putting the fetus at risk for respiratory and neurological disorders.

Cephalopelvic/Fetopelvic Disproportion

Cephalopelvic/fetopelvic disproportion is usually diagnosed when labor does not progress, although in rare cases it may be diagnosed prior to labor. It may relate to pelvic diameters that are too small (most common with android and platypelloid pelvic types) or due to contractures of the pelvic inlet (<10 cm anteroposterior diameter or <12 cm transverse diameter), contracted midpelvis, or contracted outlet (<8 cm interischial tuberous diameter). Rarely is this disproportion caused by excessive fetal size as most fetuses are within normal size and weight limits. Usually, labor is extended and premature rupture of the membranes occurs, increasing danger of cord prolapse. The fetal head is often markedly molded and continued pressure can cause neurological injury or even death of the fetus if the labor continues and the fetus cannot be delivered, but when labor fails to progress, the mother is usually given a Cesarean section (within 2 hours of labor onset) to prevent further injury to the fetus.

Fetal Malpresentation

Military

The head is erect and neck not flexed. This poses little problem because flexion often occurs as the head descends.

Brow

The neck is extended so that the brow presents first. This presentation may relate to SGA, LGA, hydramnios, and uterine or fetal anomalies. Brow presentation, with the largest diameter (about 13.5 cm), increases fetal mortality because of birth trauma, which can include compression of the neck and cerebrum, and tracheal and laryngeal damage. Cesarean delivery or vaginal delivery with episiotomy is usually required.

Face

The neck is severely extended so that the face presents first (about 9.5 cm diameter). This often prolongs labor and may result in increased edema of the fetus and trauma to the neck and internal structures. The neonate usually has bruising in the facial skin. Cesarean section is generally required.

Breech

This occurs in 4% of births and is frequently related to early labor and delivery (25% are at 25 to 26 weeks). Frank breech (buttocks presentation with legs extended upward) is most common, but single or double footling breech or complete breech (buttocks presentation with legs flexed) can occur. Breech presentation is most common with placenta previa, hydramnios, fetal anomalies, and multiple gestations. Cord prolapse is more likely. Head trauma may occur because molding does not occur, and the head can become entrapped. Mortality and morbidity are reduced with Cesarean section, especially with low or high fetal weight, hyperextension of neck (>90°), fetal anomalies, and pelvic disproportion. Version may be attempted, in which pressure is placed on the fetus externally, in attempt to move the fetus from breech position to a head-down position. This must be done before contractions begin and the fetal head is engaged. If unsuccessful, Cesarean section is the recommended and safest mode of delivery.

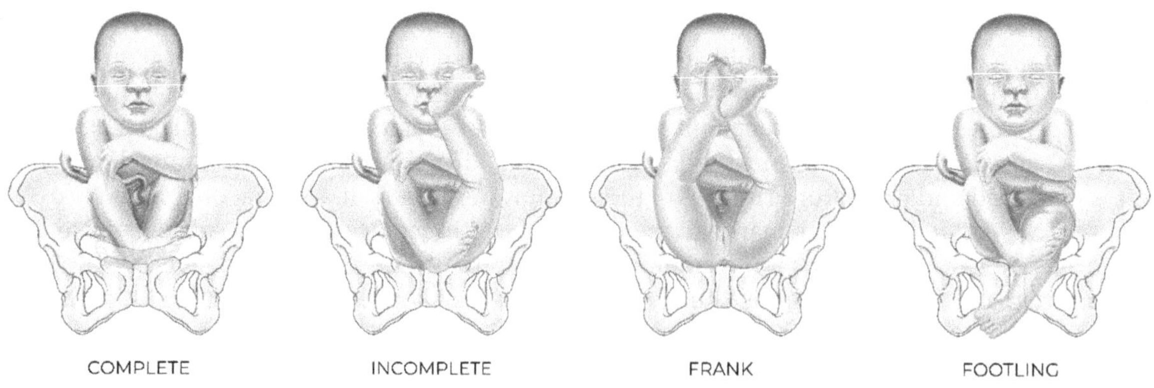

Shoulder

This transverse lie poses extreme risk of uterine rupture. The fetus cannot be delivered, and Cesarean section is required.

COMPOUND

This is when there are two presenting parts, such as the head and a hand, increasing the chance of laceration. With fetal distress or uterine dysfunction, a Cesarean section is required.

MECONIUM IN AMNIOTIC FLUID

When meconium is present in the amniotic fluid, the following considerations should be taken following birth to avoid meconium aspiration syndrome:

- If the infant is crying and showing no signs of distress (known as being vigorous), current NRP guidelines no longer recommend suctioning. Visible drainage can be wiped away with a cloth.
- If the infant shows signs of respiratory distress in the presence of meconium-stained fluid, NRP guidelines now recommend using a bulb suction as the first attempt to restore ventilation, suctioning the mouth before the nose. Deep suctioning risks the possibility of causing a vagal response that can result in dangerous arrhythmias.
- If respiratory distress continues despite these non-invasive efforts, intubation is indicated. Only if an airway obstruction is suspected (all efforts to ventilate the infant are not resulting in chest rise) should the trachea be suctioned with a large catheter within the endotracheal tube, attached to wall suction.

Once the airway has been adequately suctioned and cleared, the stomach may need to be suctioned as well in order to prevent the regurgitation of the swallowed meconium. Meconium that is swallowed and then regurgitated can be aspirated into the lungs.

PLACENTA PREVIA AND ABRUPTIO PLACENTAE

Placenta previa: Implantation of the placenta is over or near the internal cervical os. Women with placenta previa have increased incidences of hemorrhage in the third trimester. In infants, placenta previa is associated with poor growth, anemia, and increased risk of congenital anomalies in their central nervous systems, heart, respiratory and gastrointestinal tracts. Placenta previa may also cause premature birth with associated neonatal complications of prematurity.

Abruptio placentae: The placenta prematurely detaches, partially or completely, from the uterus. Abruptio placentae is related to maternal hypertension, and incidence increases with cocaine abuse. Partial detachment interferes with the functioning of the placenta, causing intrauterine growth restriction. Severe bleeding occurs with total detachment. Common fetal complications are preterm labor, hypoxia, and anemia. Fetal mortality is about 25% with partial detachment and 100% with complete. Irreversible brain damage may occur with fetal hypoxia, and neurological deficits occur in about 14% of survivors.

VASA PREVIA

Vasa previa is an abnormality where at least one of the fetal blood vessels lies across the internal cervical os. The fetal umbilical vein and arteries lie unprotected on the membrane wall on their way to the placenta. This predisposes the fetus to hemorrhage if one of the vessels is injured during membrane rupture that occurs spontaneously or artificially. The FHR reacts immediately to the vessel damage and death occurs in 56% of all cases. An immediate cesarean section is indicated. Diagnosis may be made prenatally by transvaginal Doppler ultrasound or routine ultrasound that examines placental cord insertion. A planned cesarean increases the fetal survival rate to 97%.

Abnormal Placental Implantation

Defective decidua basalis is thought to be the cause of abnormal adherence of the placenta to the uterine wall. This is more common when there has been a previous cesarean section or when placenta previa is present. It is diagnosed when manual removal of the placenta fails and surgical intervention is performed. There is a high risk of maternal hemorrhage and hysterectomy may be necessary. Three varieties are recognized:

- **Placenta accreta**: The decidual basalis is absent so the placenta grows directly into the myometrium of the uterine wall. Only a portion or all of the placenta's cotyledons may be adherent to the uterine wall in this way. This is the most common variety.
- **Placenta increta**: Trophoblastic cells invade the myometrium of the uterine wall.
- **Placenta percreta**: Trophoblastic cells penetrate through the uterine wall and invade other organs in the vicinity such as the bladder.

Uterine Rupture and Dehiscence

The uterine wall may **separate** at the site of a previous scar. If the fetal membranes stay intact and the fetus stays in the uterus, a **dehiscence** has occurred. When the uterine wall **ruptures** and part or the entire fetus extrudes into the peritoneal cavity, death can quickly occur in the fetus and mother without rapid cesarean section. Symptoms of both can include sharp, tearing uterine pain, FHR decelerations, vomiting, fainting, vaginal bleeding, tachycardia, hypotension, and shock. Factors associated with uterine rupture include uterine hyperstimulation, previous uterine surgery, use of prostaglandins, multiparity, abdominal traumatic injury, and fundal pressure.

Uterine Inversion

Inversion is the turning inside out of the uterus. It can be caused by fundal pressure and traction on the umbilical cord. It can also occur during uterine atony, with large fetuses or short umbilical cords, from adherent placental tissues, and from the use of oxytocin. It can also occur spontaneously without obvious cause. Sometimes only the fundus inverts (partial inversion) and other times the fundus protrudes through the cervical opening (complete inversion).

Inversion may be **visualized** or **occult**. There is sudden severe pelvic pain, hemorrhage, and hypotension. There will be a firm mass below the cervix felt by bimanual exam. The uterus must be immediately replaced manually prior to delivery of the placenta. Tocolytics or general anesthesia may be required to do this. IV fluids and blood are given to replace blood loss as needed. Antibiotics and a nasogastric tube may also be needed.

Prolapsed Umbilical Cord

A prolapse of the umbilical cord occurs when the umbilical cord precedes the fetus in the birth canal and becomes entrapped by the descending fetus. An **occult cord prolapse** occurs when the umbilical cord is beside or just ahead of the fetal head. About half of prolapses occur in the second stage of labor and relate to premature delivery, multiple gestation, polyhydramnios, breech delivery, and an excessively long umbilical cord. Some cases are precipitated by obstetric interventions, such as amniotomy, external eversion, and application of scalp electrode for monitoring. As contractions occur and the head descends, this applies pressure to the umbilical cord, occluding blood flow and causing hypoxia and bradycardia. The decrease in blood flow through the umbilical vessels can cause impaired gas exchange, and if pressure on the cord is not relieved, the fetus can suffer severe neurological damage or death. **Management** includes elevating the presenting part off the cord, having the mother elevate her knees to the chest, and preparing for C-section.

Velamentous Cord Insertion

Velamentous cord insertion is an abnormality in which the cord inserts into the membranes rather than the middle of the placenta, traveling through the chorion and amnion to reach the placental margin, leaving exposed vessels unprotected by Wharton's jelly. This can cause shearing of the blood vessels during delivery, leading to hemorrhage. Additionally, the exposed vessels are vulnerable to compression, which can result in fetal anoxia. Velamentous cord insertion is most common with placenta previa and multiple gestations. While incidence is only about 1% for singletons, the incidence increases to almost 9% with twins, so the nurse must be alert for indications. Velamentous cord insertion is associated with about 25% of spontaneous abortions. Velamentous cord insertion may result in vasa previa if the velamentous vessels are lower than the presenting part because they may rupture, causing the fetus to exsanguinate, especially during onset of labor or amniotomy. Indications of velamentous cord insertion include excessive bleeding and fetal distress. Treatment includes careful monitoring and cesarean.

AFI, Oligohydramnios, and Polyhydramnios

The **AFI** is determined by measuring the biggest pockets of amniotic fluid in all four of the uterine quadrants and adding the measurements together. The **normal index** is 5-24 cm, depending on which week of gestation the measurements are taken. Amniotic fluid volume increases during pregnancy to 1,000 mL by 36 weeks of gestation, then slowly decreases over the next 4 weeks.

- **Oligohydramnios** is defined by an AFI of 5 cm or less. It is linked with fetal urinary tract anomalies. The fetus is threatened by the risk of amnion adhesions that can cause amputation of body parts and pressure that can cause deformities of the musculoskeletal system, especially club foot. Cord compression and fetal distress can occur during labor and delivery.
- **Polyhydramnios** is defined by an AFI over 24 cm. It can occur acutely or over time. One-third of these cases are associated with fetal anomalies of the CNS or GI systems, maternal diabetes, or multifetal gestation. More severe polyhydramnios increases the risk of perinatal death.

Amniotic Fluid Embolism

Amniotic fluid embolism (AKA anaphylactoid syndrome of pregnancy) occurs when amniotic fluid enters the mother's circulatory system, such as may occur during cesareans and labor and delivery, during which small tears in the lower uterine segment or cervix allow amniotic fluid to enter maternal circulation. In most mothers, this poses no problem, but some mothers have an anaphylactoid response that can include hypotension, pulmonary edema, cyanosis, coagulopathy, dyspnea, seizures, and cardiac arrest for the mother as well as fetal distress.

- The **initial phase** usually includes cardiovascular collapse with severe pulmonary vasoconstriction, which results in inability of the heart to transfer blood from the right to the left and marked oxygen desaturation with neurological injury. Uterine hypertonus and lack of blood flow to the uterus occurs.
- The **second phase**, if the mother survives the first, usually includes lung injury and coagulopathy.

Treatment includes immediate CPR, circulatory support, and blood and blood components as needed. If undelivered, emergent delivery is critical to save the infant.

Methods of Delivery

Vaginal Delivery

Expulsive Period

During the **expulsive period of delivery**, the mother will need to be coached to achieve effective pushing effort. Two types of pushing are effective: open glottis physiologic pushing and closed glottis (Valsalva) pushing. The mother should be coached on the method most effective for her. During crowning, the mother should be instructed to "pant like a puppy." The integrity of the perineum needs to be taken into consideration. Most mothers would like to avoid an episiotomy if at all possible; however, there are several factors that may make an episiotomy necessary:

- Fetal malposition
- Anticipation of the delivery of a large baby
- Possibility of shoulder dystocia, where the anterior shoulder cannot pass below the symphysis pubis
- Poor elasticity of the perineal tissue
- Difficulty in maintaining adequate control of the patient's expulsive efforts

Delivery of the Placenta

The **placenta** will generally deliver 5-30 minutes after delivery of the fetus. The mechanism of **placental separation** starts with the change in the size of the uterus and then proceeds with the formation of a hematoma between the placenta and uterine wall, the separation of the placenta, the descent of the placenta through the lower uterine segment and vagina, and then expulsion. Signs and symptoms of placental separation include a sudden increase in vaginal bleeding, lengthening of the umbilical cord, and the rising of the uterus in the abdomen. Management of placental delivery includes obtaining cord blood samples after the cord is clamped, inspecting the cord for the number of vessels, and avoiding uterine massage and cord traction until the placenta is separated. Pushing by the mother may assist in expulsion of the placenta. If membranes follow the placenta, hold the placenta and carefully roll it over and over until the membranes separate and are delivered. This helps prevent retained membranes.

Perineal Lacerations

The four types of perineal lacerations are described below:

- **First degree**: The perineal skin and the mucous membranes of the vagina are torn.
- **Second degree**: The perineal skin and vaginal mucous membranes are torn as well as the fascia and muscle of the perineum.
- **Third degree**: The perineal skin, vaginal mucous membranes, and fascia and muscle of the perineum are torn and the tear extends into the rectal sphincter.
- **Fourth degree**: The perineal skin, vaginal mucous membranes, and fascia and muscle of the perineum are torn, the tear extends into the rectal sphincter, and the inner lumen of the rectum is exposed.

Operative Delivery

Forceps-Assisted Birth

Forceps-assisted birth utilizes a variety of specialized tools to assist with the birth of the fetus by providing traction and a method of rotating the fetal head into proper occiput-anterior position. Most forceps are used with the fetus in the head-down position and the forceps positioned on the sides of the head.

- **Outlet forceps application** can be used when the perineum is bulging, the scalp is visible between contractions, or the sagittal suture is not >45 degrees from midline. The fetal skull must be at station +2 or below.
- **Midforceps application** requires that the head be engaged with the leading edge above +2 station.
- **High forceps** are no longer used.

Indications for forceps-assisted birth include conditions that pose a risk to the mother or fetus and are relieved by birth. Maternal risks of forceps-assisted birth include infection, cervical and birth canal lacerations, extension of episiotomy, anal sphincter injury, and weakening of pelvic floor muscles. Neonatal risks include bruising and edema of face, caput succedaneum, cephalhematoma, transient low Apgar score, retinal hemorrhage, ocular trauma, Erb's palsy, and elevated bilirubin.

Vacuum-Assisted Birth

Vacuum-assisted birth utilizes a soft suction cup attached to a suction pump that creates negative pressure of 50-60 mmHg. The suction cup is applied to the **occiput** of the fetus, and traction is applied with contractions. Suction use should be limited to 20-30 minutes, with scalp trauma more likely after 10 minutes of use. If the suction cup dislodges more than 3 times, its use should be discontinued. Indications include prolonged second stage of labor or nonreassuring heart pattern. Vacuum-assisted birth may also be used if the mother is too fatigued to push. Neonatal risks include scalp lacerations, subdural hematoma, cephalohematoma, intracranial hemorrhage, subconjunctival hemorrhage, Erb's palsy, sixth and ninth cranial nerve trauma, retinal hemorrhage, and death. A caput forms on the neonate's head, but this should subside in 2-3 days. Maternal risks include perineal trauma, lacerations, pain, and infection.

Cesarean Section

Cesarean sections are done if there is increased risk of uterine rupture, maternal hemorrhage, dystocia, fetal-pelvic disproportion, breech presentation, active herpes infection, and emergent situations such as fetal distress or impending maternal death. Regional anesthesia (spinal, epidural) is associated with lower mortality than general anesthesia, so it is the preferred anesthetic approach. Additionally, there is less fetal depression, reduced risk of maternal pulmonary aspiration, and an opportunity to provide neuraxial analgesia for postoperative pain relief. Regional anesthesia must provide a T4 sensory level, which causes a high sympathetic blockade. In some cases, general anesthesia may be administered for Cesarean section, although the risks to the mother are intensified, so general anesthesia is usually limited to emergent situations in which the mother or fetus is at risk. Reasons for Cesareans are:

- Fetal distress during the second stage of labor
- Tetanic uterine contractions
- Patient confused, uncontrollable, and unable to cooperate (such as psychiatric patients)
- Inverted uterus
- Retained placenta
- Breech extraction or other position requiring version and extraction

VBAC

There has been decreasing interest in **vaginal birth after Cesarean section (VBAC)** with only 10% attempting it in recent years, but many mothers are able to undergo vaginal delivery after a Cesarean section without complications. Risks include hemorrhage and uterine rupture (1%). Women who attempt vaginal birth have a 60-80% success rate. Below are the guidelines for vaginal delivery after Cesarean.

- A woman with one previous Cesarean section and a low transverse uterine incision should be advised to try vaginal birth. A woman with 2 or more previous Cesarean sections may attempt vaginal birth.
- In all cases, a physician, an anesthesiologist, and adequate staff must be present and available throughout labor to provide a Cesarean section if necessary.

Contraindications to attempting a VBAC are:

- T or classic incision
- History of myomectomy
- Contracted pelvis
- Obstetrical complications precluding vaginal birth
- Inadequate facilities or staff to provide emergency Cesarean section if it is needed

Delayed Cord Clamping

Practice since the 1950s has been to clamp the umbilical cord within about 15 seconds of birth, but recent research indicates benefits to delayed cord clamping to 30-60 seconds with some recommending 2-5 minutes to allow increased blood to flow to the newborn (approximately 80 mL within the first minute and 100 mL in the first three) as well as fetal stem cells and immunoglobulins. Benefits to the term infant include increased hemoglobin and improved iron status for the first few months of life. Benefits to preterm infants include lower rates of intraventricular hemorrhage and necrotizing enterocolitis. Delayed cord clamping is contraindicated in infants that require positive pressure ventilation or if mothers are hemodynamically unstable. While there are some concerns that the infant may develop polycythemia, studies have not supported this; however, there is some increase in jaundice and the need for phototherapy. Delayed cord cutting does not appear to increase risk of maternal hemorrhage.

Maternal Postpartum Assessment, Management and Education

Physiologic Changes and Physical Assessment

Cardiovascular and Respiratory System Changes

The **cardiovascular system** remains fairly stable after delivery. Blood pressure readings are usually within normal limits for the mother. Decreased BP may indicate physiological adaptation to decreased intrapelvic pressure, but can also indicate hemorrhage. Orthostatic hypotension is common for the first few hours postpartum. Elevated BP may indicate preeclampsia. A slow heart rate (puerperal bradycardia) of 50-70 bpm is common from days 6-10 because of decreased strain on the heart, decreased blood volume, and increased stroke volume. Tachycardia may result from excessive blood loss or prolonged labor.

The **respiratory system** adapts to pregnancy by increased minute ventilation (primarily an increase in tidal volume with normal respiratory rate). By the time of delivery, **functional residual capacity (FRC)** and residual volume have decreased because of the pressure of the uterus against the diaphragm. The FRC returns to normal within about 1-2 weeks, while other respiratory changes usually return to baseline within 6-12 weeks.

Urinary and Gastrointestinal System Changes

Urinary system changes in the postpartal period include:

- Increased bladder capacity
- Possible urinary retention due to edema of tissues surrounding the urethra
- Decreased sensitivity to bladder filling and fluid pressure
- Increased urinary output (puerperal diuresis) for 12-24 hours

Combined, these put the woman at risk for **excessive bladder distension** and **residual urine**. Anesthetic blocks may inhibit neural function and cause difficulty voiding, as well as bladder distension. If the mother received oxytocin as a uterotonic, this causes an antidiuretic effect, and the bladder tends to fill rapidly. Because the ureters and renal pelvis dilate during pregnancy, the mother is at increased risk of infection for about 6 weeks postpartum. Hematuria, which may be an indication of infection, may be overlooked because of lochia.

Gastrointestinal system changes include a lack of **muscle tone** and slow **motility** from lasting effects of progesterone, which can lead to constipation. Concerns about opening an episiotomy may cause mothers to delay elimination, but bowel movements are usually not painful. A stool softener is recommended for the first few days postpartum.

Hematological System Changes

Most women lose 200-500 mL of **blood** during vaginal delivery and 700-1000 mL with Cesarean section. There is approximately a 3-point drop in hematocrit (1 mg/dL drop in hemoglobin) with every 500 mL of blood loss, so both **hemoglobin** and **hematocrit** fall after delivery, resulting in **anemia** in up to 50% of new mothers. Hemoglobin and hematocrit usually return to prelabor levels within 2-6 weeks. Coagulation factors are activated during pregnancy, putting mothers at increased risk of thromboembolism, although early ambulation and activity reduces incidence. The sedimentation rate is elevated for about a week after delivery because of increased plasma fibrinogen levels. The white blood cell count elevates and may increase to 30,000 in the days after delivery without indicating infection. However, a WBC increase of >30% in a 6-hour period may indicate infection. Vasomotor changes may cause women to have chills immediately after delivery, but this does not indicate infection.

Postpartum Uterine Involution

The normal uterus weighs about 70-100 g and has a capacity of 5 mL. During pregnancy, the uterus increases in weight to 1000 g with a capacity of 5000 mL. After delivery, the weight of the uterus decreases to 500 g by the end of the first week, 300 by the second, and 100 by the third. **Uterine involution** (the process of the uterus returning to the pre-pregnant state) begins immediately after the placenta separates. The changes occur over the first 3 weeks, except for the placental site, which takes 6-7 weeks to heal over.

- **Estrogen and progesterone levels** drop markedly, causing cells to atrophy, reversing hyperplasia.
- **Autolysis** occurs as proteolytic enzymes are released and macrophages migrate to the uterus.
- The **spongy layer of decidua** sloughs off as lochia.
- The **basal layer of decidua** separates into two layers within 48-72 hours, with the outer layer becoming necrotic and sloughing off as lochia with the inner layer providing the base for the new endometrium.

Breastfeeding accelerates uterine involution after birth and reduces the risk of hemorrhage.

Changes in Placental Site and Lochia

Placental separation occurs within 30 minutes of birth. The spongy layer of the endometrium of the uterus is lost at the same time, leaving decidual basalis. The top layer of the decidua dies and sloughs. The lower basal layer generates a new endometrium within 2-3 weeks. After separation the placental site is about 8-10 cm. This area shrinks to 3-4 cm by the end of 2 weeks postpartum. The same process occurs at the site as in the uterine walls, only more slowly. The superficial layer of the site sloughs during the first 2 weeks and new endometrium is regenerated over the next 4 weeks.

During this time, tissue sloughed by the uterus is seen as **vaginal lochia**. It is reddish in color (rubra) with clots for the first 1-3 days after birth, then turns pink (serosa) for the next 3-10 days. A yellow-whitish mucus lochia (alba) will then be seen for the next 10-14 days or longer.

Changes in Cervix, Vagina, and Pelvic Floor

The **cervix** stays dilated until the end of the first week postpartum when it is again at 1 cm. The **vagina** may be bruised at birth. By the third week, rugae are seen again in the vaginal walls. The muscles of the **pelvic floor** regain their tone by 6 weeks postpartum. Kegel exercises can help this process.

Return of Ovulation and Need for Contraception

The resumption of **ovulation** and **menses** are individual to each woman. The usual time for the first menses after childbirth is 7-9 weeks for non-breastfeeding mothers and 2-18 months for breastfeeding mothers. Ovulation may occur before the first menses but most often occurs at about 10 weeks for the non-breastfeeding mother and 17 weeks for the breastfeeding mother. Since the exact time of ovulation is unknown, a woman should receive **contraceptive information** when she is released to have sexual activity or before that time if there is doubt that she will wait a full three to four weeks to resume intercourse. Breastfeeding mothers should receive progestin-only oral contraceptives. Barrier methods may also be used safely, although effectiveness is less than oral contraceptives.

Postpartum Assessment

The postpartum assessment includes the following elements:

- **Vital signs**
  - VS should be checked every 15 minutes and evaluated in relation to baseline VS and VS prior to delivery.
  - Normal BP varies from 90/60 to 140/90.
  - Falling BP and increased pulse may indicate uterine bleeding.
  - Pulse (60-90) is usually slightly decreased from that found during labor.
  - Respirations should be relaxed and not labored, usually 12-20/min.
- **Temperature**
  - Slight elevation immediately after delivery (≤100.4 °F), but this should return to normal within 24 hours.
- **Alertness**
  - The mother should be awake, alert, responsive, and able to hold the infant.
- **Fundus**
  - Fundus is palpated to determine if it is firm, midline, and in the expected position (at the umbilicus).
  - A boggy fundus may indicate uterine bleeding.
  - Bladder distension may cause the fundus to deviate from midline.
- **Lochia**
  - Lochia should be checked every 15 minutes for signs of excess bleeding, such as copious discharge or large clots.
  - Lochia must be observed while the fundus is massaged to determine if there is free flow of blood or expulsion of clots, which may indicate hemorrhage.
  - Lochia rubra should be present with moderate amount of discharge, not to exceed 1 saturated perineal pad/hr.
- **Perineum**
  - The perineal area should be examined and the amount of swelling and bruising noted, along with the condition of episiotomy (if present) and sutures.
  - Severe perineal/rectal pain requires further examination.

- **Bladder**
  - The bladder should be palpated to determine if it is distended.
  - The mother should be given the opportunity to urinate within the first hour after delivery before catheterization is considered.
  - The mother should spontaneously urinate >100 mL clear urine with no distension noted after urination.
- **Rectum**
  - Rectum should be examined for presence of tearing or hemorrhoids.
  - No severe rectal pain should be present.
  - If hemorrhoids are present, engorgement must be reported to physician, especially if they are larger than 2 cm in size.
- **Pain**
  - Mother should have only mild pain, <3 on 1-10 scale.
  - Severe pain requires further examination to determine the cause.
  - Analgesia should be provided to control pain.
- **Legs/feet**
  - Feet and legs should be warm and pulses palpable.
  - Edema, which may have been present before delivery, should remain stable or decrease.
- **Anesthesia**
  - If the mother had an anesthetic, such as epidural or spinal, the level of anesthesia should be assessed every 15 minutes.

Wound Care

Wound care of the postpartum mother is needed if the woman has had a Cesarean, episiotomy, or lacerations. In all cases, the patient should receive analgesia as needed. **Wound care**:

- **Cesarean**: Surgi-strips or staples may be in place and the wound covered with a sterile bandage. An ice pack may be applied 15 minutes at a time to help control pain and swelling in the first 24 hours. The initial sterile bandage is usually removed after 24 hours and then the wound left open to the air or covered with light sterile gauze. The woman is usually allowed to shower after 24 hours. The wound should be routinely checked to make sure it is intact and healing.
- **Episiotomy/Lacerations**: The suture line should be checked frequently for signs of infection, hematoma, or separation. Ice packs may be applied 15 minutes at a time for the first 24 hours to reduce swelling and pain. After 24 hours, warm Sitz baths for 20 minutes 2-4 times daily are usually advised, and the woman is cautioned to tighten buttocks muscles when sitting down to avoid stress on suture lines.

Pain Assessment and Control

Assess the location, intensity, frequency, and type of pain present. **Uterine pain** occurs with assessment, cramping, and massage. Slow, deep breathing and relaxation can help the mother through this pain. Be sure your hands are warm during palpation and massage to decrease comfort. Administer analgesia as ordered and teach the mother the side effects and how to take the medicine when she goes home.

Perineal pain may be relieved by analgesics and anesthetic sprays used when pericare is performed following toileting. Ice packs are also helpful in the first 24-48 hours to decrease edema and inflammation. Apply moist heat via a sitz bath after the first 48 hours have passed.

The accumulation of intestinal gas also causes pain in the postpartum period. The use of rocking and ambulation will help. The mother should avoid gas-producing foods until the GI tract motility resumes normal functioning.

Cesarean Section Management

Postoperative Assessment

The initial assessments of the mother who has had a **Cesarean** and of the neonate are similar to those for vaginal birth, but the mother also must recover from a surgical procedure and anesthesia. These assessments constitute standard **postoperative care** during the first hour postpartum:

- **VS** are checked every 5 minutes until stable, then every 15 minutes for one hour, and finally every 30 minutes until the mother is released from the recovery area.
- **Abdominal dressing and perineal pad** are checked every 15 minutes for bleeding for the first hour; fundus gently palpated with a hand supporting the area of the incision.
- **IV oxytocin** is administered to promote contraction of the uterine muscles.
- If general anesthesia was administered, the patient should be positioned on her side and **turned** every 2 hours for 24 hours.
- If epidural or spinal anesthesia was administered, level of **anesthesia** should be checked every 15 minutes.
- **Intake and output** are monitored, and urine checked for signs of blood (indicating bladder trauma).
- **Analgesia** should be administered as needed to control pain.

Postoperative Care

The mother who has had a **Cesarean** birth has both routine postpartum and surgical needs. The mother should deep-breathe and cough (while supporting the abdomen with a pillow) and use an **incentive spirometer** every 2-4 hours during the daytime for the first few days. The mother should sit on the side of the bed within 12 hours of surgery and ambulate within 24 hours. **Pain management** with PCA, oral, and parenteral medications and/or relaxation techniques helps the mother to ambulate and care for her infant. Epidural analgesia may continue for 24 hours after delivery and must be monitored carefully. Flatus and abdominal distension are common complaints, so the mother should avoid carbonated beverages and drinking through straws. Taking an antiflatulent (Mylicon), turning frequently, rocking, or lying on the left side may help to expel gas. The mother should be encouraged to breastfeed but may be more comfortable sitting with the baby supported by a pillow or lying on her side to prevent pressure on the incision.

Common Postpartum Medications

NSAIDs

Non-steroidal anti-inflammatory drugs (NSAIDs) include cyclooxygenase (COX) inhibitors that block COX enzymes that develop with inflammation and with precancerous/cancerous tissues. COX enzymes form these prostanoids:

- **Prostaglandins**: Cell growth, inflammatory reactions, sensitivity to pain, platelet aggregation/disaggregation, and hormone and calcium regulation
- **Prostacyclin**: Platelet aggregation and vasodilation
- **Thromboxane**: Platelet aggregation and vasoconstriction

COX inhibitors are used as anti-inflammatory, analgesic, and antiplatelet drugs. Some drugs, such as ibuprofen and aspirin, block both COX-1 and COX-2 enzymes (non-selective inhibitors). Aspirin should be used with caution in the postpartum period because of increased risk of bleeding. Non-selective NSAIDs are associated with irritation of gastric mucosa because of inhibition of COX-1, which has a protective effect on gastrointestinal mucosa. Other drugs, such as celecoxib, block only COX-2 enzymes (selective inhibitors). These tend to have fewer adverse gastrointestinal effects, but they have been implicated in increased risk for cardiovascular disease and thrombus formation. COX-2 NSAIDs specifically target inflammation.

Acetaminophen

Acetaminophen is an antipyretic and non-opioid analgesic suitable for **mild to moderate pain**. Acetaminophen reduces fever by acting on the hypothalamic heat-regulating center to cause vasodilation and increased perspiration to dissipate heat. Acetaminophen is especially indicated for those who are sensitive to aspirin or at increased risk of bleeding. Acetaminophen may relieve musculoskeletal pain, but it lacks the anti-inflammatory action of NSAIDs.

- Oral adult dose: 1,000 mg 3-4 times daily, not to exceed 4 g/day
- Pediatric dose (0-3 months): 40 mg 4-5 times daily

Acetaminophen should be used cautiously with impaired hepatic function, alcoholism, and pregnancy as well as during lactation. While side effects are uncommon if recommended doses are adhered to, adverse effects may include headache, chest pain, dyspnea, hepatic toxicity, jaundice, acute renal failure, methemoglobinemia, hemolytic anemia, rash, and fever. Women should be cautioned not to exceed the recommended dose and to avoid multiple analgesic preparations as some others may contain acetaminophen.

Antibiotic Medications

Antibiotics may be classified according to their chemical nature, origin, action, or range of effectiveness. There are hundreds of antibiotics. **Broad-spectrum antibiotics** are useful against both gram-positive and gram-negative bacteria. **Medium-spectrum antibiotics** are usually effective against gram-positive bacteria, although some may be effective against gram-negative as well. **Narrow-spectrum antibiotics** are effective against a small range of bacteria. Antibiotics are bacteriocidal, meaning they function by killing the bacteria by interfering with its biological functions, or bacteriostatic, meaning they prevent reproduction of bacteria. The main classes of antibiotics are described here:

- **Macrolides**: Medium-spectrum antibiotics that prevent protein production by bacteria and are primarily bacteriostatic, but may be bactericidal at high doses. They may be irritating to the gastric mucosa, but are less likely to cause allergic responses than penicillins or cephalosporins. Macrolides include erythromycin (E-Mycin), clarithromycin (Biaxin), and azithromycin (Zithromax).
- **Penicillins**: Medium-spectrum antibiotics, which may be combined with beta-lactamase inhibitors. They are bacteriocidal, causing breakdown of the bacterial cell wall. Penicillins may cause severe allergic reactions in sensitive individuals. Penicillins include penicillin, ampicillin, and amoxicillin.
- **Cephalosporins**: Medium-spectrum antibiotics effective against gram-negative organisms. They are bacteriocidal and inhibit cell wall synthesis. They are divided into different "generations" according to antimicrobial properties, with succeeding generations having a more powerful effect against resistant strains. First generation includes cephazolin (Kefzol), cephalexin (Keflex), and cephradine (Velosef). Second generation includes cefaclor (Ceclor), cefuroxime (Zinacef), and loracarbef (Lorabid). Third generation includes cefotaxime (Claforan), cefixime (Suprax), cefpodoxime (Vantin), ceftazidime (Fortaz), and cefdinir (Omnicef). Fourth generation includes cefixime (Maxipime).
- **Polymyxins**: Narrow-spectrum antibiotics effective against gram-negative organisms. They interfere with the cell membrane of bacteria and are bacteriocidal. Polymyxins have both neurotoxic and nephrotoxic properties and are not used unless other antibiotics are ineffective. They must be given intravenously. Polymyxins include Polymyxin B Sulfate.
- **Fluoroquinolones**: Broad-spectrum antibiotics that inhibit bacterial reproduction and repair of genetic material in the bacterial DNA. Drugs include ciprofloxacin (Cipro), levofloxacin (Levaquin), and ofloxacin (Floxin).
- **Sulfonamides**: Medium-spectrum with action against gram-positive and many gram-negative organisms, as well as plasmodium and toxoplasma. Some people are sensitive and may develop an allergic response. Resistance to sulfa drugs is widespread. Sulfa drugs interfere with folate synthesis and prevent cell division, so they are bacteriostatic. Sulfonamides include cotrimoxazole (Bactrim) and trimethoprim (Proloprim).
- **Tetracyclines**: Broad-spectrum antibiotics, which are also used for rickettsia- and psittacosis-producing agents. Tetracyclines include tetracycline, doxycycline (Vibramycin), and minocycline.
- **Aminoglycosides**: Effective against gram-negative bacteria. They interfere with protein production in the bacteria and are bacteriocidal. Aminoglycosides cannot be taken orally. They are often given in conjunction with other classes of antibiotics, such as penicillin. Aminoglycosides include gentamicin (Garamycin), tobramycin (Tobrex), neomycin, and streptomycin.

> **Review Video: Antibiotics: An Overview**
> Visit mometrix.com/academy and enter code: 165628

Vasodilators and Antihypertensive Medications

Postpartum hypertension is at its highest risk during days 3-6 postpartum. This hypertension may be a continuation of pregnancy-induced hypertension or chronic hypertension, or may be new onset. While often times postpartum hypertension spontaneously resolves without medical intervention within a few weeks of child birth, if it persists or if it is acutely severe, pharmacologic interventions may be indicated.

Calcium Channel Blockers

Calcium channel blockers are primarily arterial vasodilators that may affect the peripheral and/or coronary arteries. They are indicated in severe postpartum hypertension (≥160/110 mmHg) or in the case of persistent postpartum hypertension that is not severe, but not self-resolving. Side effects include lethargy, flushing, abdominal and peripheral edema, and indigestion. **Dihydropyridines**, such as nicardipine (Cardene), are primarily arterial vasodilators that affect both coronary and peripheral arteries and are used to treat acute hypertension. Nicardipine is recommended in the cases of both severe postpartum hypertension (parenterally) and non-severe persistent hypertension (orally).

Beta-Blockers

Beta-blockers, such as, labetalol, slow the heart rate, reduce hypertension, prevent dysrhythmias, and reverse ventricular remodeling, but should not be used during decompensation and should be monitored carefully for those with airway disease, uncontrolled diabetes, slow or irregular pulse, or heart block. Labetalol is recommended parenterally in cases of severe postpartum hypertension.

Diuretics

Diuretics increase **renal perfusion and filtration**, thereby reducing preload and decreasing peripheral and pulmonary edema, hypertension, CHF, diabetes insipidus, and osteoporosis. There are different types of diuretics: loop, thiazide, and potassium-sparing. Diuretics are rarely used during pregnancy.

Loop Diuretics

Loop diuretics inhibit the reabsorption of sodium and chloride (primarily) in the ascending loop of Henle. They also cause increased secretion of other electrolytes, such as calcium, magnesium, and potassium, and this can result in imbalances that cause dysrhythmias. Other side effects include frequent urination, postural hypotension, and increased blood sugar and uric acid levels. They are short-acting and are therefore less effective than other diuretics for control of hypertension.

- **Bumetanide** (Bumex) should be avoided while breastfeeding. High doses may suppress lactation.
- **Ethacrynic acid** (Edecrin) should be avoided while breastfeeding.
- **Furosemide** (Lasix) is used for the control of congestive heart failure as well as renal insufficiency. It may suppress lactation, but is recommended if emergent diuresis is needed in the postpartum mother.

Thiazide Diuretics

Thiazide diuretics inhibit the reabsorption of **sodium and chloride**, primarily in the early distal tubules, forcing more sodium and water to be excreted. Thiazide diuretics increase secretion of **potassium and bicarbonate**, so they are often given with supplementary potassium or in combination with potassium-sparing diuretics. Thiazide diuretics are the first line of drugs for treatment of hypertension. They have a long duration of action, 12-72 hours, depending on the drug, so they are able to maintain control of hypertension better than short-acting drugs. They may be given daily or 3-5 days per week. There are numerous thiazide diuretics, and considerations must be made for the lactating mother:

- **Chlorothiazide** (Diuril): Low doses do not interfere with lactation.
- **Bendroflumethiazide** (Naturetin): Shorter-acting diuretics are usually preferred, but low doses should not interfere with lactation.
- **Chlorthalidone** (Hygroton): This drug may suppress lactation and may accumulate in the infant.
- **Trichlormethiazide** (Naqua): Large doses may suppress lactation.

Side effects include dizziness, lightheadedness, postural hypotension, headache, blurred vision, and itching, especially during initial treatment. Thiazide diuretics cause sensitivity to sun exposure, so patients should be counseled to use sunscreen.

Potassium-Sparing Diuretics

Potassium-sparing diuretics inhibit the reabsorption of sodium in the **late distal tubule and collecting duct**. They are weaker than thiazide or loop diuretics, but do not cause a reduction in potassium level; however, if used alone, they may cause an increase in potassium, which can cause weakness, irregular pulse, and cardiac arrest. Because potassium-sparing diuretics are less effective alone, they are often given in a combined form with a thiazide diuretic (usually chlorothiazide), which mitigates the potassium imbalance. Typical side effects include dehydration, blurred vision, nausea, insomnia, and nasal congestion, especially in the first few days of treatment.

- **Spironolactone** (Aldactone) is a synthetic steroidal diuretic that increases the secretion of both water and sodium and is used to treat congestive heart failure. It may be given orally or intravenously. By itself, it does not usually affect lactation and has minimal effects on the infant.
- **Eplerenone** is similar to spironolactone but has fewer side effects, so it may be used with patients who can't tolerate the other drug.

Review Video: Diuretics
Visit mometrix.com/academy and enter code: 373276

GI Motility (Laxative) Drugs

Bulk Formers

Bulk formers have high fiber content and both soften stool and create more formed stools. These include products such as Metamucil, Citrucel, and FiberCon, which are usually added to liquids, because without adequate fluids, they can increase constipation. These can be safely used while breastfeeding.

Lubricants

Lubricants include both oral mineral oil and glycerin suppositories. They coat the stool, preventing fluid absorption and keeping the stool soft. Mineral oil absorbs fat-soluble vitamins and should be avoided, but glycerin suppositories pose no risk.

Saline

Saline products include Milk of Magnesia and Epsom salt, which contain ions (such as magnesium phosphate, magnesium hydroxide, and citrate) that are not absorbed through the intestines and draw more fluid into the stool. The magnesium in the preparations also stimulates the bowel. People with impaired kidney function should avoid magnesium products, and saline laxatives should be used infrequently to avoid dependence. Epsom salt often has a purging effect and is rarely used. Milk of Magnesia in small doses may be used during breastfeeding.

Stimulants

Stimulants increase intestinal motility, moving the stool through the bowel faster and reducing the absorption of fluids so the stool remains softer. Common ingredients include cascara in Castor Oil, senna in Senokot, and sennosides in Ex-Lax. Stimulants work quickly and are effective, but can result in electrolyte imbalance, abdominal distension, and cramping. Chronic use may cause a cycle of constipation and diarrhea. Stimulant suppositories, such as Dulcolax, are also available. Large doses of stimulant laxatives may be excreted in the milk and can cause diarrhea in the infant.

Metoclopramide (Reglan)

Metoclopramide (Reglan) is used to reduce nausea and vomiting from a wide range of causes. It is also a prokinetic drug that increases gastrointestinal contractions and promotes faster gastric emptying, so it is used for heartburn, GERD, and diabetic gastroparesis. Infants receive <10% of the dose through breastfeeding with little effect. Metoclopramide may increase milk supply by increasing serum prolactin. It may cause depression, so care must be used with postpartum women.

Stool Softeners

Stool softeners include emollients, such as Colace, and Phillip's Liqui-Gels. They use wetting agents such as docusate sodium to increase liquid in the stool, thereby softening it. They should not be used with mineral oil because of increased absorption of the oil through the intestines. Stool softeners are safe to use while breastfeeding.

Hyperosmotics

Hyperosmotics contain materials that are not digestible and serve to retain fluid in the stool. Products such as Kristalose and MiraLax soften the stool. These may result in increased abdominal distension and flatus, especially initially. There are 3 types of hyperosmolar laxatives: lactulose, polymer, and saline. Lactulose types use a form of sugar and work similarly to saline laxatives, but more slowly, and may be used for long-term treatment. Salines empty the bowels quickly and are used short-term. Polymers contain polyethylene glycol, which retains fluid in the stool and is used short-term.

Combination

Use two or more types together, such as stool softener with stimulant (short-term only).

Common Problems and Complications

Urinary Problems

Bladder retention, the inability to initiate urine flow or completely empty the bladder, is common after delivery because of **periurethral edema**. **Dysuria** is usually transitory. Mothers should be encouraged to try to urinate within the first hour after delivery. The mother should empty the bladder at least every 4-6 hours, and the bladder should not be palpable. Warm water poured over the perineum or a warm shower may help relax muscles enough to promote urination. The time and amount of voiding should be recorded. Normal volume for each urination is 300-400 mL. Smaller amounts may indicate dehydration or incomplete bladder emptying, which may be verified by ultrasound. Repeated catheterization (more than twice in 24 hours) should be avoided. If the mother is still unable to urinate after straight catheterizations, then an indwelling catheter with prophylactic administration of ampicillin may be considered.

Constipation

Slowed GI motility often results in constipation in the postpartum period, especially if the mother is reluctant to bear down because of an episiotomy. If the mother holds a clean pad against the episiotomy and applies firm pressure while bearing down, this may alleviate discomfort. Adequate fluids and dietary fiber help promote evacuation. Stool softeners are often prescribed, but laxatives (other than fiber laxatives) and enemas should be avoided if possible.

Hemorrhoids

Pressure on veins in the rectum and anus during pregnancy and delivery may cause hemorrhoids. Usually, these begin in the days after delivery, but constipation may worsen them, so measures used to prevent constipation may help promote healing. Sitz baths and application of witch hazel pads may relieve discomfort. Other comfort measures include anesthetic ointments, manual replacement of hemorrhoids, and side-lying position.

Afterpains

With a first pregnancy, the uterus usually remains contracted after delivery, but with subsequent pregnancies or complications, such as polyhydramnios or retention of clots or placental tissue, the uterus may alternate between contraction and relaxation, causing severe cramp-like afterpains in the 2-3 days after delivery. If the mother receives oxytocin to stimulate contractions, this may increase discomfort. Breastfeeding naturally stimulates release of oxytocin, so nursing may cause afterpains. **Analgesic agents** such as acetaminophen or ibuprofen an hour before nursing and at bedtime may relieve discomfort.

Perineal Edema/Pain

Bruising and swelling of the perineum are common because of birth trauma, although excessive bruising may indicate hematoma. Small hematomas resolve over time, but large collections of blood may need to be drained. Gentle palpation of an episiotomy incision should cause minimal tenderness. If the incision is warmer than surrounding tissue, or redness or indurated areas appear, these changes may indicate an infection that requires antibiotics. Swelling may be reduced by applying an ice pack. A sitz bath may relieve perineal discomfort after episiotomy.

Spinal Headaches Following Spinal Block

Spinal headaches may occur following a spinal block for delivery when **cerebrospinal fluid (CSF)** leaks from the meninges, usually within a few hours up to 48 hours. The headaches may persist for a few hours to over a week. Sitting and standing results in pain from the reduced volume of CSF creating traction on pain-sensitive CNS structures. Some women experience associated dizziness, nausea, and vomiting. Spinal headache can be prevented and treated by keeping the woman flat in the supine position for several hours and increasing hydration. Some find relief from administration of caffeine, a vasoconstrictor. If the pain is severe or persistent, an epidural blood patch is applied to the epidural space. (A small volume of blood is obtained from the mother via venipuncture [without coagulation] and then injected into the epidural space at the same site.) Relief is usually achieved immediately. If pain persists after the blood patch, then further testing and evaluation are needed to determine another cause, such as cerebral thrombosis.

Obstetrical Lacerations

Risk factors for **obstetrical (vaginal/perineal) lacerations** include fetal macrosomia, precipitous labor and delivery, fetal malpresentation, and forceps- and vacuum-assisted delivery. Lacerations often occur in the **anterior vaginal wall** near the urethra but are usually superficial and heal without intervention. Longitudinal lacerations are most common with forceps- or vacuum-assisted delivery and occur in the upper or middle third of the vagina, often extending into underlying tissue and posing the risk of hemorrhage. Tearing may be prevented by allowing labor to progress slowly, delivering in side-lying position, avoiding assisted delivery, and utilizing an episiotomy if tearing appears imminent. **Classifications** of obstetrical laceration:

Degree	Description
First	Laceration of vaginal mucosa or perineal skin but not underlying tissues
Second	Laceration extends to underlying subcutaneous tissues but not rectal sphincter or rectal mucosa
Third	Laceration extends through rectal sphincter but not rectal mucosa
Fourth	Laceration extends through rectal mucosa

Hunger and Thirst

Mothers often feel very hungry after giving birth and may enjoy a light meal. If the mother had a C-section, she may be limited to clear liquids initially but should be progressed to a **regular diet** as soon as possible.

Because fluids are lost during delivery, the mother often experiences marked **thirst**, alleviated by providing ample **oral fluids** to replace those lost. If the mother had a C-section and is receiving IVs, the rate of replacement must be adequate.

Chill

Postpartum chills immediately after delivery is common and may relate to neurological or vasomotor changes. The mother experiences uncontrollable shivering that typically subsides an hour or two after delivery. The mother should be covered with a warmed **blanket** and offered warm **liquids**.

Diaphoresis

Perspiration increases during the postpartum period to help eliminate excess fluid and waste products, and the mother may wake up drenched in sweat at night. The mother should be provided with a dry gown and linens and protected from chilling.

Flatulence

The GI tract is sluggish after birth because of hormonal changes and decreased muscle tone. Flatulence is common, especially after C-section. This is alleviated by early ambulation, turning from side to side, avoiding carbonated beverages, and taking antiflatulent medications.

Fatigue/Sleep Disturbance

Fatigue is common after delivery, but it sometimes becomes chronic and is associated with **sleep disturbance**. Because the baby must be fed around the clock, the mother is rarely able to sleep more than 3 hours at a time. During this period, the mother should be encouraged to nap frequently when the infant sleeps. Family support is critical. If the mother is breastfeeding, she can pump and have someone else give an occasional feeding.

Postpartum Blues

Adjustment reaction with depressed mood, more commonly referred to as **postpartum blues,** is a mild depression that occurs in 50-80% of women after childbirth. Onset is usually ≤5 days postpartum and duration is typically 2-3 days, but it may persist for up to 10 days in some women. Symptoms include mild insomnia, anger, mood swings, fatigue, irritability, impaired concentration, depressed affect, and frequent episodic tearfulness. The cause is not clear but may relate to changes in hormones and psychological adjustments to parenting. Because mothers often are discharged on the first or second day postpartum, symptoms may not appear until after discharge, so mothers and family should be advised about the symptoms and encouraged to seek help if the symptoms persist, suggesting a more serious depression. About 20% of women experiencing postpartum blues progress to **postpartum depression**. Mothers should be reassured and supported during this period.

Care of the Mother with HIV/AIDS

Mothers infected with **HIV/AIDS** who are **asymptomatic** prior to pregnancy usually have no added risk for acceleration of their disease, but increased risk occurs if the **CD-4 count** was already low. Because about half of neonatal infections occur during birth and delivery, the HIV/AIDS mother may have an elective C-section at 38 weeks. Routine care should be provided, always using standard precautions to avoid contact with blood or other body fluids. The mother is at increased risk of postpartum hemorrhage, urinary and endometrial/pelvic infections, and poor wound healing, and requires careful evaluation for complications. The mother should be educated about all aspects of her disease and its implications and about the need for follow-up care for both her and her infant. Mothers should be advised not to breastfeed as the virus may be transmitted through human breast milk. Prior to discharge, the mother should receive referrals to social agencies that can provide support.

Lactation and Newborn Nutrition

Digestion and Absorption

Digestion is the processes by which food is converted into chemicals that are used by the body. These processes are immature at birth and most don't function until 3-6 months. Digestion begins in the mouth as milk is mixed with saliva, but salivary amylase, which begins the digestion of starch, has little effect on milk because milk passes into the esophagus and stomach quickly. Protein digestion begins in the stomach where hydrochloric acid acts on curds formed by the enzyme renin. The curds slow the progress of the milk to allow digestion. Pancreatic and liver enzymes further digest protein and fat in the small intestine. Infants cannot adequately absorb fat until 4-5 months or complex carbohydrates until 4-6 months. Simple carbohydrates break down into glucose and monosaccharides and fat into fatty acids and glycerol. Trypsin levels are sufficient to convert proteins into polypeptides and amino acids. **Absorption**, the transfer of digestive end products (electrolytes, vitamins, fluids, nutrients) into the circulation, takes place primarily in the small intestine and is facilitated by villi.

Nutritional Needs

Caloric Requirements of Neonates

The caloric needs of a neonate (pre-term or term) depend on postnatal age, activity, current weight, growth rate, thermal environment, and route of nutritional intake. Cold stress increases caloric requirements. Infants who receive parenteral nutrition need fewer calories, as they do not have any fecal loss, and the nutrients are not absorbed by the gastrointestinal tract. These are the general requirements for adequate growth:

- **Full-term infant**: 100-120 cal/kg/day
- **Premature infants**: 110-160 cal/kg/day
- Infants who are recovering from **surgery** or have a **chronic illness**, such as bronchopulmonary dysplasia (BPD): ≤180 cal/kg/day

Most human breast milk and unfortified formulas supply 20 calories per ounce. To ingest 120 cal/kg/day, an infant needs to ingest 6 ounces/kg/day of unfortified formula or human breast milk. Special formulas designed for premature infants and fortifiers that can be added to human breast milk provide higher calorie contents per ounce (22-24 calories per ounce).

Protein Requirements

Neonates require adequate **protein** to sustain growth, with intake requirements depending on gestational age. A positive nitrogen balance exists when the intake of protein meets or exceeds the infant's requirements. A negative protein balance occurs when protein is provided in inadequate amounts, leading to catabolism (muscle breakdown). Generally, the USDA recommends newborns through 6 months of age receive 9.1 g/day of protein. Premature neonates have higher protein requirements relative to body weight than do full term infants:

- **Full term**: 2.0-2.5 g/kg/day
- **Preterm**: 3.5-4.0 g/kg/day

Preterm infants should be started on parenteral nutrition supplemented with protein as soon as possible to avoid negative protein balances. Special formulas designed for premature infants are available with elevated protein contents. Human breast milk fortifiers are also available to enhance the protein levels and caloric content of human breast milk for premature infants although the content of human breast milk adjusts automatically for the needs of preterm infants.

CARBOHYDRATE AND FAT REQUIREMENTS

Nutritional requirements of carbohydrates and fats vary according to whether a neonate is full-term or preterm and the type of feeding (human breast milk, enteral, parenteral).

Lactose is the primary **carbohydrate** in human breast milk. A full-term neonate requires 60 g of carbohydrate daily for the first 6 months of life according to the USDA, and a preterm neonate requires 12-14 g/kg/day. Preterm infants may require supplemental glucose via infusion, starting at 6 mg/kg/min, and increased daily by 1 mg/kg/min, up to 12-13 mg/kg/min until blood glucose levels are stabilized and can be maintained by the neonate. Lactose is metabolized into galactose and glucose, the main energy source for the brain. Human breast milk is approximately 40% carbohydrates. Inadequate intake may result in hypoglycemia, while excess intake may result in weight gain and hyperglycemia.

Fats provide the primary energy source for neonates and should comprise at least 30% of calories but no more than 54%. Fat intake needs are 31 g/day for full-term neonates, according to the USDA, and 5-7 g/kg/day for preterm neonates. Because preterm neonates are more susceptible to essential fatty acid deficiency, they should be closely monitored, and administered IV 20% emulsion lipids (0.5-1.0 g/kg/day) if necessary, until stabilized. Fats provide energy for the body and contribute to the development of the CNS and tissue growth. Excess fat may contribute to weight gain, impaired cholesterol metabolism, and later cardiac morbidity. Deficiency may result in impaired development and dermatitis (from lack of adequate fatty acids).

VITAMINS

Nutritional requirements of vitamins are generally met with human breast milk or formula in the healthy neonate. Daily vitamin requirements vary according to the neonate's condition and whether preterm or term. **E**=Enteral, **P**=Parenteral.

Vitamin	Preterm/Term	Notes
A	**E**:700-1500/1250 IU **P**: 700-1500/2300 IU	**Deficiency**: Vision impairment/blindness, impaired growth, depressed immune system **Excess**: Poor feeding, weight loss, fever, diarrhea
C	**E**: 20-60/30-50 mg **P**: 35-50/80 mg	**Deficiency**: Impaired brain development, weakness, bleeding **Excess**: Diarrhea, skin irritation, GI upset
D	**E**: 400/300 IU **P**: 120-260/400 IU	**Deficiency**: Impaired skeletal growth, calcium malabsorption **Excess**: Hypercalcemia, dehydration, cardiac and renal impairment, bone loss, hearing impairment
E	**E**: 6-12/5-10 IU **P**: 2-4/7 IU	**Deficiency**: Peripheral neuropathy, retinopathy, IVH, spinocerebellar impairment, hemolytic anemia **Excess**: GI upset, bleeding
K	**E**: 0.05/0.2 mg **P**: 0.06-0.1/0.05 mg	**Deficiency**: Bleeding **Excess**: Hemolysis, hyperbilirubinemia
Vitamin B1 (Thiamine)	**E**: 0.2-0.7/0.3 mg **P**: 0.8-0.8/1.2 mg	**Deficiency**: Cardiovascular and neurological damage **Excess**: rash, tachycardia, irritability
Vitamin B2 (Riboflavin)	**E**: 0.3-0.8/0.4 mg **P**: 0.4-0.9/1.4 mg	**Deficiency**: Thyroid hormone insufficiency, stomatitis, hepatic and neurological impairment, anemia **Excess**: Vomiting, hypotension
Vitamin B3 (Niacin)	**E**: 5-12/5 mg **P**: 5-12/7 mg	**Deficiency**: GI upset, diarrhea, cognitive impairment **Excess**: Flushing, hives, hepatic impairment

Vitamin	Preterm/Term	Notes
Vitamin B6 (Pyridoxine)	E: 0.3-0.7/0.3 mg P: 0.3-0.7/1.0 mg	**Deficiency**: Impaired development of neurological system, seizures **Excess**: Peripheral nerve damage, respiratory distress, hypotonia, lethargy, GI upset
Vitamin B12 (Cobalamin)	E: 0.3-0.7/0.3 mg P:0.3-0.7/1.0 mg	**Deficiency**: Vomiting, diarrhea, hypotonia, lethargy, anemia, megaloblastic anemia **Excess**: Skin irritation, diarrhea, tachycardia, poor sleeping

MINERALS

Daily mineral requirements vary according to the neonate's condition and whether preterm or term. **E**=Enteral, **P**=Parenteral.

Minerals	Preterm/Term	Notes
Biotin	**E:** 6-20/10 mcg **P:** 6-13/20 mcg	Deficiency: Hypotonia, seizures, skin disorders, hearing loss, conjunctivitis, lethargy Excess: Hyperglycemia
Calcium	**E:** 210-250/130 mg/kg **P:**60-90/60-80 mg/kg	Deficiency: Jitteriness, irritability, stridor, tetany, high-pitched cry, seizures, and cardiac dysfunction Excess: Vomiting; constipation, hypertension, hypotonia, lethargy, seizures
Chloride	**E:** 2-3/2-3 mEq/kg **P:**2-3/2-3 mEq/kg	Deficiency: Weakness, lethargy, irritability, impaired absorption of iron and vitamin B_{12} Excess: Metabolic acidosis
Chromium	**E:** 2-4/2 mcg/kg **P:** 0.2/0.2 mcg/kg	Deficiency: peripheral neuropathy, impaired glucose tolerance, muscle weakness, loss of weight Excess: Skin irritation
Copper	**E:** 100-150/75 mcg/kg **P:** 20/20 mcg/kg	Deficiency: Hypochromic anemia, bone demineralization, neutropenia Excess: Gastroenteritis, hepatic injury
Folate (Folic acid)	**E:** 50/25-50 mcg **P:** 40-90/140 mcg	Deficiency: Lethargy, pallor, tachycardia, low weight, general weakness Excess: GI upset, poor sleeping
Iodine	**E:** 4/7 mcg/kg **P:** 1.0/1.0 mcg/kg	Deficiency: Intellectual disabilities, hypothyroidism, thyroid enlargement Excess: Abdominal pain, fever, hypothyroidism, skin irritation
Iron	**E:** 1-2/1-2 mg/kg **P:** 0.09-0.2/0.1-0.2 mcg/kg	Deficiency: Anemia, lethargy, impaired development Excess: GI upset, tachycardia, hyperpnea, hypotension, seizures, coma, liver failure
Magnesium	**E:** 8-15/7 mg/kg **P:** 4-7/5-7 mg/kg	Deficiency: Tetany, seizure, coma, tachycardia, ventricular arrhythmias, respiratory depression Excess: Hypotonia, hyporeflexia, constipation, hypotension, apnea, vasodilatation/flushing
Manganese	**E:** 10-20/85 mcg/kg **P:** 1.0-1.0 mcg/kg	Deficiency: Weakness, hearing impairment Excess: Impaired iron absorption
Molybdenum	**E:** 2-3/2 mcg/kg **P:** 0.25/0.25 mcg/kg	Deficiency: Inability to metabolize sulfites, seizures Excess: growth restriction, diarrhea

Minerals	Preterm/Term	Notes
Phosphorus	**E:** 112-125/45 mEq/kg **P:**40-70/40-45 mEq/kg	Deficiency: Impaired bone metabolism, muscle weakness, tremors, seizures, impaired immune response Excess: GI upset, tachycardia, hyperreflexia, tetany
Potassium	**E:** 2-3/2-3 mEq/kg **P:** 2-3/2-3 mEq/kg	Deficiency: Cardiac arrhythmias, ileus, and lethargy Excess: Cardiac arrhythmias (bradycardia, tachycardia, VF)
Selenium	**E:** 1.3-3/1.6 mcg/kg **P:** 1.5-2/2.0 mcg/kg	Deficiency: Impaired immune response Excess: Diarrhea, lethargy, respiratory depression
Sodium	**E:** 2-4/2-3 mEq/kg **P:** 2-3.5/2-3 mEq/kg	Deficiency: Apnea, irritability, twitching, weight gain, and seizures Excess: weight loss, irritability, lethargy, fever, seizures (late)
Zinc	**E:** 800-1000/830 mcg **P:** 400/250 mcg	Deficiency: Impaired growth, impaired immune response, dermatitis Excess: Vomiting and diarrhea, neurological damage

Human Breast Milk

Human breast milk is the food of choice for newborn infants. **Colostrum**, produced during the first few days after birth, is scant, thick, yellowish, and high in protein and antibody content. Colostrum stimulates the passage of meconium. **Transitional milk** (days 3-14) is thinner and white, with a composition closer to that of mature milk. By the second week, most mothers produce 23-27 ounces of bluish-white **mature human breast milk**. Most neonates nurse every 1-3 hours for 20-40 minutes. Benefits of human breast milk are as follows:

- Human breast milk provides appropriate amounts of carbohydrate, protein, fat, vitamins, minerals, enzymes, and trace elements.
- It contains maternal antibodies that help bolster the infant's immature immune system.
- Breastfed babies have reduced risks of eczema, asthma, obesity, and elevated cholesterol later in life.
- Breastfeeding enhances the bond between the mother and the infant by physical contact and promotes recognition of communication signals.
- The maternal cost is an extra 500 calories a day and extra water.
- It eliminates the possibility of kidney damage caused by incorrectly mixed formula.

Composition

Human breast milk has immunologic benefits that formulas lack, resulting in decreased morbidity in breastfed infants. Human breast milk contains these important substances:

- **Antibodies**: Secretory IgA to provide protection from respiratory, enteric, and viral pathogens
- **Primary nutrients:** Protein with whey-to-casein ratio of 60:40 (including IgM, IgG, lactoferrin, lysozyme, casein [40%], and fibronectin), carbohydrate (about 40% of total calories), and fat (free fatty acids)

The following are **secondary nutrients:**

- Nucleotides
- Vitamins A, C, D, E; vitamin D content ≤25 IU/L; supplement if ≤2 months of age
- Enzymes: anti-inflammatory and antibacterial properties, including lipase, which breaks down fat
- Growth factors
- Hormones: prolactin, cortisol, thyroxine, insulin, and erythropoietin
- Cells: beta-lymphocytes, macrophages (90%), neutrophil, T-lymphocytes, cytokines, interleukin 1b, 6, 8, 10, 12 (both inflammatory and anti-inflammatory properties)

FEEDING

FEEDING CUES

The infant gives a number of feeding cues to show hunger. Mothers should be taught to recognize these cues, as it's more difficult for a frantically hungry baby to latch on. These are some indications that the infant is hungry:

- Licking the lips
- Sucking motions of the mouth
- Rooting or bobbing of the head
- Keeping hands in fists
- Bringing hands near mouth or face
- Turning the head toward and trying to suck on a finger stroking the baby's cheek or lower lip
- Crying (usually the last indication)

Infants who are consistently not receiving adequate nutrition usually appear sleepy and listless. They often stop gaining weight or lose weight. Skin turgor may be poor. Urinary output and stools decrease. The infant may appear disinterested in nursing. On the other hand, an infant who is satisfied usually stops sucking and may turn the head away from the breast or resist nursing. The infant will appear relaxed and may doze. Some infants take short breaks while nursing and then resume.

Early Feeding Cues

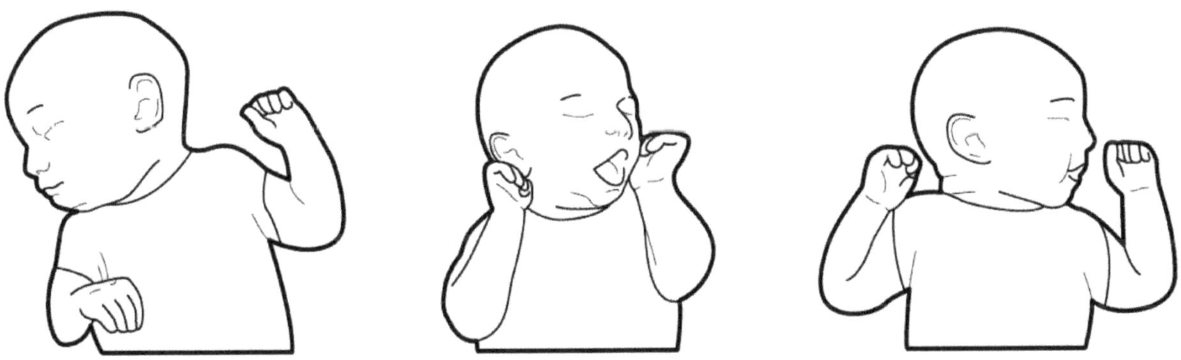

Mid-Active Feeding Cues

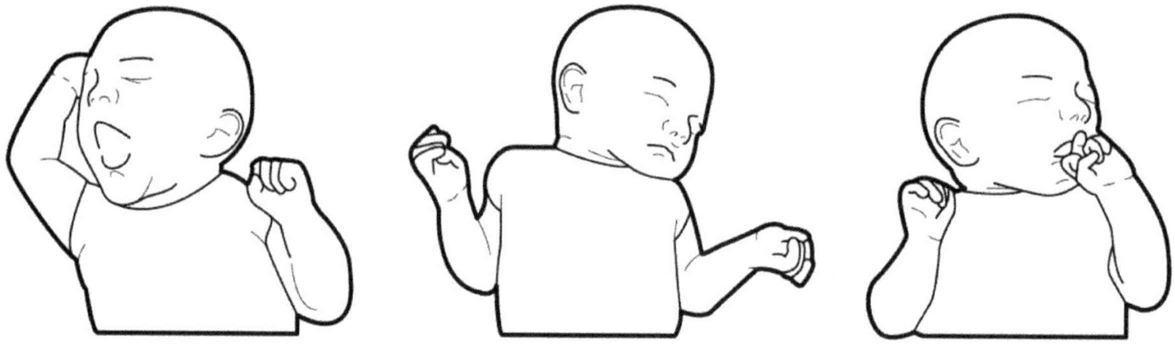

Late Feeding Cues

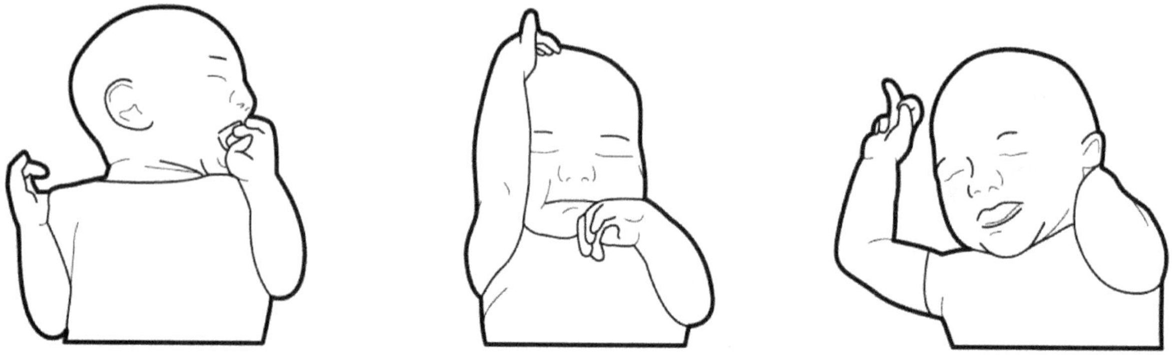

Breastfeeding Frequency and Duration

Most infants initially nurse every 1-3 hours, but during **growth spurts** (2-3 weeks, 6 weeks, 3 months, and 6 months), the infant may nurse every half to one hour for 2-3 days, stimulating the breasts to increase production. Nursing usually takes 20-45 minutes, with 15-20 minutes on each side. Nursing should begin on the last breast used. Infants may nurse more frequently in the late afternoon and evening. Infants should be fed every 3 hours until they regain their birth weight, even if the infant must be awakened. Infants vary in **demand schedules**. Some eat 5-10 times over a 3-hour period and then sleep for about 4 hours. The schedule is less important than assuring that the child nurses **8-12 times** every 24 hours and appears satisfied. By 8-12 weeks, infants begin sleeping longer at night. Some may sleep through the night at 4 months, while others continue to nurse at night.

Latching On and Let-Down

Once the infant is in position, the mother should grasp the breast using a C-hold or U-hold (to make the breast firmer) and lean toward the baby, guiding the nipple toward the infant's mouth. Brushing the nipple against the infant's mouth usually causes the infant to open the mouth and lunge toward the breast. Then, the mother guides the nipple into the infant's mouth while pulling the infant toward the breast. The infant's lower lip should be low on the areola so the baby **latches** on to both the areola and the nipple.

Proper Latch

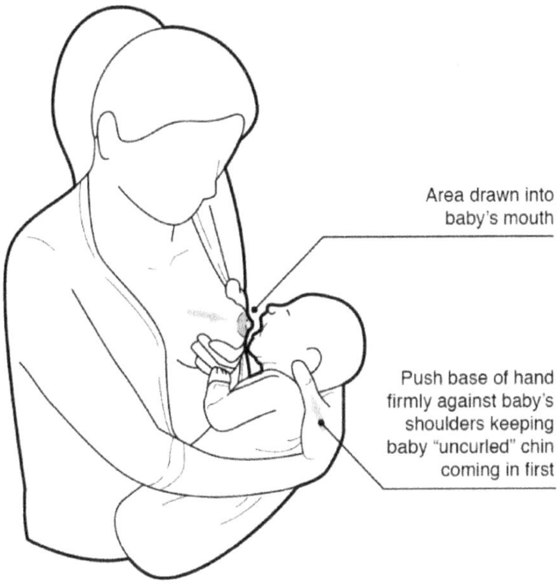

C-Hold

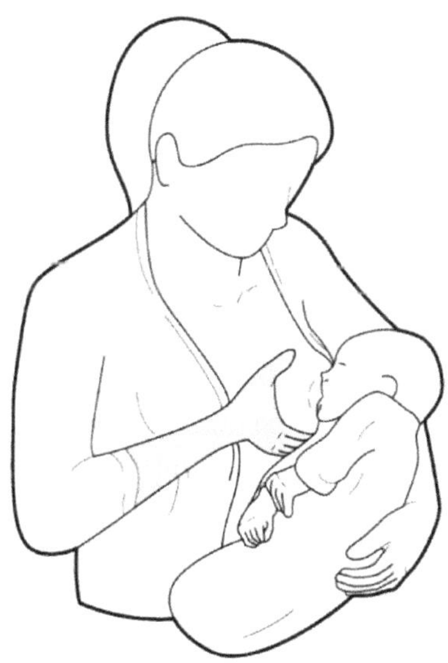

U-Hold

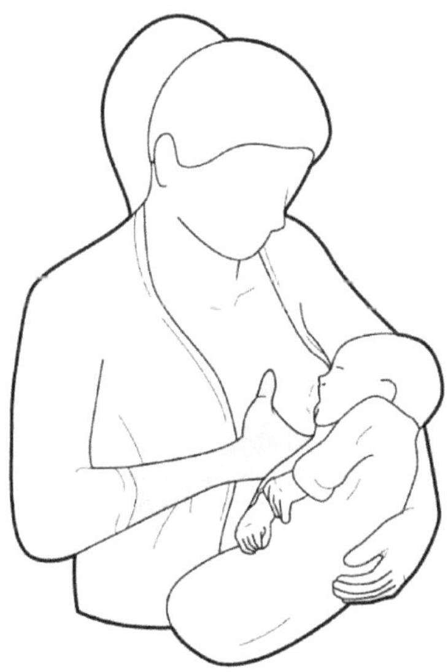

Suckling stimulates nerves in the areola and nipple, increasing production of prolactin and oxytocin, which in turn stimulate contraction of cells about the areola, causing milk to be ejected in a **"let-down"** (milk-ejection) reflex, which is sometimes associated with a tingling sensation, usually within a few minutes of nursing. It may take up to 2 weeks before letdown is efficient.

Problems Associated with Latch-On

Most problems associated with latch-on result from poor maternal technique and are easily resolved with demonstration and support:

- **Infant latches on to the end of the nipple,** resulting in pain and limited milk flow: The mother should learn to brush the nipple against the infant's lips until the baby opens the mouth completely before inserting the nipple.
- **Infant's mouth on just the nipple and not the areola**: The mother should use a C-hold or U-hold to guide the nipple into the infant's mouth, making sure that most of the areola (1.0-1.5 inches) is covered by the infant's mouth.
- **Inverted nipples**, making latching on difficult: If the nipple is so flat that the infant cannot easily latch on, using a silicone nipple shield for the first few minutes may help to elongate the nipple, at which point the shield should be removed because the shield doesn't allow adequate breast stimulation, and the infant must work harder to suckle.

Nipple Shields

Silicone nipple shields, which fit over the mother's nipple and areola, are sometimes used if a mother's nipples are inverted or flat, but they should not be used with cracked nipples if the mother can tolerate feeding. The breast does not receive adequate stimulation if the infant feeds with the shield in place, so milk production decreases and the baby may not be able to get adequate nutrition. Also, because the silicone nipple feels different from the breast, the infant may be reluctant to wean from the shield. If it is absolutely necessary to use a nipple shield for a flat or inverted nipple, it should be used only for the first few minutes, as even a flat nipple will usually elongate during that time. Then the rest of the feeding can be done without the shield.

Suck-Swallow Sequence

A neonate usually **sucks** and then **swallows** when the mouth becomes full. Each suck usually fills the mouth, a **suck to swallow ratio** of 1:1. Infants do not breathe while swallowing, so a 1:1 ratio means the child must breathe quickly, resulting in a rapid suck-hold breath and swallow-breathe sequence. During a swallow, the soft palate rises to block access to the nasal passages, the larynx rises, and the epiglottis covers the airway to prevent aspiration. If milk flow is inadequate, the child may need to suck twice for each swallow (2:1). If the flow is too fast, the child may need to swallow twice or more for each suck (1:2) and some milk may run down the pharynx and into the airway, resulting in aspiration. Or, the child may need to swallow so rapidly there is no time to breathe, and apnea may occur. A newborn usually sucks twice a second for about a minute and then about once per second as the milk flow increases.

Expressing and Storing Human Breast Milk

A mother can **express and store milk** for her infant if the infant is unable to nurse or if she must be separated from the infant. The most efficient method is to use a **bilateral electric breast pump**. The **pulsatile electric pump** provides adequate stimulation in the early postpartum period to establish and maintain the mother's milk supply, usually emptying the breasts within 15-20 minutes. If the child is not nursing, the pump should be used at least 8 times in each 24-hour period. Other methods of expressing milk include manual expression and use of a hand pump. Electric pumps usually have collection systems, so the milk flows into a bottle that can be used for feeding. Human breast milk can be stored for later use using the following guidelines:

- **Room temperature**: 4 hours
- **Refrigerated**: ≤4 days (best used within 48 hours)
- **Frozen**: 3-4 months in a separate-door freezer-refrigerator, and 6 months in a deep freezer at 0 °F

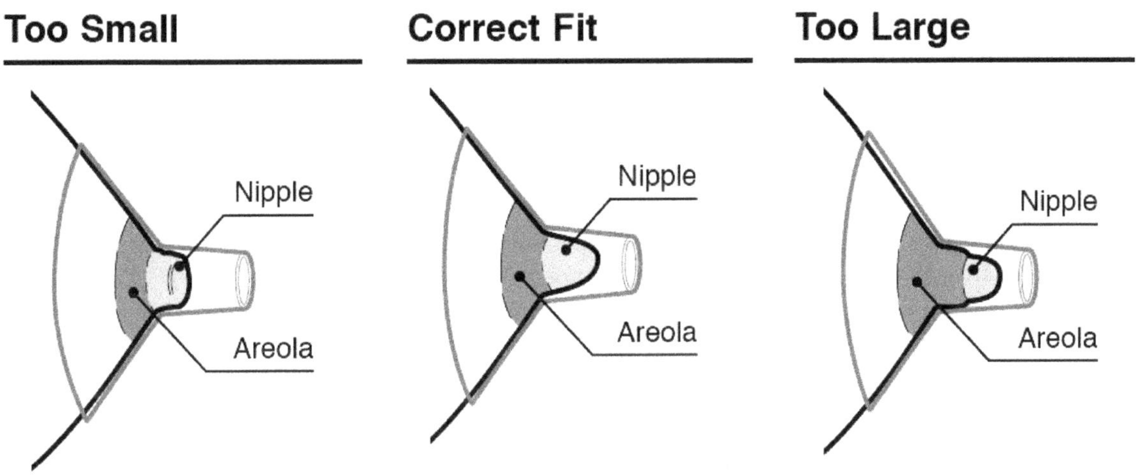

Supplemental Nursing System

Supplemental nursing systems allow the mother to provide supplemental nutrients or medication to the infant while breastfeeding. A typical system has a container for the liquid supplement and a tubing system with a tubing clamp to adjust flow. The tubing is taped to the breast and the end extends about 2-3 mm past the end of the nipple on the top, so the baby encloses both the nipple and the tubing in the mouth when nursing. The tubing should be under the baby's upper lip. Once the baby begins to nurse, the clamp is released so the supplement begins to flow. The bottom of the container is usually positioned level with the breast or slightly lower, so the child must suckle in order to gain the supplement. If the container is higher than the breast, the solution may flow too freely and may choke the child.

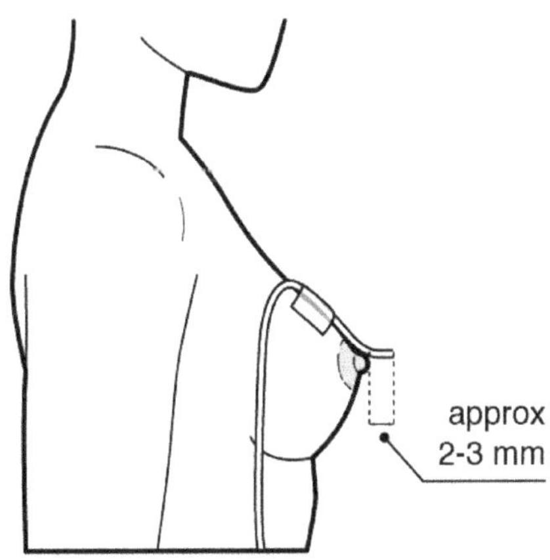

Donor Milk

While the mother's milk is most highly recommended for her newborn's nutrition, some mothers are not able to express sufficient milk for newborn growth and development. Low birth weight infants may also need more human breast milk than available. In these instances, the first recommendation for supplemental nutrition is donor milk, followed by formula. **Donor milk** has an association with lower rates of gut disorders (such as necrotizing enterocolitis) and other infections. Donor milk is generally collected by hospitals and nonprofit milk banks that receive human breast milk donations from mothers that overproduce milk. These mothers have been approved by their physician, by the infant's physician, and through a screening process to ensure the milk is safe to donate.

Infant Formulas

A wide variety of infant formulas are available, but there are 3 primary types:

- **Cow-milk-based formulas** (Enfamil, Similac, Good Start): These are appropriate for most infants. These are enriched with various components, including vitamins, minerals, iron, tyrosine, phenylalanine, and carnitine.
- **Soy-based formulas** (Isomil, Soyalac, ProSobee, Nursoy): These are appropriate for infants with primary lactose deficiency or galactosemia and those allergic to cow-milk-based formulas.
- **Therapeutic formulas** (Nutramigen, Pregestimil): Many preparations are available to meet special needs.

Formula may be purchased in ready-to-feed bottles or cans that require no preparation, liquid concentrate, or powder. Concentrate and powder require the addition of water, so a clean water supply and the ability to measure correctly are necessary to avoid inadequate or unsafe nutrition. Babies who are bottle-fed with formula usually feed less frequently than those who are breastfed. Neonates usually take 2-3 ounces of formula every 3-4 hours. Neonates require approximately 2.5 ounces of formula for each pound (0.5 kg) of weight within each 24-hour period.

Nutritional Value of Full Term Formula and Preterm Formulas

The nutritional value of full term formula and preterm formulas is discussed below:

- **Carbohydrates**: One gram of carbohydrates provides 3.4 calories. Carbohydrates provide approximately 1/3 of the caloric content in infant formulas. Lactose is the predominant carbohydrate. Premature infants may be deficient in the enzyme lactase (enzyme that breaks down lactose), so premature infant formulas utilize lesser amounts of lactose, combined with glucose polymers.
- **Lipids**: One gram of fat provides 9 calories. Lipids supply approximately 2/3 of the caloric content in infant formulas. Common sources of lipids include palm, soybean, coconut, and safflower oils. Premature infant formulas have a higher percentage of fat supplied as medium-chain triglycerides (MCT). MCTs can be absorbed without pancreatic lipase or bile salts that are deficient in premature infants.
- **Proteins**: One gram of protein provides 4 calories. Proteins provide less than 5% of the caloric content in infant formulas. Proteins provide amino acids that are used as building blocks for muscle and other tissues. Preterm formulas have higher protein content than term formula to help meet the increased growth requirements of preterm infants.

Special Preterm Formulas

Preterm formulas are designed with the special requirements of the premature infant in mind. These infants often have an increased caloric requirement to meet growth expectations. **Preterm formulas** differ from full-term formulas because they provide:

- 24 cal/oz as opposed to the 20 cal/oz found in human breast milk and in formulas for full-term infants.
- Increased levels of protein, vitamins, and minerals, particularly increased amounts of vitamin D, calcium, and phosphorus to prevent osteopenia of prematurity.
- Less lactose than term formulas, so they are less likely to cause diarrhea.

Human breast milk can be **fortified** with the addition of human breast milk fortifiers to achieve the same results. Infants are typically switched to a transitional or cow milk-based formula prior to discharge.

Fat-Soluble Vitamins in Formulas

Vitamins found in formulas are organic nutrients required in small amounts to maintain growth and normal metabolism. **Fat-soluble vitamins** include:

- **Vitamin A:** Important for growth and development of tissues as well as proper functioning of the immune system. Vitamin A supplementation in extremely low birth weight infants has been shown to reduce the incidence of bronchopulmonary dysplasia.
- **Vitamin D:** Required for adequate calcium and phosphorus absorption. Vitamin D deficiency leads to rickets (soft bones, bowed legs).
- **Vitamin E:** An antioxidant that is limited in preterm infants, making them susceptible to developing hemolytic anemia without proper supplementation.
- **Vitamin K:** Important in the clotting process. Infants receive an injection of Vitamin K shortly after birth to prevent hemorrhagic disease of the newborn.

Excessive fat-soluble vitamins A and D are toxic because they accumulate in adipose tissue and the liver. Water-soluble vitamins include thiamine (B_1), riboflavin (B_2), niacin (B_3), pantothenate (B_5), pyridoxine (B_6), cobalamin (B_{12}), C, biotin, and folic acid. Excessive water-soluble vitamins are excreted in the urine.

Enteral Feeding

Enteral (tube) feeding provides nutrition to infants with a functioning gastrointestinal tract but the inability to take an adequate amount of milk/formula orally. Ideally, human milk is provided for enteral feedings because it provides antimicrobial factors (IgA, leukocytes, complement, lactoferrin, lysozyme) lacking in formula. However, preterm infants don't grow at adequate rates on human milk alone, so human milk is usually supplemented with formula that contains additional carbohydrates, protein, fatty acids, vitamins, and minerals. Enteral feeding is indicated in infants requiring endotracheal intubation, or weak infants with an inability to suck, swallow, gag, or coordinate these activities (<34-36 weeks). Feedings may be continuous or intermittent (over 30 to 60 minutes). Feedings should be given slowly and tube position checked frequently to prevent aspiration. If feedings must be prolonged, oral aversion and gastroesophageal reflux may occur, so gastrostomy tube placement may be done. Oral feedings must be introduced slowly once per day, then once per 8 hours, every third feeding, every other feeding, and finally every meal.

Procedure

A feeding tube for enteral feeding should be measured (tip of ear to midpoint between xiphoid process and umbilicus) and marked before insertion. The infant should be swaddled and supine. Oral tubes are used for infants <1 kg and those with NCPAP, on a ventilator, or with a high need for oxygen. Nasal tubes are used for infants >1kg or those taking oral feedings or with a strong gag reflex. Short-term tubes (polyvinyl chloride) are changed every 24-72 hours and long-term tubes (polyurethane) every month. Prior to feeding, stomach contents are aspirated for assessment but then re-instilled to prevent electrolyte loss unless blood, bile, stool, or thick mucus is in aspirate. Feeding should be by gravity flow 5-8 inches above infant, usually over 30 minutes for intermittent feeding, and the tube should be cleared with 1-2 mL water at end. For continuous feeding, the placement of the tube and residual milk/formula should be checked every 2 hours. Usually, a 4-hour amount of milk/formula feeding is hung at one time.

Gavage Feeding

Gavage feeding per a nasogastric or orogastric tube is indicated for neonates who are preterm, critically ill, or unable to adequately swallow to obtain sufficient nutrition. Calories and nutrition provided are based on gestation, development, and laboratory findings (such as electrolytes). Typical caloric feedings:

- Preterm, 24-34 weeks: 15-20 g/kg/day.
- Preterm, 33-36 weeks: 14-15 g/kg/day.
- Full-term, 37-40 weeks: 7-9 g/kg/day.
- Full-term 0-3 months of age: 30 g/day.

Non-nutritive sucking should be provided during gavage feeding with the mother/caregiver holding the neonate with skin-to-skin (kangaroo care) contact during feeding if possible. The neonate has increased risk of gastroesophageal reflux if fed in the supine position, so prone or left lateral position with head elevated to 30 degrees during feeding is preferred. Additionally, one hour after feeding, position the neonate in the right lateral position for one hour followed by the left lateral position to facilitate gastric emptying.

Bolus vs. Continuous Feedings

Bolus gavage feedings are generally administered over a 15-30-minute period while continuous feedings are administered over a number of hours. There is not yet consensus as to which method is better and study results are often conflicting on the effects of each type, such as which method is most likely to increase apneic periods. Bolus feedings are generally more common but continuous feedings are becoming more popular and require less direct nursing time. Intermittent feedings are usually done with gravity flow and require constant attendance during feeding, but continuous feedings are usually provided with an automatic pump.

Bolus feedings:

- Simulates normal feeding patterns
- May cause metabolic instability
- Increases risk of gastroesophageal reflux
- May overwhelm immature GI system
- May improve splanchnic oxygenation

Continuous feedings:

- Improves feeding tolerance
- Promotes metabolic stability
- Decreases risk of gastroesophageal reflux
- May result in increased weight gain
- May increase risk of bacterial contamination
- May result in fat separation and decreased fat intake

Trophic Feedings

Trophic feedings (also called minimal enteric nutrition) are very small enteral feeds given soon after birth to extremely premature infants not expected to tolerate enteral feeds for several weeks. Studies have shown that trophic feeds prevent atrophy of the gut and enhance gastrointestinal maturation and small intestine motility. They may also protect the preterm infants from developing necrotizing enterocolitis (NEC). Trophic feeds can be started within 24-48 hours of birth in stable infants. The fluids of choice are colostrum, human milk, or preterm infant formula. Trophic feedings are non-nutritive (not designed to add significant calories or nutrition to the infant). Typical volumes are 1-2 mL/kg per feeding, with a total volume not to exceed 15 mL/kg/day.

Total Parenteral Nutrition

A preterm or compromised infant may not tolerate enteral feedings for several weeks, so the infant's nutritional needs are met with IV **total parenteral nutrition** (TPN). The goals of TPN are to:

- Provide normal metabolism
- Support growth without significant morbidity
- Prevent essential fatty acid deficiency
- Balance nitrogen
- Prevent muscle wasting (catabolism)

TPN is started after birth. Dextrose provides the majority of calories, but to avoid elevated blood glucose levels, dextrose is administered at 6mg/kg/min and increased to 10-12 mg/kg/min over several days. The infant's serum glucose is monitored regularly for hyperglycemia. Protein content is slowly increased over several days to 3-3.5 g/kg/day. Lipids, required for calories and the absorption of fat-soluble vitamins like A, D, and E, are started at 0.5 g/kg/day and increased to 3-3.5 g/kg/day. Other components of TPN include sodium, potassium, calcium, phosphorus, magnesium, trace elements, and vitamins. TPN may be administered through a peripheral IV line for <one week and a central line for longer periods.

Intravenous Lipids

Intravenous lipids are an important component of total parenteral nutrition (TPN) because they provide essential fatty acids, a concentrated calorie source (9 calories per gram of fat), and improve delivery of fat-soluble vitamins to infants who cannot tolerate enteral feeds. General guidelines for the administration of IV lipids are to start with 0.5/g/kg on the third day of life and advance slowly to a final administration rate of 3-3.5/g/kg/day by 7-10 days. Delivery of IV lipids should be continuous over 18-24 hours each day. Serum lipid levels should be monitored for hyperlipidemia. Potential **complications** include:

- Risk of kernicterus in infants with elevated unconjugated bilirubin (Free fatty acids displace bilirubin from albumin binding sites. Infusion of lipids should be at the lower level in infants with elevated unconjugated bilirubin.)
- Exacerbation of chronic lung disease
- Exacerbation of persistent pulmonary hypertension

TPN Complications

Complications of total parenteral nutrition (TPN) result from the presence of the intravenous access (usually a central line) and the development of cholestasis. Both of these events are more common in infants receiving TPN for longer than 2-3 weeks. The longer an infant receives TPN, the more likely complications will occur. Consequences of prolonged venous access include sepsis, thrombophlebitis, and extravasation of fluid into soft tissue with possible tissue necrosis. Premature infants have an immature hepatobiliary system. One hypothesis for the development of cholestasis is that a lack of fat in the duodenum leads to biliary stasis. Infants requiring TPN are often very ill, may have episodes of shock, or require surgical interventions, all of which contribute to the development of TPN-associated cholestasis. Jaundiced infants show an elevated direct bilirubin in blood serum. Treatment usually involves the discontinuation of TPN, along with the slow introduction of enteral feeds (if possible).

Supplementary or Complementary Feeding

Supplementary or complementary feeding with breastfed babies is usually discouraged because it may weaken the suckling reflex or cause the child to lose interest in breastfeeding, especially if a bottle is offered before breastfeeding is well established. To breastfeed, the child must latch on differently to the breast than to a bottle nipple, with the mouth opened more widely for the breast. Additionally, the tongue moves front to back when nursing (expressing milk) and up and down (squeezing the nipple) when feeding from a bottle. Changing from one to the other can be confusing for the infant, and some cannot adjust. Once the infant nurses well, usually after about 4 weeks, mothers who want to pump for supplementary feedings may try to slowly introduce the bottle. Neonates do not need water and should not be given juice or sugar water.

Dietary Supplements

Dietary supplements include:

- **Human milk fortifiers**: HMFs are added to human milk to improve nutritional values. Contains nutrients (protein, carbohydrates, fats), vitamins, and minerals. Some fortifiers are derived from cow's milk and others from human milk. Human milk fortifiers are generally used for preterm and VLBW (very low birth weight) neonates.
- **Glucose polymers**: Glucose polymers are derived from starches (such as rice and tapioca) and are alternatives to glucose used as nutritional supplements to increase carbohydrate intake. Glucose polymers and lactose are commonly found in formulas intended for preterm neonates.
- **Medium chain triglycerides**: This nutritional supplement is provided to preterm neonates in order to increase fat absorption to promote growth.
- **Probiotics**: Live bacteria and yeast supplements are added to feedings of preterm neonates to reduce the risk of necrotizing enterocolitis.

Iron Supplementation

The premature infant is especially susceptible to iron deficiency because of the lack of maternal iron transfer during the third trimester and the multiple blood samplings that occur with the extensive monitoring of the premature infant. To minimize the risk of iron deficiency anemia, premature infants fed human milk should be started on **iron supplementation** once they receive full enteral feeds. Studies have shown that premature infants fed a premature formula have better iron stores when that formula is supplemented with 15 mg/L of iron compared to those receiving formula with only 3 mg/L of iron. All formula-fed term infants should receive iron-fortified formulas. Breastfed term infants should be given iron supplementation when they are several months old.

Carnitine Supplementation for Premature Infants

Carnitine is a quaternary amino acid that is synthesized from methionine and lysine in the liver and kidney. Carnitine aids in the metabolism of long chain fatty acids by helping to transport them across the mitochondrial membrane. Carnitine is present in human milk and formulas in sufficient amounts. Infants who are born premature have low tissue stores of carnitine, as much of it is transferred to the fetus during the third trimester. Symptoms of carnitine deficiency include increased episodes of apnea, decreased muscle tone, and poor growth. Infants who are not being enterally fed and are receiving TPN may benefit from supplementation with carnitine because it makes them better able to metabolize fats.

Complications of Breastfeeding

Engorgement

Production of milk sometimes outstrips demand in the first 2-3 days as the mother is starting to nurse, and the breasts become **engorged** (enlarged, taut, and painful). The mother should be reassured that this is normal and can be relieved, as new mothers may feel they should stop nursing or be afraid they are doing something wrong. Nursing frequently (every 2-3 hours) and gently massaging the breast toward the nipple during nursing should reduce engorgement. If the areola is hard, some milk should be manually expressed to soften the areola before the infant latches on. Breast pumps and heat (except in a shower) may increase engorgement. Cold compresses, acetaminophen, or ibuprofen may provide relief. Engorgement usually recedes within 24-48 hours.

Insufficient Milk

Only about 1.5% of women are physiologically unable to produce **sufficient milk** for an infant. In almost all cases, the mother is simply not nursing correctly or frequently enough to stimulate milk production.

Blocked Milk Duct

A palpable, localized lump or an area of hard, swollen erythematous tissue usually indicates a **blocked duct**. Causes include nursing the baby in the same position or wearing a constricting or poorly-fitting bra. Painful, blocked ducts generally open within 24-48 hours, with symptoms receding, as opposed to mastitis which tends to worsen. Massaging the affected area while breastfeeding, manually expressing the breast during a warm shower, applying heat to the area, and using a breast pump to completely empty the breast after feeding may alleviate the blockage. Additionally, while breastfeeding on the affected side, the infant should be positioned so the chin points toward the blocked area, usually using the football position. If blockage is not alleviated, blocked milk ducts may progress to mastitis.

Mastitis

Indications that the breast has become infected (**mastitis**) with bacteria include induration, swelling, erythema, increasing fever, and acute pain. Without prompt treatment, painful abscesses may form. The infected area may be localized, sometimes appearing similar to blocked milk duct, or generalized, encompassing the whole breast. The mother may have chills and flu-like symptoms before obvious inflammation of the breast. Usually, the mother becomes infected from the infant, most commonly with *Staphylococcus aureus,* so breastfeeding does not endanger the neonate. Treatment includes antibiotics, usually penicillin G, dicloxacillin, or erythromycin, and nursing, pumping, or expressing on the affected side to prevent abscess formation. Applying heat or massaging the breasts in a warm shower may increase circulation. Pain relief includes alternating warm and cold compresses, and acetaminophen or ibuprofen.

Cracked Nipples

Nipples often become sore when the mother begins breastfeeding, but this typically lessens in a few days. However, **cracked nipples** may lead to infection. These are some of the causes:

- The baby latching on improperly to just the nipple and not the areola
- Use of drying lotions or soaps
- Use of a breast pump with too much suction
- Monilial infection from thrush in the baby's mouth

Sometimes changing the baby's **position** or rotating positions during nursing may reduce discomfort. Nursing should begin on the least sore nipple, as the infant nurses more strongly at first. The breasts should be cleansed only with water and a small amount of human milk applied to the nipple after nursing, unless the baby has thrush. One hundred percent USP modified **lanolin** (Lansinoh or PureLan) applied to the nipples may promote healing. It does not need to be removed for breastfeeding. Acetaminophen or ibuprofen may be taken 30 minutes before nursing. Nipple shields should be avoided if possible, as they interfere with latching on.

Psychosocial Issues

FAMILY TYPES

Some of the different types of families are described below:

- **Nuclear**: This **husband-wife-children** model was once the most common family type but is no longer the norm. In this model, the husband is the provider, and the mother stays home to care for the children. This makes up only about **7%** of current American families.
- **Dual career/dual earner**: This model, where **both parents work**, is the most common in American society, including about **66%** of two-parent families. One parent may work more than another, or both may work fulltime. Income disparities may affect family dynamics.
- **Childless**: **10-15%** of families have no children because of **infertility** or **choice**.
- **Extended**: These may include **multigenerational families** or **shared households** with friends, parents, or other relatives. Childcare responsibilities may be shared or primarily assumed by an extended family member, such as a grandparent.
- **Extended kin network**: Two or more nuclear families live close together, share goods and services, and support each other, including sharing childcare. This model is common in the Hispanic community.
- **Single-parent**: This is one of the fastest-growing family models. Typically, the mother is the single parent, but in some cases, it is the father. The single parent may be widowed, divorced, or separated, but more commonly, has never married. In cases of divorce or abandonment, the child may have minimal or no contact with one parent, often the father. Single parents often face difficulties in trying to **support and care for a child** and may suffer **economic hardship.**
- **Stepparent**: Because of the high rate of divorce, stepparent families are common. This can result in **stress** and **conflict** when a new child enters the picture. There may be jealousy and resentment on the part of siblings and estranged family members. In some cases, families work together to achieve harmony and provide added support to children.
- **Binuclear/co-parenting**: In this model, children share time between two primarily nuclear families because of **joint custody agreements.** While this may at times result in conflict, the child benefits from having a continued relationship with both parents.
- **Cohabiting**: **Unmarried heterosexual couples** live together. The relationships within this model may vary, with some similar to the nuclear family. In some cases, people are in committed relationships and may avoid marriage because of economic or personal reasons. A planned child may strengthen the relationship, but an unplanned child may cause conflict.
- **Gay/lesbian**: Whether gay and lesbian couples marry or cohabit, they create families in non-traditional ways. For example, lesbian couples may use sperm donors. Gay couples often adopt. Children in these families may face social pressures because of their parents' lifestyles.

Maternal Attachment Process

By the time of birth, most mothers have developed an emotional connection with their infants and demonstrate a number of typical steps in the **maternal attachment process**.

- **Touching**: The mother usually begins by lightly touching the infant's extremities with her fingertips and running her palm over the baby's trunk. This exploration of the infant can proceed very quickly in minutes, or be more tentative and take days. Early skin-to-skin contact with the infant tends to accelerate this process.
- **En face positioning**: The mother increases the amount of face-to-face eye contact with the infant, typically holding the infant close to her face and responding to eye contact by speaking in a sing-song, high-pitched tone (baby talk).
- **Responding**: The mother tends to respond verbally to sounds the infant makes.

Initially, the mother may feel separate and distant from the child, especially if she doesn't feel an immediate bond, and she should be reassured that these feelings are normal.

Acquaintance

During the acquaintance period, the first few days, responding helps the mother to recognize **clues** the child is giving about needs, such as hunger. The mother's ability to respond to those needs strengthens the bond and helps her gain confidence in her parenting ability. During this time, the infant is also learning to recognize **routines**, such as nursing when held toward the breast.

Mutual Regulation

During this phase, which may vary in duration, the mother is learning to **balance** the needs of the infant against her own needs, and she may have some negative feelings, such as resenting her lack of sleep or feeling frustrated by the infant's crying. The mother may be afraid to express any negative feelings, fearful that people will think she is a "bad" mother, but these feelings are normal and are likely to continue until the mother and infant reach a mutual balance. The ability of the mother and infant to recognize each other's cues and respond to them is termed **reciprocity**.

Maternal Attachment/Bonding Assessment

Assessment of maternal attachment/bonding should be done prior to discharge so that any issues and needed interventions can be discussed. In doing the assessment, the nurse evaluates the mother's:

- Progression in touching and face-to-face eye contact with extended times and indications of attraction, such as verbally responding to the infant and cuddling the infant. If there has been no progression, the nurse should assess contributing environmental, cultural, and social factors that may be interfering.
- Consistency in caring for the infant and seeking knowledge about and validation of her infant care; adjusting care to the needs of the infant. Sensitivity to infant's needs, such as recognizing discomfort or hunger quickly and exhibiting pleasure at infant's response to her efforts.
- Pleasure in the infant, expressed by calling the infant by name, noting family traits/characteristics, showing overt happiness. If the mother shows displeasure or apathy, this may indicate poor attachment, but might also indicate that the mother is experiencing pain or weakness.

Paternal Attachment

Paternal attachment, referred to as engrossment, occurs in many ways similar to maternal attachment. The father may feel pride and wonderment at the child and develop a strong sense of nurturing. Early and frequent contact with the infant promotes engrossment, so the nurse should ensure that the father is not overlooked after delivery but is able to hold, touch, and respond to the child as soon as possible.

Sibling and Family Attachment

Siblings should be allowed to visit the mother and infant as early as possible and be encouraged to hold or care for the infant as appropriate for their ages. Siblings sometimes feel left out or overshadowed by the new infant, so it's important that the parents take time to talk to the siblings and give them attention as well. Grandparents and other family members also form attachments to the infant and should be included.

Sibling Responses/Interventions

If there are abnormalities or complications with the neonate, this may cause stress to the **siblings**. Younger children may be hostile and older children ashamed. They may feel guilty about their responses, and they may feel neglected as parents go through the stages of grief and are unable to provide the support that the siblings need. In some cases, parents may express their concern by focusing their anxiety on one of the siblings, becoming hypercritical. In these cases, staff may need to intervene by discussing observations with the parents and encouraging other family members to provide support to the siblings. Parents' groups that involve the entire family can be very helpful. Whenever possible, children should be included in education and demonstrations and encouraged to ask questions. Age-appropriate books and other materials that explain medical conditions and treatments should be available for siblings.

Preparation of Siblings for Birth of Infant

Preparation of siblings prior to the birth of an infant can decrease anxiety and sibling rivalry by helping the children feel that they are participants in the process and are valued. Children should be prepared for physical changes in the mother, changing family dynamics, and infant care. Formal classes may be available for children ages 3-12 to help them identify and express their concerns, and to teach them about pregnancy and childcare. Booklets, books, and videos are also available. The parent or teacher may use dolls to demonstrate childcare and allow the children to practice holding and caring for the baby. When possible, children should have contact with an infant, such as that of a friend or family member. Children may help to decorate the infant's room or prepare a welcome gift, such as a drawing or toy. Children should be told who will care for them during labor and delivery and should visit the mother and infant as soon after delivery as possible.

Barriers to Parent-Infant Interaction

There are many **barriers to parent-infant interaction**, especially with preterm infants or those with genetic disabilities or birth defects that require prolonged hospitalization or treatment. Barriers include:

- **Physical separation**: When the infant cannot be held or fed, when the child is transported to a different facility outside of the area, or when the mother is discharged and the infant remains hospitalized, attachment can be difficult to form.
- **Lack of clear understanding of handicaps or developmental problems**: Lack of infant response is sometimes interpreted as rejection, and parents may be frightened by abnormalities.
- **Attitude of medical staff**: Negative attitudes may cause the parent to grieve rather than attach to the child. Staff members need to encourage the parents to become involved in the child's care and to provide stimulation. Staff often needs to demonstrate care to parents, who may be intimidated by the infant's condition and medical needs.
- **Environmental overload**: The equipment (alarms, ventilators, monitors) and environmental constraints (no chairs) may overwhelm parents.

Cultural/Lifestyle Factors Affecting Family Integration

Values

Values based on attitudes, ideas, and beliefs often connect family members to common **goals**. However, these values may be influenced by many **external factors**, such as education, social norms, and attitudes of peers, other family, and coworkers, so values may change and impact family integration.

Roles

In some families, roles are clearly defined by **gender** and **task** (homemaker and breadwinner), but the roles blur or are **shared** in many families, and in some cases, the father becomes the primary caregiver while the mother works. Other common roles include peacemaker, nurturer, and social planner. How these roles are perceived and actualized affects the manner in which a child is integrated into the family.

Decision-Making

Family power structures vary widely, but in many families, **power** rests with one person who makes ultimate decisions and whose opinions affect other family members. In cultures with a strong emphasis on tradition, power often lies with the father, a grandparent, or another family member. However, it should not be assumed that the families of a given cultural background will always have the same power structure. Instead, power may be **shared** or it may rest with either the mother or the father.

Socioeconomic

Employment trends, marriage rates, and economic trends all affect **family integration**. Many people have become unemployed and are unable to support their families, resulting in severe **stress**, which may be exacerbated by the arrival of a new child. The divorce rate is high, leaving many parents with inadequate funds to support a child. Even if both parents are employed, the cost of living continues to escalate, including the cost of caring for a child.

Mother Relinquishing Child for Adoption

A mother relinquishing her child for **adoption** may have feelings of ambivalence and sadness. Many who relinquish their infants for adoption are young and unmarried. Adoptions may be closed or open, so procedures will vary. In some open adoptions, the adoptive parent(s) may accompany the mother and participate in the birth, with the birth mother relinquishing the child immediately after birth. In this case, the adoptive parents should be treated as the actual parents of the child, while staff should recognize the needs of the birth mother and provide for her emotional and physical support. In other cases, the child is first relinquished to an agency, such as Social Services, which then places the child. If possible, prior to the birth, the birth mother should indicate how she wants to handle the birth. Some want to hold and spend time with the child; others do not. The birth mother should be in a single room, rather than with other mothers, to protect her privacy.

Types of Grief

Anticipatory grief occurs when a child is diagnosed with a terminal illness. The parent begins to mourn over the loss of the child before he or she expires.

Delayed grief occurs when the grieving process is postponed months to years after the loss of a child. Initially, the parent may not be able to grieve appropriately because of an inability to cope, or the pressing need to care for other family members.

Incongruent grief occurs when the mother and the father are out of sync in their grieving process, creating a source of stress and conflict in the marriage. It may be due to the differences in how men and women grieve:

- **Women** are often more expressive about their loss and more emotional. They are more likely to look for support from others.
- **Men** often grieve in a more solitary and cognitive manner. They are generally more oriented to fact-gathering or problem-solving.

Incongruent grief may also exist because the **bond** that develops between a pregnant woman and the developing fetus is unique and generally very intense. The mother's bond begins before the birth of the child, while the father often forms a strong bond after the birth of the child.

Factors That Influence Grieving Families

The emotions that individuals and families experience with the loss or severe illness/disability of an infant are varied and dependent on many **factors that influence grief**:

- **Cultural influences**: Different cultures have their own practices and beliefs concerning sickness, death, and dying, and varying rituals and ceremonies for processing loss.
- **Family system**: The family's composition, the roles of its various members, and its economic circumstances affect its expression of grief. A large family with extended community support processes grief differently from a single mother living far from home.
- **Siblings**: The impact on other children in the family must be considered, in addition to the impact on the parents.
- **History of loss**: Many diseases have a genetic component, and this may not be the first child to be affected.

Minimizing Dilemmas Surrounding Severe Illness of an Infant

Dealing with neonates who are severely ill and not likely to survive is distressing to the staff responsible for their care. Caregivers can have dilemmas concerning adequate pain control, do not resuscitate (DNR) status, the family's cultural norms and religious beliefs that differ from their own, or grieving parents. Studies have shown that formal palliative care teams can help with issues that families face and with staff concerns. Specific procedures that may help staff deal with dying neonates include:

- Formal training in palliative care
- Assigning nurses who are comfortable with administering palliative care to dying neonates whenever possible
- Debriefing meetings shortly after a traumatic death or event to allow staff concerns to be discussed
- Consistent procedures established concerning organ donation

Interventions for Specific Circumstances

Parents may need extra support in circumstances that lead to grief:

- **Chronic sorrow**: If grief is prolonged and the individual does not seem to be able to move forward, the individual should be encouraged to talk about feelings and express grief openly and to seek outside support, such as a therapist or support group.
- **Death of a twin or other multiple**: The parents should be allowed to hold the child if possible and encouraged to name the child, talk about the child, and express feelings of loss. Some parents may want to keep a tangible memory, such as a clipping of hair or a handprint or footprint of the child. Some may benefit from a support group.
- **Repeated obstetric loss** (recurrent abortion, still birth, preterm delivery): The losses should be acknowledged by those caring for the parents ("I'm so sorry…") and the parents encouraged to express feelings about their loss.

Helping Families Deal with Their Dying Infant

The loss of an infant is an incredibly difficult time for families. In order to provide **compassionate care for the grieving family**, follow these steps:

- Recognize and acknowledge their emotions.
- Provide a private area for family members to gather.
- Allow the family members to take pictures or gather other mementos of the infant (identification bracelets, etc.).
- Discuss possible end-of-life care.
- Acknowledge that the grieving process can be a lifelong process and that each individual experiences grief in a different manner.
- Ensure the family is aware of counseling services provided by the hospital.
- Give the family contact information for local grief support groups.

Review Video: The Five Stages of Grief
Visit mometrix.com/academy and enter code: 648794

Pathologic/Complicated Grief Responses

Pathologic/Complicated grief occurs when the grieving process does not become resolved over time. The person continues to have intrusive thoughts and severe emotions for a period of greater than 6 to 12 months and typically has sleep disturbances, shows lack of interest in activities, withdraws from others, and feels severely lonely. With complicated grief, the person is at risk of comorbidities, such as depression and PTSD. **Types of complicated grief** includes:

- **Absent**: The person shows little emotion or response to grief but may experience a delayed grief reaction months or years later.
- **Chronic**: Prolonged grief that persists for years with little resolution, often associated with a codependent relationship.
- **Conflicted**: The person has ambivalent feelings about the deceased and may have little emotion initially but may feel delayed and increased grief associated with feelings of guilt.
- **Traumatic**: Associated with traumatic loss that did not allow any time to prepare. Some may react with anger or guilt.

Palliative Care for Children

Palliative care is providing pain relief and comfort to the neonate who is not responding to current methods of treatment and has a poor prognosis. The goal of palliative care is to achieve the best possible quality of life for the patient and his or her family. Consider the cultural and spiritual beliefs of the family during this difficult time. In its *Policy Statement of Palliative Care for Children,* the American Academy of Pediatrics recommends the following guidelines:

- Respect for the dignity of patients and family
- Access to compassionate and competent care
- Support for the caregivers
- Improved professional and social support
- Continuing improvement through research and education
- The availability of an interdisciplinary pediatric palliative care team 24 hours a day

Ethical Issues

Ethical Principles

Autonomy is the ethical principle that the individual has the right to make decisions about his or her own care. In the case of children or patients with dementia who cannot make autonomous decisions, parents or family members may serve as the legal decision maker. The nurse must keep the patient and/or family fully informed so that they can exercise their autonomy in informed decision-making.

Justice is the ethical principle that relates to the distribution of the limited resources of healthcare benefits to the members of society. These resources must be distributed fairly. This issue may arise if there is only one bed left and two sick patients. Justice comes into play in deciding which patient should stay and which should be transported or otherwise cared for. The decision should be made according to what is best or most just for the patients and not colored by personal bias.

Beneficence is an ethical principle that involves performing actions that are for the purpose of benefitting another person. In the care of a patient, any procedure or treatment should be done with the ultimate goal of benefitting the patient, and any actions that are not beneficial should be reconsidered. As conditions change, procedures need to be continually reevaluated to determine if they are still of benefit.

Nonmaleficence is an ethical principle that means healthcare workers should provide care in a manner that does not cause direct intentional harm to the patient:

- The actual act must be good or morally neutral.
- The intent must be only for a good effect.
- A bad effect cannot serve as the means to get to a good effect.
- A good effect must have more benefit than a bad effect has harm.

Nursing Code of Ethics

There is more interest in the **ethics** involved in healthcare due to technological advances that have made the prolongation of life, organ transplants, prenatal manipulation, and saving of premature infants possible, sometimes with poor outcomes. Couple these with healthcare's limited resources, and **ethical dilemmas** abound. Ethics is the study of **morality** as the value that controls actions. The American Nurses Association Code of Ethics contains nine statements defining **principles** the nurse can use when faced with moral and ethical problems. Nurses must be knowledgeable about the many ethical issues in healthcare and about the field of ethics in general. The nurse must help a patient to reveal their values and morals to the health care team so that the patient, family, and team can resolve moral issues pertaining to the patient's care. As part of the healthcare team, the nurse has a right to express personal values and moral concerns about medical issues.

Bioethics

Bioethics is a branch of ethics that involves making sure that the medical treatment given is the most morally correct choice given the different options that might be available and the differences inherent in the varied levels of treatment. In the health care unit, if the patients, family members, and the staff are in agreement when it comes to values and decision-making, then no ethical dilemma exists; however, when there is a difference in value beliefs between the patients/family members and the staff, there is a bioethical dilemma that must be resolved. Sometimes, discussion and explanation can resolve differences, but at times the institution's ethics committee must be brought in to resolve the conflict. The primary goal of bioethics is to determine the most morally correct action using the set of circumstances given.

Ethical Decision-Making Model

There are many ethical decision-making models. Some general guidelines to apply in using ethical decision-making models could be the following:

- Gather information about the identified problem
- State reasonable alternatives and solutions to the problem
- Utilize ethical resources (for example, clergy or ethics committees) to help determine the ethically important elements of each solution or alternative
- Suggest and attempt possible solutions
- Choose a solution to the problem

It is important to always consider the **ethical principles** of autonomy, beneficence, nonmaleficence, justice, and fidelity when attempting to facilitate ethical decision-making with family members, caregivers, and the healthcare team.

Ethical Assessment

While the terms *ethics* and *morals* are sometimes used interchangeably, ethics is a study of morals and encompasses concepts of right and wrong. When making **ethical assessments,** one must consider not only what people should do but also what they actually do, as these two things are sometimes at odds. Ethical issues can be difficult to assess because of personal bias, which is one of the reasons that sharing concerns with other internal sources and reaching consensus is so valuable. Issues of concern might include options for care, refusal of care, rights to privacy, adequate relief of suffering, and the right to self-determination. Internal sources might include the ethics committee, whose role is to make decisions regarding ethical issues. Risk management can provide guidance related to personal and institutional liability. External agencies might include government agencies, such as the public health department.

Ethical Analysis of a Situation

Assessment of the situation is done to reveal the ethical, legal, and professional **conflicts** that are present. Those who are involved are identified, including the patient, family, and healthcare personnel. The decision maker is determined if it is not the patient. Information about the situation is collected to determine medical facts about the disease and condition of the patient, options for treatment, and nursing diagnoses. Any pertinent legal information is included. The patient and family's cultural, religious, and moral values are determined. Possible courses of action are listed and compared in terms of outcomes for the patient using the utilitarian or deontological theory of ethics. Professional codes of ethics are also applied. A decision is made and evaluated as to whether it is the most morally correct action. Ethical arguments for and against the decision are given and responded to by the decision maker.

Professional Boundaries

Gifts

Over time, patients may develop a bond with nurses they trust and may feel grateful to the nurse for the care provided and want to express thanks, but the nurse must make sure to maintain professional boundaries. Patients often offer **gifts** to nurses to show their appreciation, but some adults, especially those who are weak and ill or have cognitive impairment, may be taken advantage of easily. Patients may offer valuables and may sometimes be easily manipulated into giving large sums of money. Small tokens of appreciation that can be shared with other staff, such as a box of chocolates, are usually acceptable (depending upon the policy of the institution), but almost any other gifts (jewelry, money, clothes) should be declined: "I'm sorry, that's so kind of you, but nurses are not allowed to accept gifts from patients." Declining may relieve the patient of the feeling of obligation.

Sexual Relations

When the boundary between the role of the professional nurse and the vulnerability of the patient is breached, a boundary violation occurs. Because the nurse is in the position of authority, the responsibility to maintain the boundary rests with the nurse; however, the line separating them is a continuum and sometimes not easily defined. It is inappropriate for nurses to engage in **sexual relations** with patients, and if the sexual behavior is coerced or the patient is cognitively impaired, it is **illegal**. However, more common violations with adults, particularly elderly patients, include exposing a patient unnecessarily, using sexually demeaning gestures or language (including off-color jokes), harassment, or inappropriate touching. Touching should be used with care, such as touching a hand or shoulder. Hugging may be misconstrued.

Attention

Nursing is a giving profession, but the nurse must temper giving with recognition of professional boundaries. Patients have many needs. As acts of kindness, nurses (especially those involved in home care) often give certain patients extra attention and may offer to do **favors**, such as cooking or shopping. They may become overly invested in the patients' lives. While this may benefit a patient in the short term, it can establish a relationship of increasing **dependency** and **obligation** that does not resolve the long-term needs of the patient. Making referrals to the appropriate agencies or collaborating with family to find ways to provide services is more effective. Becoming overly invested may be evident by the nurse showing favoritism or spending too much time with the patient while neglecting other duties. On the other end of the spectrum are nurses who are disinterested and fail to provide adequate attention to the patient's detriment. Lack of adequate attention may lead to outright neglect.

Coercion

Power issues are inherent in matters associated with professional boundaries. Physical abuse is both unprofessional and illegal, but behavior can easily border on abusive without the patient being physically injured. Nurses can easily **intimidate** older adults and sick patients into having procedures or treatments they do not want. Regardless of age, patients have the right to choose and the right to refuse treatment. Difficulties arise with cognitive impairment, and in that case, another responsible adult (often the patient's child or spouse) is designated to make decisions, but every effort should be made to gain patient cooperation. Forcing the patient to do something against his or her will borders on abuse and can sometimes degenerate into actual abuse if physical coercion is involved.

Personal Information

When pre-existing personal or business relationships exist, other nurses should be assigned care of the patient whenever possible, but this may be difficult in small communities. However, the nurse should strive to maintain a professional role separate from the personal role and respect professional boundaries. The nurse must respect and maintain the confidentiality of the patient and family members, but the nurse must also be very careful about **disclosing personal information** about him or herself because this establishes a social relationship that interferes with the professional role of the nurse and the boundary between the patient and the nurse. The nurse and patient should never share secrets. When the nurse divulges personal information, he or she may become vulnerable to the patient, a reversal of roles.

Newborn Assessment and Management

Transition to Extrauterine Life

Neutral Thermal Environment

A neutral thermal environment (NTE) is a place in which the infant's body temperature is maintained within a normal range without alterations in metabolic rate or increased oxygen consumption (i.e., environmental temperature in which oxygen consumption and glucose consumption are lowest). Infants who are in an NTE are not utilizing energy to maintain their body temperature in the normal range. Just because an infant has a normal body temperature does not mean he/she is in an NTE. The infant may still be utilizing mechanisms, such as non-shivering thermogenesis, to maintain body temperatures, as evidenced by increased oxygen consumption and poor weight gain over time. Charts are commercially available that outline the appropriate NTE for infants based on current weight and birth weight.

Heat Transfer Mechanisms

There are four heat transfer mechanisms to consider when caring for a neonate, especially a premature one:

- **Conduction**: The transfer of heat between solid objects of different temperatures in contact with each other. Heat is transferred from the body of the infant to a cold surface it may come into contact with, such as a scale. Care should be taken to make sure the scales are warmed before use. Conduction can also be used to warm the infant by placing a warmed blanket next to the skin.
- **Convection**: The transfer of heat through air currents moving around and across an infant's body. Incubators use convection of warm air being pumped into the incubator to keep an infant warm. Heat can be lost this way if a cool draft is allowed near the infant.
- **Radiation**: Heat transferred between two objects not in contact with each other. This is the transfer of heat through emission of infrared rays. Radiant warming beds use this mechanism to warm the infant. Heat loss occurs when an infant is in an incubator and the walls of the incubator are cooler than body temperature. The neonate in an incubator with this situation will lose body heat through radiation from its body to the cooler walls despite the warm air being pumped in.
- **Evaporation**: Loss of heat occurs when moisture evaporates from the surface of the skin. Evaporation is the result of the conversion of liquid into a vapor and is a major concern at birth, as a wet infant can experience a 3-degree drop in body temperature in only about 10 minutes. Thus, it is critical to dry the neonate at birth and to replace wet linens with warm, dry ones.

Evaporative Heat Loss and Humidity Related to Preterm Infants

Evaporative heat loss occurs when moisture vaporizes from the skin of an infant. In infants born younger than 31 weeks gestation, **evaporative heat loss** is greatly enhanced by the poor keratinization of the infant's skin. Poor keratinization makes skin highly permeable, which promotes both fluid and heat loss. This permeability decreases 7-10 days after birth. The amount of evaporation is dependent on the relative humidity of the environment. The more **humid the environment**, the more that evaporation and its associated heat loss are suppressed. A dry environment promotes evaporative heat and fluid loss through the skin. An incubator with humidity controls should be used for infants who are vulnerable to evaporative heat loss. Infants prone to temperature instability should be kept in a highly humid environment.

Cold Stress/Hypothermia

Signs of Cold Stress

Cold stress/hypothermia in the neonate is a body temperature measurement of less than 36.5 °C rectally with associated symptoms. Preterm neonates are especially vulnerable to cold stress, as they have limited ability to intrinsically create or conserve body heat. They do not shiver, have limited ability to constrict superficial blood vessels and have limited amounts of both subcutaneous and brown fat. **Signs of cold stress** include:

- Body is cool to touch
- Central cyanosis and acrocyanosis
- Mottling of skin
- Poor feeding, weak suck, increased gastric residuals, and abdominal distension
- Bradycardia
- Shallow respirations with tachypnea
- Restlessness and irritability
- Apnea
- Lethargy and decreased activity
- Weak cry
- Hypoglycemia
- Central nervous system depression with hypotonia
- Edema

Risk Factors in Preterm Infants

Preterm infants have not yet developed many of the features that full term infants use to help protect them from heat loss. The characteristics that make premature infants especially **vulnerable to cold stress** include:

- Larger surface area to body mass ratio that allows for quicker transfer of body heat to the environment
- Decreased amounts of subcutaneous fat that provides insulation from heat loss
- Decreased amounts of brown fat used for non-shivering thermogenesis
- Immature skin that is not completely keratinized is more permeable to evaporative water and heat loss
- Inability to flex the body to conserve heat
- Limited control of skin blood flow mechanisms that conserve heat

Non-Shivering Thermogenesis

Non-shivering thermogenesis (NST) is the major route of rapid increase of body temperature in response to cold stress in the term neonate. NST is the oxidation of brown fat to create heat. Brown adipose tissue contains a high concentration of stored triglycerides, a rich capillary network, and is controlled by the sympathetic nervous system. Brown fat cells have a rich supply of mitochondria that are unique, in that when fat is metabolized ATP is not produced, but instead heat is created. Temperature regulation is controlled by the posterior hypothalamus. When a cold body temperature is detected, the posterior hypothalamus responds by triggering the adrenal glands to release norepinephrine and the pituitary gland to release thyroxine. Both norepinephrine and thyroxine stimulate NST. Brown adipose production begins around 26-28 weeks of gestation and continues until 3-5 weeks after delivery. Premature infants have limited amounts of brown fat and limited ability to create heat via NST.

Thermoregulation to Treat Hypothermia

There are a number of steps in the treatment of hypothermia:

1. Determine if the cause of hypothermia is from an abnormal physiological process in the infant or from environmental conditions.
2. Rewarm the infant slowly, as rewarming too rapidly may result in apnea or hypotension.
3. Maintain the ambient temperature at 1.0-1.5 °C higher than the infant's temperature. Oxygen consumption is not elevated when the difference between the skin temperature and the environmental air temperature is less than 1.5 °C.
4. Increase the air temperature by approximately 1 °C every hour until the infant's temperature is in the normal range and stable.
5. Warm IV fluids with a blood-warming device prior to infusion, to enhance warming of the child.
6. Closely monitor the infant's blood glucose levels, vital signs, and urinary output during rewarming.

Hyperthermia

Hyperthermia (rectal temperature greater than 37.0 °C) can be caused by excessive heat from an external source (such as a radiant warmer set too high) or internally from a hypermetabolic state (such as a fever):

External heat source	Hypermetabolic
Core temperature < skin temperature	Core temperature > skin temperature
Skin warm and flushed	Skin cool to touch

Infants who are physiologically competent attempt to cool themselves when hyperthermia is caused by an external heat source by an extended posture, diaphoresis, and flushed, warm skin. Hyperthermia in the neonate can cause increased metabolic demands, vasodilatation, and increased fluid loss. An increased metabolic demand leads to an increased oxygen requirement, hypoxia, cyanosis, and breathing irregularities, such as tachypnea. Increased glucose consumption leads to hypoglycemia and its associated signs (jitteriness, lethargy, vomiting, or seizures). Peripheral vasodilatation helps cool the infant but may cause tachycardia and hypotension. Increased fluid losses contribute to tachycardia and hypotension. Signs of shock may develop with lethargy and decreased urine output. Dehydration may also cause electrolyte abnormalities.

Minimizing Heat Loss

At delivery, minimize heat loss while evaluating the newborn by following these steps:

- Dry the infant thoroughly (including hair) to minimize evaporative heat loss and remove wet towels.
- Place a cap on the infant's head, as the head is the most significant area of heat loss.
- When the infant is to be weighed, cover the scales with a warm cloth to minimize conductive heat loss.
- Place the infant in a warm environment such as:
  - Skin-to-skin contact with the mother and covered with a warm blanket.
  - Bundled in warm blankets and given to the mother to hold.
  - Underneath a preheated warmer for further evaluation or resuscitation.

Minimizing heat loss is especially important if the newborn is premature or has intrauterine growth restriction, but full-term newborns also suffer if they become chilled.

Kangaroo Care

Dr. Edgar Ray invented kangaroo care in the late 1970's in Bogotá, Colombia, when morbidity and mortality rates rose in his NICU, but he had limited technological resources. **Kangaroo care** consists of placing the infant, after drying and warming, in minimal clothing in an upright position on the mother's bare chest between her breasts. This allows for skin-to-skin contact with the infant's head next to the mother's heart. A precipitous drop was noted in premature infant mortality after this method of care was instigated. The concept is to provide the neonate with closeness similar to that experienced with the mother while in the womb. Kangaroo care is maintained for as long as the neonate allows. Preterm infants attached to ventilators and IV infusions also benefit from kangaroo care. There are physiological and psychological benefits for both the neonate and the mother. Enhanced bonding between the neonate and the mother, shorter hospital stays, low cost, and decreased morbidity and mortality are all documented benefits.

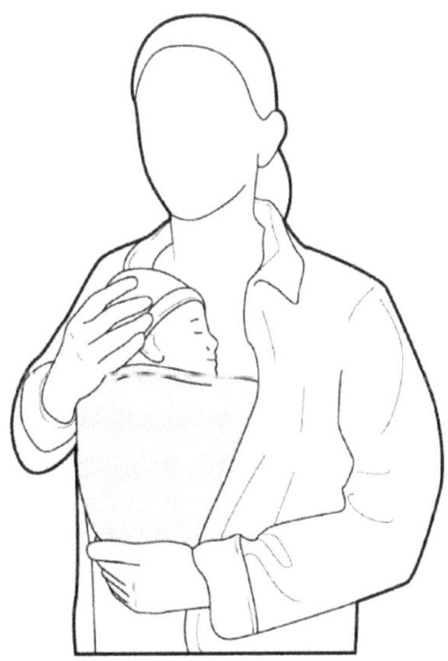

The following are specific **benefits** of kangaroo care for the mother, the neonate, and the institution:

- **Mother's benefits**:
  - Enhanced bonding with the infant
  - Increased production of milk with higher rates of successful breastfeeding
  - Increased confidence in caring for the infant
  - Increased opportunity for teaching and assessing maternal care by nursing staff
- **Neonate's benefits:**
  - Regulation of temperature, heart and respiratory rates
  - Calming effect with decreased stress
  - Decreased episodes of apnea
  - Increased weight gain
  - Enhanced bonding with the mother
  - Fewer nosocomial infections
- **Institutional benefits**:
  - Earlier discharge from hospital
  - Decreased morbidity and mortality (especially in developing countries)
  - Decreased use of financial resources

Incubators

The goal of placing an infant in an incubator is to provide a neutral thermal environment (NTE) that places minimal stress on the infant. Most incubators are rigid, box-like structures like an isolette, in which an infant is kept in a controlled environment to receive medical care. The infant is allowed to grow and mature here before being transitioned to the more "uncontrolled" environment of an open crib. Features that incubators possess that enhance the production of an NTE include a heater, a fan to circulate warmed air, and a humidity control system. They also usually have a way to increase the oxygen content of the environment and ports to allow for nursing care without removing the infant. A servo-control is used in conjunction with a temperature-sensing thermistor that is attached to the infant to help regulate the infant's temperature within a set range. Some incubators may have double walls that lessen radiant heat loss. Infants who are in need of close monitoring are not placed in an incubator but instead are placed under a radiant warmer with minimal covering. This allows the nurse to monitor the infant's skin color and breathing patterns more closely.

Radiant Warmers

Radiant warmers are devices that provide overhead heat directly to the infant. Radiant heaters provide an area for direct observation and free access to the infant, which is very useful in the initial evaluation and resuscitation (if necessary) of the newborn or for procedures such as intubation or line placement. Radiant heat devices work best if the room temperature is kept above 25 °C. Two **problems related to radiant warmers** include:

- Promote dehydration if an infant is placed under them for a prolonged amount of time, especially if the infant is premature
- Risk overheating the infant or cause first-degree burns

Temperature sensors must be appropriately placed and the infant's temperature monitored frequently to ensure the infant is not being over or under heated.

SKIN TEMPERATURE PROBES

Skin temperature probes are often used to monitor the temperature of the infant in an isolette or radiant warmer. Incorrect placement of the probe can alter the reading, causing the warming device to deliver too much or too little heat. The temperature probe should not be placed over a bony area of the body or over an area where brown adipose tissue is abundant. Brown adipose tissue is abundant around the neck, the midscapular region of the back, and the mediastinum and organs in the thoracic cavity, kidneys, and adrenal glands. A common probe placement area for an infant who is supine is over the liver. If the probe is not making good skin contact, it will indicate that the infant is cold, and the warmer will deliver increased amounts of heat, possibly causing hyperthermia. If the probe is underneath the infant, it may indicate an artificially warm temperature and decrease heat to the infant, causing hypothermia.

SERVOCONTROL

The servocontrol is a **thermistor probe** used to monitor the temperature of the infant in an incubator or radiant warmer. The servocontrol is essentially the automatic thermostat that adjusts the environmental temperature in response to the infant's body temperature. Typically, the infant's temperature should be maintained at 36.0-36.5 °C. Incorrect placement of the probe can alter the reading, causing the warming device to deliver too much or too little heat. The servocontrol should avoid a bony area of the body or an area where brown adipose tissue is abundant (neck, midscapular region, mediastinum, and organs in the thoracic cavity, kidneys, and adrenal glands). If the infant is supine, the probe is placed on the abdomen at the midpoint between the xiphoid process and the umbilicus. If prone, the probe is placed over either flank. If in a radiant warmer, a special foil shield should protect the probe. As mentioned above, the probe must make proper skin contact, and the nurse should be sure that is not reading artificially warm or artificially cool. An incorrect reading can put the infant at risk for hyperthermia or hypothermia.

Physical Assessment

Physical Assessment

The neonate should undergo three different types of physical assessment:

- **Immediate**: The first examination is done in the delivery room to determine the need for resuscitation or other intervention. This includes the APGAR assessment.
- **1-4 hours after birth**: The second examination includes gestational age assessment, which must be completed within 24 hours for accuracy, and brief physical assessment to determine if there are any problems that might place the infant at risk. This includes assessment of respiratory and cardiac status, cord color, skin color, and movement. The Modified Ballard scoring system is often used.
- **≥24 hours after birth (or prior to discharge)**: The final examination should include a complete physical and behavioral assessment that includes all systems and evaluation of reflexes. All weights and measurements are taken and reviewed. This exam requires observation, palpation, and auscultation. In some cases, instead of a separate examination at 1-4 hours, only this complete physical examination is completed.

Rapid Assessment

The infant should be given a rapid assessment within seconds of birth to determine if the infant is at term, if the amniotic fluid is clear, if there is muscle tone, and if there are respirations or crying. If any of these conditions are not met, then the child should be placed under radiant heat and further resuscitation done. The basic **steps to resuscitation** include:

- Warming the infant after drying
- Positioning the infant and clearing the airway if necessary
- Stimulating and repositioning the infant

The child should be evaluated throughout the initial procedures:

- **Respirations**: Rate and character of respirations should be noted as well as observation of chest wall movement.
- **Heart rate**: Should be >100 bpm, assessed with stethoscope or at the base of the umbilical cord.

APGAR Delivery Room Assessment

Dr. Virginia Apgar developed the **APGAR** test in 1952. APGAR stands for **A**ppearance, **P**ulse, **G**rimace, **A**ctivity, and **R**espiration. The APGAR is the first test given to a newborn. It is used as a quick evaluation of a newborn's physical condition to determine if any emergency medical care is needed and is administered 1 minute and 5 minutes after birth. The test is administered more than once, as the baby's condition may change rapidly. It may be administered for a third time 10 minutes after birth if needed. The baby is rated on the five subscales and the scores are added together. A total score of ≥7 is a sign of good health.

SCORING CHART

Sign	0	1	2
Appearance (Skin Color)	Cyanotic or pallor over entire body	Normal, except for the extremities	Entire body normal
Pulse (Heart Rate)	Absent	<100 bpm	>100 bpm
Grimace (Reflex Irritability)	Unresponsive	Grimace	Infant sneezes, coughs, and recoils
Activity (Muscle Tone)	Absent	Flexed limbs	Infant moves freely
Respiration (Breathing Rate and Effort)	Absent	Bradypnea, dyspnea	Good breathing and crying

Review Video: Newborn APGAR Score
Visit mometrix.com/academy and enter code: 253451

APPEARANCE, WEIGHT, MEASUREMENTS, AND VITAL SIGNS

The neonate's general appearance, measurements, and VS should be evaluated:

- **Head**: disproportionately large for body
- **Body**: long
- **Extremities**: short and in flexed position (Feet are usually dorsiflexed after breech birth.)
- **Hands**: clenched
- **Neck**: short and chin resting on chest
- **Abdomen**: prominent
- **Hips**: narrow
- **Chest**: rounded
- **Weight**: 2500-4000 g (average about 3400); physiologic weight loss is 5-10% for full term and up to 15% for preterm
- **Length**: 45-55 cm (average 50 cm)
- **Head circumference**: 32-38 cm (usually 2 cm greater than chest circumference)
- **Chest circumference**: 30-36 cm
- **Temperature**: Temperature drops rapidly (skin temperature falls 0.3 °C/minute) after birth with exposure to ambient room temperature but stabilizes within 8-12 hours. Temperature is usually measured by axillary method (for 3 minutes) and ranges from 36.3-37.0 °C.
- **Blood pressure**: 56-77/33-50 mmHg
- **Pulse**: 120-160 bpm awake; 100 bpm asleep; 180 bpm crying
- **Respiration**: 30-60 per minute

Cardiac Rates

Normal cardiac rates can vary widely from one neonate to another, so it's important to understand the normal range in order to determine if the infant has an abnormal pulse. Rates will also vary depending upon whether the infant is awake, sleeping, or active. Pulse rate should be taken with a stethoscope, because the pulse may be difficult to palpate or count accurately manually. The neonatal **point of maximal intensity (PMI)** is located at the intersection between the 4th intercostal space and the midclavicular line (versus the adult PMI located at the 5th intercostal). Additionally, this allows for assessment of heart murmurs.

Newborn infant:

- At rest: 100-180
- Asleep: 80-160
- Active/sick: ≤220

1-12 weeks:

- At rest: 100-220
- Asleep: 80-200
- Active/sick: ≤220

Monitoring of heart rate is particularly important as alterations of heart rate occur with periods of apnea. A period of apnea is usually followed by decreased heart rate, as well as decreased oxygen saturation. Respiratory rates should be monitored as well as heart rate. **Color** should be noted. Pink coloring indicates good perfusion. Generalized mottling or central cyanosis should be investigated further.

Blood Pressure

Normal blood pressure values for **term infant**:

- Systolic: 56-77 mmHg
- Diastolic: 33-50 mmHg
- MAP: 42-60 mmHg
- Hypertension: Systolic >90 and diastolic >60.

In a **preterm infant**, normal systolic and diastolic values will vary depending on the gestational age and size of the infant. A preterm infant should have a mean arterial pressure that is a number matching the gestational age in weeks of that infant. For example, an infant born at 28 weeks gestation should have an MAP of 28 mmHg. Hypertension in this instance would be systolic >80 and diastolic >50.

Proper **fit of the blood pressure cuff** is imperative to obtain an accurate reading. One must measure the width of the infant's arm in the area that the cuff will be applied. The cuff should be approximately 25% wider than this measurement. A cuff too small results in a BP reading too high and a cuff too large results in a BP reading too low.

Heart Sounds

S1

S1 is the heart sound heard as the mitral and tricuspid valves close at the beginning of the contraction of the ventricle (systole). S1 is easiest to hear if the stethoscope is placed at the fourth intercostal space while the infant is supine and calm. If the S1 heard is louder than normal, that means **cardiac output** and **blood flow** are higher than normal. The conditions that can cause this are:

- Patent ductus arteriosus
- Ventricular septal defect
- Tetralogy of Fallot

If the S1 heard is softer or quieter than normal, this is an indication of **lowered cardiac output**, which could be caused by these problems:

- Congestive heart failure
- Myocarditis

S2

S2 is the sound heard when the pulmonic valve and the aortic valve close at the end of the contraction of the ventricles (systole). S2 is easiest to hear at the upper left border of the sternum. S2 is normally split, as the aortic valve closes slightly ahead of the pulmonic valve. In the presence of a cardiac defect, the S2 split becomes wider (the difference in time between the closing of the aortic and pulmonic valve becomes greater). Conditions that cause a **widened S2 split** include:

- Atrial septal defect
- Tetralogy of Fallot
- Pulmonary stenosis
- Ebstein anomaly

Conditions that cause **no split** in the S2 (the two valves close at the same time or one is not closing) include:

- Pulmonary or aortic atresia
- Aortic or pulmonary stenosis
- Persistent pulmonary hypertension

Peripheral Pulses

Peripheral pulses, usually palpated at the brachial or femoral arteries, are graded according to strength. Peripheral pulses may be difficult to palpate in a neonate and should not be relied upon for cardiac assessment. Pulses should always be verified by auscultation:

- 0 = absent
- 1+ = weak
- 2+ = weak to average
- 3+ = strong
- 4+ = bounding

Weak pulses are noted in conditions that cause a decrease in cardiac output. Some of these conditions include:

- Any defect resulting in obstructed blood flow leaving the left ventricle
- Failure of the heart muscle itself
- Shock

Bounding pulses (4+) are noted when there is too much blood coming from the aorta. Some of the conditions that would cause this are:

- Patent ductus arteriosus
- Aortic insufficiency
- Shunts

Respiratory Rate of Neonate and Breath Sounds Found on Auscultation

The average **respiratory rate** for newborns is about 35 to 40 (ranging from 30 to 60) times per minute. Tachypnea (>60/min) may occur within the first hour after birth and during the second period of reactivity, but it should not be prolonged. While mild substernal retractions may occur during the first hour, they should not persist, and movement of the chest should be symmetric (asymmetry may indicate pneumothorax). Nasal flaring may also occur during the first hour, but continued flaring may indicate inadequate oxygenation. After birth, the **lungs should be auscultated anteriorly and posteriorly** with almost all lung fields clear. However, during the first hour or two after birth, some fluid may remain in the lungs, so fine rales may be noted. If the newborn was delivered by Cesarean, more fluid may remain in the lungs, so the rales may sound coarse. If the breath sounds are absent (apneic periods of more than 20 seconds) or diminished, breathing is labored, seesaw respirations are evident, or expiratory grunting occurs, these are indications of respiratory distress.

Chest and Respiratory Assessment

The neonate's chest and respiratory status should be evaluated by observation and auscultation. The chest should be symmetric and the ribs flexible. The xiphoid process may protrude slightly. Breasts are sometimes engorged, and the nipples may secrete small amounts of white fluid. Accessory nipples may be noted. Pulmonary function assessment should include anterior and posterior auscultation. Abdominal movement should synchronize with respirations. Periodic breathing is common, but apneic periods should be <20 seconds or they can result in cyanosis or bradycardia. The **Silverman-Anderson Index** is used to evaluate respiratory status. A score of 0 indicates normal findings, and higher scores indicate respiratory distress.

Characteristic	0	1	2
Chest/Abdomen	Rise together with inspiration	Rising abdomen with sinking or lagging upper chest	See-saw movement
Intercostals	No retraction	Minimal retraction	Pronounced retraction
Xiphoid Process	No retraction	Minimal retraction	Pronounced retraction
Nasal Flaring	None	Minimal flaring	Pronounced flaring
Grunt (Expiratory)	None	Grunt heard with auscultation	Audible grunt

Gastrointestinal Assessment

As the neonate breathes, air enters the **GI system**—first the stomach and then the intestines—within 2-12 hours and enters the colon within 24 hours. Bowel sounds are usually present within 30-60 minutes of birth. The stomach has a capacity of about 50-60 mL and empties intermittently, usually beginning a few minutes after feeding begins and continuing for 2-4 hours after; however, because of immaturity of the cardiac sphincter, the neonate may regurgitate the first few feedings. If regurgitation becomes continuous, further evaluation is indicated. Infants produce little saliva until the salivary glands mature in about 3 months. Term neonates usually pass **meconium** within 8-24 hours, although they may not do so for 48 hours. First meconium is thick, dark, and tarry. **Transitional stools** for the next few days are usually brown to green, after which the child should pass normal stools. Stools of breastfed babies are usually yellow-gold and mushy, and those of formula-fed babies are pale yellow and pasty.

Abdominal and Rectal Assessment

The **abdomen** should be soft, symmetric, and rounded. A distended abdomen with engorged vessels may indicate GI abnormalities. Bowel sounds (present about an hour after birth) should be auscultated prior to palpation. The liver is usually palpable 1-2 cm below the right costal margin, and the tip of the spleen may be palpable in preterm infants only in the left lateral upper quadrant. It should not extend >1 cm below the costal margin. The umbilical cord should be white or blue-white, with two umbilical arteries and one umbilical vein observed and no discharge or bleeding. The presence of only one umbilical artery is associated with GI/GU congenital anomalies. Green/yellow discoloration may indicate meconium staining. The abdomen should be examined carefully for hernias while the infant is at rest and crying.

The **rectal area** should be examined to determine if the anus is present and patent. Meconium is usually passed within 24 hours of birth. Soft swelling in the femoral area may indicate hernia or undescended testicle.

Genitourinary Assessment

Genitourinary assessment requires evaluation of **urinary output**. Many neonates void immediately after birth, although the small amount of urine may be overlooked. About 92% void within 24 hours and 99% by 48 hours. Neonates with **edema** may have higher urinary output as edema recedes. In the first 2 days, most infants void 2-6 times daily, with an output averaging about 15 mL/kg/day. After this, the infant should urinate 5-25 times per day, with volume increasing to 25 mL/kg/day. Urine may appear cloudy because of mucus, and initial voidings have high **specific gravity**, but specific gravity returns to normal levels when the child feeds. Pink stains, referred to as "brick dust spots" often show on the diapers, but these **urate deposits** are of no concern. Female infants may exhibit **pseudomenstruation**—slight bleeding—as maternal hormones are withdrawn.

Male Genitalia Assessment

Male genitalia should be carefully examined to determine if they are clearly male or ambiguous:

- **Penis**: The normal penis is usually about 2.5-3.5 cm long and 1 cm wide with the urinary meatus at the distal end in the glans. Displacement of the urethra is found with epispadias/hypospadias. Micropenis may indicate congenital anomaly. The urethral opening should not be inflamed. The foreskin should adhere to the glans and is tight (if uncircumcised). Small white cysts are sometimes evident on the prepuce.
- **Scrotum**: Skin may be loose/hanging or tight/small with normal slightly darkened skin color and extensive rugae. A large scrotum should be examined by transillumination for hydrocele. If the skin is red and shiny, this may indicate orchitis. Discoloration (bruising) may be present with breech presentation.
- **Testes**: Should be descended and 1.5-2.0 cm in diameter, but may not be in scrotum and may be retractile (moving into the upper scrotum or inguinal canal on stimulation).

Female Genitalia Assessment

Female genitalia should be assessed to determine if there are indications of gender ambiguity, as enlarged clitoris and micropenis may be similar in appearance:

- **Mons**: The labia majora should be symmetric and should cover the clitoris and labia minora in full-term and post-term infants although the labia minora and clitoris are exposed with preterm infants. The urinary meatus should be positioned below the clitoris. Bruising of the labia majora may be evident after vaginal birth.
- **Clitoris**: The clitoris is enlarged in the neonate, and bruising and edema may occur with breech birth. Hypertrophy may indicate hermaphroditism.
- **Vagina**: The vaginal opening should be evident (0.5 cm). Hymenal tag may be observed in the vagina. White or pink-tinged vaginal discharge is common for 2-4 weeks after birth. An imperforate hymen may be indicated by suprapubic mass or mass between labia majora.

Skin Assessment

Skin colors vary with race, but all should be pink-tinged to some degree, as skin pigmentation is slight after birth. Skin characteristics include:

- **Birthmarks**: Dark-skinned infants may have **Mongolian spots** on the buttocks and dorsal area. **Nevus flammeus** (port-wine stain) is a demarcated unraised red-purple lesion caused by capillaries below the epidermis. **Nevus vasculosus** (strawberry mark) is a capillary hemangioma and is a raised, demarcated dark red lesion.
- **Acrocyanosis**: Slight cyanosis of the hands and feet during the 2-6 hours after birth, especially if chilled. Color returns rapidly when skin blanched.
- **Mottling**: Common for hours to weeks after birth and may relate to long periods of apnea/chilling.
- **Harlequin sign**: Deep color on one side of body only for 1-20 minutes; usually transient.
- **Erythema toxicum**: Perifollicular lesions (1-3 mm) white or yellow with pustule appears suddenly over body (except palms and soles); usually transient, cause unknown.
- **Milia**: Small raised white spots on face from exposed sebaceous glands; transient.

Skin Appearance of Neonate

Newborns' skin appearance depends on the development and thickening of their dermis, epidermis, and vernix caseosa. When skin develops during week 15 of gestation, it is initially thin and translucent. By week 20, vernix caseosa production begins. Vernix is a thick, waxy substance secreted by the sebaceous glands and mixed with sloughed-off skin cells, often described as "cheesy." The stratum corneum (protective top layer of the epidermis) develops from weeks 20-24. The epidermis continues to develop and thicken, and is able to form a water barrier by week 32. Near term, the vernix washes away and the skin becomes more wrinkled without its protection:

Gestational Age	Skin Appearance
24-26 Weeks	Translucent, red, many visible blood vessels, and scant vernix
35-40 Weeks	Deep cracks, no visible blood vessels, and thick vernix
42-44 Weeks	Dry, peeling skin, no vernix, and loss of subcutaneous fat

Musculoskeletal Assessment

The **musculoskeletal system** should be assessed for muscle tone. Maintenance of fetal position or limp tone may indicate hypoxia, CNS abnormalities, or hypoglycemia. Joint movement should be spontaneous with good muscle tone. Spasticity or floppiness indicates cerebral palsy or other disorders. Jitteriness may indicate hypoglycemia or hypocalcemia.

Extremities should be short, flexed, and able to move symmetrically through range of motion, but without full extension. Arms/legs should be equal in length with feet and hands of normal size (5 digits each). Feet should be flat. Hips should abduct to >60°. Cyanosis or clubbing of nails indicates cardiac anomalies, and yellow-green discoloration indicates meconium staining.

The **back and spine** are examined with the infant in a prone position. The spine should be straight, without a sacral or lumbar curve, which develops only after the child begins to sit. Obvious anomalies, such as spina bifida, and indications of a pilonidal dimple, skin lesions, or tufts of hair that may indicate abnormalities should be noted. C-shaped spine may indicate spina bifida occulta, and lumbar lordosis may indicate myelomeningocele.

Assessment of Muscular Tone

Determining the quality of **muscle tone** in a neonate is an important part of neuromuscular assessment. The child is placed supine with the head in neutral position and the LRN nurse moves body parts (arms, legs, head) to determine if the muscle tone is flaccid, jittery, or hypertonic. Neonates are slightly hypertonic so that some resistance should be felt to movement, such as when moving a leg or straightening an arm. Tone should be symmetric. The extremities are usually flexed and legs abducted to the abdomen. This assessment allows the LRN nurse to differentiate common fine tremors or jitteriness found in neonates from seizure activity or nervous system disorders that cause muscular twitching. Normal fine tremors are usually halted by holding or flexing the extremity while seizure activity or twitching does not resolve in this way.

Assessment of Neonatal Reflexes

Reflex	Eliciting Reflex	Normal Response	Discussion
Palmar Grasping	Stroke the infant's palm.	The infant responds by grasping the finger.	Grasp reflex is stronger in premature infants and fades away at 2 to 3 months of age. Absence indicates CNS deficit or muscle injury.
Rooting	Stroke the side of the infant's cheek.	The infant turns the head in the direction of the touch, and opens mouth to feed.	Rooting reflex helps the infant find and latch onto the mother's breast.
Sucking	Touch the infant's mouth.	The infant sucks.	Premature infants may have an absent or weak suck reflex, as it usually develops around week 32 of gestation. Weak or absent reflex indicates CNS deficit or depression.
Moro (Startle)	Make a loud sound or give the infant a gentle jolt.	The infant extends arms, legs, and neck, then pulls back arms and legs. May also cry.	Moro reflex disappears at 5 to 6 months of age. Asymmetric response indicates peripheral nerve injury, or fracture of long bones, clavicle, or skull.
Blinking	Flash light at eyes.	Eyelids close.	Absence or delay may indicate cerebral palsy, hydrocephalus, and developmental delay.
Tonic Neck (Fencing)	With infant supine, turn head to one side.	Extremities flex on opposite side and extend on same side.	May be incomplete immediately after birth and should diminish by 4 months. Persistence >4 months may indicate neurological abnormalities.
Babinski (Plantar)	Stroke the lateral aspect of the sole from heel to ball of foot.	Hyper-extension of all toes.	Persists until ≤2 years, after which the toes flex.
Trunk Incurvation (Galant)	With infant prone, stroke down one side of the spine (1 inch from spine).	Pelvis turns to stimulated side.	Absence indicates CNS depression or lesion of spinal cord. Should disappear by 4 months.
Tongue Extrusion	Touch tip of tongue.	Neonate pushes tongue out of mouth.	Continuous or repetitive extrusion indicates CNS abnormalities or seizure activity.

Stepping Reflex

If a newborn is held upright with the feet touching a horizontal surface, the contact should make the infant lift one foot and then the other, giving the appearance of walking. This reflex promotes the development of muscles and usually disappears by 4 months. If this reflex is missing, then may be an indication that the infant has a motor nerve defect or other neurological abnormality.

Anal Wink

The anocutaneous reflex is the reflexive contraction of the anus in response to gentle stroking or stimulation of the skin around the rectum. It occurs in both females and males. Pulling the penis elicits the response in males as well; at one time, this response was believed indicative of sexual abuse, but that has been disproved. Failure of this response indicates that there in an interruption in the reflex arc in the sensory or motor nerves.

Assessing Motor Development

Pull-to-Sit

This test, also known as the head lag test, is conducted with the infant lying in supine position. The infant's arms are grasped with the elbows slightly flexed and the infant pulled into sitting position. The head should be observed carefully as it may lag behind the trunk but should not be completely flexed backward. When the infant reaches the sitting position, the infant should be able to at least briefly bring the head into upright position. If the head consistently lags, this may be an indication of cerebral injury and/or neurobehavioral abnormalities.

Truncal Tone

This test is used to assess hypotonia/floppy infant syndrome. The infant is suspended face down by the abdomen and draped over the examiner's hand. A normal response is for the infant to straighten the back, flex the limbs, and straighten the head while an abnormal response is for the infant to hang in place with the head down and the extremities extended. An abnormal response may indicate CNS disorders or neuromuscular disorders. The most common cause of hypotonia is hypoxic-ischemic encephalopathy.

Eyes, Nose, Neck, and Throat Assessments

The appearance and movement of the **face** should be symmetric in the neonate and a number of different characteristics examined:

- **Eyes**: Usually blue to blue/gray with white to bluish-white sclera. Small conjunctival hemorrhages and transient strabismus or squint may be evident. Pupils should be equal and reactive. Red retinal reflex should be present. Tears are usually absent during crying. Eye blink test causes lids to close.
- **Nose**: Infants usually breathe through their nose and should be able to breathe easily if mouth is closed. If not, the child should be examined for choanal atresia. Sense of smell is determined if the infant turns toward milk source or away from strong smells, such as alcohol.
- **Neck**: The infant should be able to hold head up slightly while prone, but the head lags when lifted from the supine position because of weak muscles. Neck rigidity may indicate injury to sternocleidomastoid injury.
- **Throat**: The palate should be highly arched, mucous membranes moist, and uvula midline (if bifid, this can indicate submucosal cleft). The infant should exhibit the sucking, rooting, gag, and extrusion reflexes.

Mouth Assessment

The mouth should be carefully examined with a gloved finger pressing against the tongue to open the mouth:

- **Lips**: Should be pink, normal-shaped, and symmetric. Thin upper lip with smooth philtrum and short palpebral fissures may indicate fetal alcohol syndrome.
- **Sucking**: Sucking (symmetrical) should occur if lips are touched. Asymmetric movement of the mouth may indicate injury to facial nerve.
- **Gums**: Examined for precocious teeth and Epstein's pearls (keratin-containing cysts).
- **Tongue**: Examined for ridge of frenulum tissue on underside (tongue-tied), although this is not clipped and evidence of protrusion or hypertrophy, which can indicate various disorders, such as Down syndrome and hypothyroidism. Bluish swelling of the frenulum may indicate mucus/salivary gland retention cyst.
- **Mucus membranes**: Examined for color and moisture as cyanosis may indicate respiratory distress and dryness or dehydration. Excessive salivation and drooling may indicate esophageal atresia. White patches on mucus membranes/tongue indicate infection with *Candida albicans.*

Structures of the Ear

The **tympanic membrane** is the eardrum, a thin, semitransparent membrane that separates the external auditory canal from the middle ear. Sound waves cause the membrane to vibrate, transmitting sounds to structures in the middle ear. Three **auditory ossicles** help to transmit the vibrations from the ear drum to structures in the inner ear. These three bones are named the malleus (hammer), incus (anvil), and stapes (stirrup) and are connected to each other by synovial joints. The **cochlea** (snail shell) is located in the inner ear and translates vibrations received from the auditory ossicles into signals that are transmitted to the brain via the vestibulocochlear nerve (cranial nerve VIII).

The following are **structures of the external ear**:

- **Pinna**: All the structures that make up the external ear
- **Helix**: The outermost, curved portion of the ear, which is posterior/superior and has a folded edge
- **Antihelix**: 'C' shaped cartilage that runs on the inside of the helix, separated from the helix by a scooped-out section, called the scapha
- **Tragus**: Small projection just anterior to the external auditory ear canal
- **Antitragus**: Lower cartilaginous portion of the concha, just superior to the fleshy lobe of the ear
- **Concha**: Bowl that surrounds the external auditory canal
- **Lobe**: Fleshy lower portion of the ear that is the traditional site of ear piercing

Ear Assessment

The ears should be carefully examined for a number of different characteristics:

- **Position**: The insertion point of the top of the ear should be parallel to the inner and outer canthus of the eye. Low-set ears may relate to a number of disorders, such as trisomy 13 and trisomy 18, intellectual disability, and various other disorders.
- **Shape/size**: Ears should be proportionate to head size and symmetric.
- **Pliability**: Ears should be soft and pliable. Cartilage is lacking in premature infants, and the pinna is soft. Cartilage should be firm by 38 to 40 weeks with 2/3 of pinna curving inward.
- **Hearing**: Hearing may be initially assessed by observing response to sudden loud sound. Evoked otoacoustic emissions (EOAE) and auditory brainstem response (ABR) are used for universal hearing screening.
- **Tympanic membrane**: Usually not examined with otoscope because of occlusion with vernix and blood after birth, but should appear gray-white and vascular.

Head Assessment

Fontanels

The newborn has 8 skull bones and 14 facial bones. Their adjoining edges are bone sutures. Soft spots where the skull flexes along sutures to exit the vagina are **fontanels**. The newborn has 6 fontanels:

- Diamond-shaped anterior fontanel (AF): 2.1 cm
- Triangular posterior fontanel (PF)
- Sphenoid fontanels (2)
- Mastoid fontanels (2)

The AF is the largest and most informative during clinical examination. Fontanels **bulge** when the newborn cries, vomits, lies down, or has hydrocephalus, intracranial tumor, hemorrhage, or meningitis. Fontanels should return to normal when the NNP holds the baby head up and the infant is calm. **Depressed fontanels** indicate the newborn is dehydrated. Conditions associated with an abnormally large AF include hypothyroidism, Down syndrome, achondroplasia, rickets, and increased intracranial pressure. Infants with Down syndrome may have an extra fontanel between the AF and posterior fontanel.

Craniotabes

Craniotabes is an area of softened skull found in 30% of newborns. It is softer and more pliable than surrounding tissue and gives way when pressure is applied, as though one is pushing on a ping-pong ball. It is more commonly in premature infants, but can also be found in full-term infants. Usually, craniotabes occurs in the posterior occipital or posterior parietal bones or along the suture lines. Craniotabes is considered to be a normal finding that requires no treatment because it usually resolves by one month of age. Craniotabes may persist longer when it is positioned along a suture line. No work-up is required, but the infant should be carefully examined for indications of disease-related causes of craniotabes, including other conditions that affect bone growth or hardness, such as rickets, syphilis, marasmus, or osteogenesis imperfecta.

Caput Succedaneum and Cephalohematoma

Caput succedaneum and cephalohematoma are both examples of head molding resulting from head trauma during birthing. They can be observed during the newborn period and appear similar upon physical examination because the neonate's head is swollen:

- **Caput succedaneum** is more common. It is a collection of fluid beneath the skin, but superficial to the periosteum. It often occurs when the head presses against the dilating cervix during the birth process. Vacuum-assisted deliveries also contribute to caput succedaneum. The swelling crosses suture lines. Complications are rare. Swelling usually resolves over several days.
- **Cephalohematoma** occurs when blood vessels between the skull and the periosteum rupture, causing a subperiosteal collection of blood. The swelling appears several hours after birth. It does not cross suture lines. Complications such as anemia or hypovolemia may occur if the amount of bleeding is large. The blood will eventually be resorbed and may cause jaundice secondary to the breakdown of red blood cells.

Gestational Age Assessment

Estimating Gestational Age

Accurate determination of gestational age (GA) predicts neonatal morbidity and mortality. Compare GA with the birth weight to determine if the patient is large or small for GA. Respiratory distress syndrome affects 1% of neonates. The prognosis for a premature infant with respiratory distress who is an appropriate weight for GA (e.g., 33 weeks and 2,000 grams), is better than the prognosis for a full term, small for gestational age (SGA) baby (e.g. 40 weeks and 2,000 grams). These infants have identical birth weights, but the SGA baby is more likely to require mechanical ventilation and has a greater chance of mortality.

The obstetrician **calculates prenatal GA** throughout a pregnancy by the:

- Reported date of last menstrual period (LMP)
- Periodic physical examinations of the mother
- Ultrasound examinations of the fetus
- Date the fetal heartbeat is first heard
- Date fetal movements are first felt (quickening)

The **Modified Ballard examination** is the first comprehensive postnatal test of the neonate, and when scored correctly, it gives a very accurate estimate of the GA.

Initial Methods for Gestational Age Estimation

The initial marker for measuring gestational age is the date of the last menstrual period (LMP). Various calculators are available for this, but they are limited by both the reliability of the mother's report of the dates of her LMP and the typical variability in menstrual periods and ovulatory times. Ultrasound that utilizes various measurements of fetal dimensions is a more accurate method of estimating gestational age. Ultrasound is most accurate during the first trimester, when it has been shown to have a 95% accuracy of ±6 days. As the fetus grows, its size becomes more dependent on the environment, rather than the date of conception, making ultrasound dating during the second and third trimesters less accurate. Clinical examination by the obstetrician is less accurate in determining gestational age than ultrasound.

Modified Ballard Score Overview

The Modified Ballard Score is used to estimate **maturity and gestational age** in newborn infants. It is most reliable when performed within the first 12 hours of life. The Ballard Score was modified to include evaluation of extremely premature infants with gestational ages as low as 20 weeks (score 10) and as high as 50 weeks (score 44). It scores 6 measurements of **neuromuscular maturity** and 6 signs of **physical maturity** on a scale of -1 to +4 or +5, depending upon the category. The total score indicates the estimated gestational age for the infant.

Neuromuscular Measurements

- Observation of the **infant's posture** while lying supine indicates the total amount of muscle tone the infant possesses. Increased amounts of flexion of the elbows and knees correlates with increased gestational age.
- **Square window test** measures the resistance to stretching of extensor muscles in the infant's forearm. Increased ability for the tester to flex the infant's wrist correlates with greater gestational age.
- **Arm recoil test** measures the tone of the biceps muscle. Increased amount of arm recoil (flexion by the infant after the infant's arms are extended) correlates with greater gestational age.
- **Popliteal angle measurement** assesses the flexor tone of the knee joint. Increased resistance to flexion at the knee is associated with greater gestational age.
- **Scarf sign test** measures the tone of shoulder flexor muscles. Increased resistance to movement of the infant's arm across the chest is associated with greater gestational age.
- **Heel-to-ear test** measures the tone of pelvic girdle muscles. Increased resistance to movement of the infant's foot to its ear is associated with greater gestational age.

Physical Signs of Maturity

- **Skin**: Immature infants have thin, transparent skin. The vernix caseosa begins development at the beginning of the third trimester. Dried, cracked skin occurs as this protective coating disappears after the fortieth week.
- **Lanugo**: Fine, usually unpigmented hairs begin to appear at 24-25 weeks of gestation and thin as the neonate matures.
- **Plantar surface of feet:** Very immature infants have no creases on the soles of their feet. Creases develop first on the anterior portion, and more mature infants will have creases over the entire sole.
- **Breast buds**: These are fatty tissue underneath the areola which increase in size as the fetus matures.
- **Ears**: Increased cartilage content produces a more rigid pinna; ear recoil increases as the infant matures.
- **Genitalia**
  - **Male**: The testes descend from the abdomen into the scrotum at 30 weeks of gestation, and the scrotum develops rugae as the fetus matures.
  - **Female**: Initially, the female fetus has a large clitoris and small labia majora. As the fetus matures, the labia majora enlarge, while the clitoris shrinks.

PRETERM INFANT

A preterm infant is one born prior to 37 weeks gestational age. In the United States, preterm birth is the most important factor influencing infant mortality; preterm infants account for 75-80% of all neonatal morbidity and mortality. **Health problems associated with premature birth** include:

- Respiratory distress syndrome because of inadequate surfactant production (hyaline membrane disease)
- Hypothermia because of inadequate subcutaneous fat, small amounts of brown fat, and large skin surface area to mass ratio
- Hypoglycemia secondary to poor nutritional intake, poor nutritional stores, and increased glucose consumption associated with sepsis
- Skin trauma or infection secondary to fragile, immature skin
- Periods of apnea because of an immature respiratory center in the brain
- Intraventricular hemorrhage

The original cause of the preterm birth (such as maternal infection) may also play an integral role in the likely health problem associated with prematurity.

CHARACTERISTICS OF PRETERM INFANTS BORN AT 24-25 WEEKS

Characteristics of preterm infants born at 24-25 weeks include the following:

- **Skin**: very thin with visible veins; absent or minimal vernix caseosa as it is just beginning to be secreted at 2 weeks
- **Lanugo**: sparse
- **Feet**: smooth plantar surfaces or faint marks on the anterior surfaces
- **Areolae**: newly developing, breast bud not yet present
- **Eyes**: open
- **Ears**: no or very limited recoil
- **Posture**: immature, indicated by limited flexion of the limbs while the infant is in a supine position
- **Square window sign**: shows decreased flexion at the wrist of approximately 60-90°
- **Range of motion**: increased ROM (lone tone) when performing the popliteal angle, scarf sign, and heel to ear examinations
- **Arm recoil**: limited or no recoil

NEUROMUSCULAR CHARACTERISTICS OF FULL-TERM INFANTS

Neuromuscular characteristics of full-term infants include the following:

- **Supine resting posture**: hips, knees, and arms all flexed past 90°, indicating mature muscular tone
- **Square window**: wrist flexes to 0°, reflecting very little resistance to the extensor muscles of the wrist
- **Arm recoil**: arms recoil past 90°; contact between the infant's fist and face demonstrates mature tone in the biceps muscles
- **Popliteal angle**: <90° knee flexion
- **Scarf sign**: the arms cannot be drawn past the ipsilateral axillary line because of the mature tone of the posterior shoulder girdle flexor muscles
- **Heel to ear**: resistance is felt in the knee and hip when the heel is at the femoral crease because of the tone of the posterior pelvic girdle flexor muscles

Characteristics of Postterm Infants

Postterm infants are those born >42 weeks of gestation. Many are normal in size and appearance, but some continue to grow *in utero* and weigh >4000 g. Some may exhibit post-maturity syndrome (about 5%), which puts the infant at increased risk. **Characteristics** include:

- **Appearance**: alert (this may indicate intrauterine hypoxia)
- **Skin**: loose, dry, cracking, parchment-like, and lacking lanugo or vernix; may have meconium staining, yellow to green (indicating recent meconium release)
- **Fingernails**: long (sometimes with meconium staining)
- **Scalp hair**: long and thick
- **Body**: long and thin (fat layers absent)
- **Hypoglycemia** from nutritional deprivation
- **Hypothermia** due to decreased brown fat and liver glycogen
- **Meconium aspiration** (risk increases with oligohydramnios), increasing risk of impaired gas exchange
- **Polycythemia** as response to hypoxia, increasing risk of impaired tissue perfusion
- **Seizures** resulting from hypoxia
- **Cold stress** (lack of fat stores)
- **Congenital anomalies**

Birth Weight and Gestational Age Acronyms

These terms do not take into account the estimated gestational age of the infant:

- **ELBW (Extremely Low Birth Weight)**: birth weight of less than 1,000 g (2.2 lb)
- **VLBW (Very Low Birth Weight)**: birth weight of less than 1,500 grams (3.3 lb)

The following terms take into account the estimated gestational age of the infant in comparison to the birth weight:

- **SGA (small for gestational age)**: below the tenth percentile for gestational age
- **AGA (appropriate for gestational age)**: between the tenth and ninetieth percentiles for gestational age
- **LGA (large for gestational age)**: above the ninetieth percentile for gestational age

SGA

Small for gestational age (SGA) infants are those whose weight places them below the 10th percentile for their gestational age. SGA is also called dysmaturity and intrauterine growth restriction. SGA babies commonly aspirate meconium and have a low APGAR score, asphyxia, hypoglycemia, and polycythemia. Common **causes of SGA** include:

- Multiple gestation (twins, triplets, quadruplets)
- Constitutional SGA because both parents are small
- Many genetic defects, such as trisomy 18 (Edwards syndrome), Down syndrome, and Turner syndrome
- Placental malfunction or misplacement (inadequate fetal nutrition from reduced blood flow, sepsis, placenta previa, or abruptio placentae)
- Maternal disease (pre-eclampsia; high blood pressure; malnutrition; advanced diabetes mellitus; chronic kidney, heart, or respiratory disease; and anemia)
- Infections such as cytomegalovirus, toxoplasmosis, and rubella
- Maternal tobacco, illegal drug, or alcohol use during pregnancy
- Birth defects

LGA

Large for gestational age (LGA) infants are those whose weight places them above the 90th percentile for their gestational age. The main pathologic cause for LGA is maternal diabetes (either gestational diabetes or diabetes mellitus). Infants exposed to elevated levels of glucose produce elevated amounts of insulin, which has an anabolic effect on the developing fetus, causing macrosomia (large body). Poor control of diabetes during pregnancy generally results in a larger infant with these **common health problems**:

- Delivery complications (shoulder dystocia, clavicle fracture, prolonged vaginal exit requiring use of forceps or Cesarian section, and perinatal asphyxia)
- Abnormal blood test results (hypoglycemia developing within 1-2 hours of birth, hyperbilirubinemia, hypocalcemia, hypomagnesemia, hyperviscosity [thickened blood] secondary to polycythemia [elevated hemoglobin])
- Jaundice
- Feeding intolerance
- Lethargy
- Respiratory distress
- Birth defects

Intrauterine Growth Restriction

When a fetus does not fulfill his or her growth potential for any reason, the diagnosis is **intrauterine growth restriction (IUGR)**. Prenatal ultrasound is used to diagnose IUGR, which is associated with oligohydramnios (decreased amniotic fluid) and preeclampsia (pregnancy-induced hypertension and proteinuria). IUGR is classified as symmetric or asymmetric, based on the size of the newborn's head:

- **Symmetric IUGR**
  - Both head and body are small (growth-restricted).
  - The restriction occurs early in pregnancy.
  - Common causes are chromosomal abnormalities and infections.
- **Asymmetric IUGR**
  - The head is large in proportion to the body; the head is spared.
  - The head is normal in size for gestational age, while the body is growth-restricted.
  - Restriction occurs late in pregnancy.
  - Common causes include placental insufficiency and preeclampsia.

Clinical Laboratory Tests

Capillary Blood Sampling

Neonatal capillary blood sampling is a common procedure used to acquire small samples of blood for testing of glucose and drug levels, blood gases, electrolytes, urea, blood counts, and other screening tests. If done incorrectly, it can cause pain, trauma, and nerve damage. The lancet should be ≥2.4 mm deep. The baby should be supine. The nurse grasps the foot with one hand holding the ankle with the thumb and index finger and supporting the leg with the other fingers. The infant's heel (bottom, lateral aspect only to avoid nerves in the middle of the foot) should be cleansed thoroughly with water (not alcohol) and air-dried. The skin of the heel should be held tense until after the puncture, and then it is relaxed and the heel lightly compressed to express a drop of blood, which is collected in a capillary tube. Relaxing the pressure and then compressing again will "milk" additional drops. Pressure is applied to the puncture site until bleeding stops and then a dressing is applied.

Microbiological Testing

Neonates with exposure to microbiological agents before, during, or after birth may require **microbiological testing:**

- Blood cultures are done to isolate causative agents in order to begin appropriate antibiotic treatment.
- In some cases, microbiological testing of expressed human milk may be indicated.
- Microscopic examination of urine and urine culture may be done to identify urinary pathogens.
- Stool cultures may be done to identify GI pathogens.
- Tracheal secretions may be cultured to identify pathogens causing pneumonia, especially in infants who are ventilated. The findings should be reviewed along with chest radiographs to ensure that positive findings don't just represent tracheal colonization alone.
- Gram stain and scraping of conjunctiva may be done to identify gonococcal conjunctivitis.
- Skin culture may be indicated for the infant with a skin infection.

Clinical Laboratory Urine Tests

Urine testing includes:

- **pH** should range from 4.5 to 9.0. An alkaline (high) pH can be caused by urinary tract infections, diarrhea, or kidney infection. An acidic (low) pH may reflect lung disease, hyperglycemia, or diarrhea with dehydration.
- **Specific gravity** ranges from 1.001 to 1.040 (usually about 1.015).

About 2% of full-term infants have asymptomatic bacteriuria, but this increases to about 10% for preterm infants. However, urinalysis alone is not an effective test to determine if an infant has a urinary tract infection because the neonate's urine usually contains leukocytes (≥25/mm^3 in males and ≥50/mm^3 in females), so urine cultures of infants younger than 3 days often show poor results, even in the presence of infection. Thus, blood cultures (and in some cases cultures of CSF) are preferred if infection is suspected, as neonates are more likely to develop kidney infections and sepsis from cystitis than older infants. The most common infective agent is *Escherichia coli* although *Candida* and *Staphylococcus* are common with prolonged hospitalization.

Serum Creatinine Levels and Renal Function

Serum creatinine is a marker of renal function. Creatinine is a byproduct of creatine phosphate metabolism in muscle. **Serum creatinine levels** reflect the balance between the production of creatinine and its clearance by the kidneys. Creatinine is filtered by the kidneys and generally not reabsorbed by the tubules, so it is a good indicator of the glomerular filtration rate (GFR). Elevated serum creatinine at birth may reflect elevated maternal levels, especially if the mother has toxemia. The serum creatinine level normally drops in the first few weeks of life. Premature infants often have a higher serum creatinine level and take longer to reach a normal level, because the GFR is lower in premature infants and immature kidneys allow creatinine to be reabsorbed across leaky tubules. Certain disease states (such as respiratory distress syndrome with mechanical ventilation) are associated with decreased GFR.

Clinical Laboratory Tests for ABGs

Arterial blood gases (ABGs) are monitored to assess the effectiveness of oxygenation, ventilation, and acid-base status and to determine oxygen flow rates. Partial pressure of a gas is that exerted by each gas in a mixture of gases, proportional to its concentration, based on total atmospheric pressure of 760 mmHg at sea level. Normal values for children include:

- Acidity/alkalinity (pH): 7.26-7.44
- Partial pressure of carbon dioxide ($PaCO_2$): 35-45 mmHg
- Partial pressure of oxygen (PaO_2): >80 mmHg
- Bicarbonate concentration (HCO_3^-): 22-28 mEq/L
- Oxygen saturation (SaO_2): >92%

The relationship between these elements, particularly the $PaCO_2$ and the PaO_2, indicates respiratory status. For example, $PaCO_2$ >55 and the PaO_2 <60 in an infant previously in good health indicates respiratory failure. There are many issues to consider. Ventilator management may require a higher $PaCO_2$ to prevent barotrauma and a lower PaO_2 to reduce oxygen toxicity. Premature infants may need lower PaO_2 to prevent retinopathy of prematurity.

Invasive Blood Gas Monitoring

Invasive blood gas monitoring options include the following:

- **Arterial blood gas (ABG)** is the most informative measurement of blood gas status. If an infant has an umbilical artery catheter, it is easily obtained by aspirating 1-2 mL of blood.
- **Venous blood gas (VBG)** is easier to obtain if an arterial catheter is not in place. In order to compare the values in the VBG with an ABG, make the following calculations:
    - Add 0.05 to the pH of the VBG.
    - Subtract 5-10 mmHg from the $PaCO_2$ of the VBG.
- **Capillary Blood Gas (CBG)** can be obtained with a heel stick, without a venous or arterial line, but the values obtained in a CBG are the least accurate and are rarely useful. The oxygen status of the neonate (reflected in the PaO_2) can be estimated by clinical evaluation of the neonate and a noninvasive pulse oximeter reading.

Review Video: Newborn Cord Blood Gases
Visit mometrix.com/academy and enter code: 188117

Clinical Laboratory Tests for Red Blood Cells

Red blood cells (RBCs or erythrocytes) are biconcave disks that contain hemoglobin, which carries oxygen throughout the body. The heme portion of the cell contains iron, which binds to the oxygen. RBCs live about 120 days in adults but this is reduced 20-25% in neonates and 50% in preterm infants. The RBCs are destroyed and their hemoglobin is recycled or excreted. **Normal values of red blood cell** count vary by age:

- Neonate: 4.1-6.1 million per mm^3
- 2-6 months: 3.8-5.6 million per mm^3

The most common disorders of RBCs are those that interfere with production, leading to various types of **anemia**:

- Blood loss
- Hemolysis
- Bone marrow failure

The **morphology** of RBCs may vary depending upon the type of anemia:

- Size: normocytes, microcytes, macrocytes
- Shape: spherocytes (round), poikilocytes (irregular), drepanocytes (sickled)
- Color (reflecting the concentration of hemoglobin): normochromic, hypochromic

Clinical Laboratory Tests for Hgb, Hct, MCV, Reticulocyte Count, and Platelets

Additional laboratory tests specific to red blood cells include the following:

- **Hemoglobin:** carries oxygen and is decreased in anemia and increased in polycythemia
    - Neonate: 14.5-22.5 g/dL
    - 2 months: 9.0-14.0 g/dL
- **Hematocrit:** indicates the proportion of RBCs in a liter of blood (usually about 3 times the hemoglobin number)
    - Neonate: 48-69%
    - 3 days: 44-75%
    - 2 months: 28-42%
- **Mean corpuscular volume (MCV):** indicates the size of RBCs and can differentiate types of anemia (For adults, <80 is microcytic and >100 is macrocytic, but this varies with age.)
    - Neonate: 95-121 μm^3
    - 0.5-2 years: 70-86 μm^3
- **Reticulocyte count:** measures marrow production and should rise with anemia
    - 0.5-1.5% of total RBCs
- **Platelets:** essential for clotting
    - 150,000-400,000
    - may increase to >1 million with iron deficiency anemia or decrease to <100,000 during acute infection

Clinical Laboratory Tests for WBCs

Leukocytes are white blood cells (WBCs). Normal total values vary according to age. The differential is the percentage of each type of WBC out of the total. The differential will shift with infection or allergies, but should return to normal values:

Item	Neonate	1 Day	2 Weeks	1 Month
WBCs (1000s/mm^3)	9.0-30.0	9.4-34.0	5.0-20.0	5.0-19.5.
Myelocytes	0%	0%	0%	0%
Neutrophils (Bands)	9.1%	9.2%	5.5%	4.5%
Neutrophils (Segs)	52%	52%	34%	30%
Lymphocytes	31%	31%	48%	56%
Monocytes	5.8%	5.8%	8.8%	6.5%
Eosinophils	2.2%	2.0%	3.1%	2.8%
Basophils	0.6%	0.5%	0.4%	0.5%

Clinical Laboratory Tests for Pituitary Hormones

The **anterior pituitary gland (adenohypophysis)** produces hormones that are critical for growth and development:

- **Growth hormone** (GH) promotes growth of bones and muscles and promotes protein synthesis and metabolism of fat but decreases carbohydrate metabolism. Normal values:
  - Cord blood: 8-40 µg/L
  - 1 day:5-50 µg/L
  - 1 week: 5-25 µg/L
- **Thyroid stimulating hormone** (TSH) stimulates secretion of thyroid hormones. Normal values:
  - 0-3 days: <20 mIU/L
- **Adrenocorticotropic hormone** (ACTH) stimulates the adrenal glands to produce glucocorticoids, androgens, and mineralocorticoids. Abnormalities can result in Cushing's disease or Addison's disease. Normal values:
  - Cord blood: 11-25 pmol/L
  - Neonate: 2-41 pmol/L

The **posterior pituitary gland (neurohypophysis)** stores hormones produced by the hypothalamus, critical to renal function. **Antidiuretic hormone (ADH)** controls the reabsorption of fluids in the kidney tubules. Changes in serum osmolality stimulate or depress ADH secretion, so values vary:

- Serum osmolality 270-280 mOsm/kg: ADH 0-1.4 pmol/L
- Serum osmolality 280-285 mOsm/kg: ADH 0.5-2.3 pmol/L
- Serum osmolality 285-290 mOsm/kg: ADH 0.9-4.6 pmol/L

Clinical Laboratory Tests for Thyroid Hormones

The **thyroid gland** produces hormones critical for metabolism and growth. They are amino acids that contain iodine and are stored in the thyroid until needed by the body. The thyroid gland takes iodide from the blood and utilizes it to produce hormones. Thyroid hormone production is controlled by the thyroid-stimulating hormone (TSH) produced by the pituitary gland and the thyrotropin-releasing hormone (TRH) produced by the hypothalamus. Together, the thyroid hormones increase metabolic rate and protein and bone turnover. They are necessary for the growth and development of the fetus and infant. Thyroid hormones include:

- **Thyroxine** (T_4) is a weak hormone that maintains the body's metabolism in a steady state.
    - Neonate: 10-36 pmol/L
- **Triiodothyronine** (T_3) is about 5 times stronger than thyroxine and can respond quickly to metabolic needs.
    - All ages: 4.0-7.4 pmol/L
- **Thyrocalcitonin** is secreted in response to serum calcium levels and reduces the serum level of calcium and phosphate by increasing deposits in bones, aiding ossification and bone development.
    - Male: <19 ng/L
    - Female: <14 ng/L

Clinical Laboratory Tests for Infants with HIV Positive Mothers

The immunological status of infants with **HIV-positive mothers** is assessed in a series of tests performed over the first two years in order to institute treatment and decrease likelihood of transmission to 2% or less.

ELISA and rapid tests are used to identify those neonates who are HIV-positive at birth. Confirmatory testing is done with the neonate's blood (not cord blood due to possibility of maternal contamination), usually using DNA PCR, which is about 99% sensitive by 1 month, but does NOT detect very recent infection (for instance, infection acquired during the birth). RNA PCR may be used for some subtypes of HIV infection.

In the United States, testing is based on identifying mothers with HIV. If the mother's status is not known, then some states require mandatory testing of the infant, but laws vary. Based on positive findings, treatment is begun within 24 hours without waiting for confirmatory test results. Subsequent testing is done at 2, 4, 12, and 18 months.

Newborn Care

Developmental Care

Developmental care is neonatal nursing that acknowledges environmental conditions and behavioral cues. Minimize noises and bright lights to decrease excessive stimuli. Observe the patient for cues regarding his or her feeding requirements and emotional state. The goal is to provide the optimum environment and treatment modalities that are the least stressful to the neonate, allowing for positive growth and development. Encourage parental involvement to foster attachment and competence in caring for the neonate. **Key components of developmental care** include:

- Observe, interpret, and respond to infant cues during care.
- Alter care based on neonatal developmental changes (e.g., the needs of a neonate at 26 weeks gestational age are different from those of one at 38 weeks gestational age).
- Time, pace, and handle the infant based on observed cues during care.
- Position infants based on their needs.
- Modify the environment based on the infant's needs.
- Foster parental participation in the care of their infant.

Neurobehavioral Development

Terms related to neurobehavioral development:

- **Habituation**: A decreasing response to repeated stimuli. For example, if a child is exposed to repeated sounds, the child will over time become used to the sound and show less reaction.
- **Motor organization**: Motor organization involves 3 different levels:
  - The spinal cord (which mediates automatic movement and reflexes)
  - The brain stem (which includes the medial descending systems that control body movement and antigravity reflexes and the lateral descending systems that control voluntary limb movements)
  - The cerebral cortex (which regulates movement)
- **State organization**: The brain has the ability to respond differently in different states or conditions, suggesting that the neonate's brain is active and not just passive.
- **Sensory/Interaction capabilities**: The ability to respond to stimuli and to interact with the environment and others. The interactions the neonate has after birth with others (dyadic interactions) help the child to learn patterns of interactions and responses.

Sleep States

Infants spend a high percentage of their time in **sleep states**. Sleep periods are divided into active sleep or quiet sleep by observing the infant's behavior:

- **Quiet sleep** is restorative and fosters anabolic growth. Quiet sleep is associated with increased cell mitosis and replication, lowered oxygen consumption, and the release of growth hormone. During quiet sleep, the infant appears relaxed, moves minimally, and breathes smoothly and regularly. The eyelids are still. The infant only responds to intense stimuli during quiet sleep.
- **Active sleep** is associated with processing and storing of information. Rapid eye movement (REM sleep) occurs during active sleep, but it is unknown if newborn infants are able to dream. During active sleep, the infant moves occasionally and breathes irregularly. Eye movements can be seen beneath the eyelids. Infants spend most of their sleep time in active sleep, and it usually precedes wakening.

Awake States

Infants have different levels of consciousness in the 4 **awake states**. Infants respond differently to outside stimuli and interaction from caregivers, depending on which state they are in:

- **Drowsy:** This is characterized by variable activity, mild startles, and smooth movement. There is some facial movement. Eyes open and close, breathing is irregular, and response to stimuli may be delayed.
- **Quiet alert:** The infant rarely moves, breathing is regular, and the infant focuses intently on individuals or objects that are within focal range, widening eyes. The face appears bright and alert, breathing is regular, and the infant focuses on stimuli.
- **Active alert:** The infant moves frequently and has much facial movement although the face not as bright and alert, eyes may have a dull glaze, breathing is irregular, and there are variable responses to outside stimuli.
- **Crying:** Characterized by grimacing, eyes shut, irregular breathing, increased movement with color changes and marked response to both internal and external stimuli.

Brazelton Neonatal Behavioral Assessment Scale

The Brazelton Neonatal Behavioral Assessment Scale is a multi-dimensional scale that is used to assess a neonate's state, temperament, and behavioral patterns. It includes the assessment of 18 reflexes, 28 behaviors, and 6 other characteristics. It is usually completed on day 3 with an attempt to elicit the most positive response, usually when the infant is comforted and in a quiet dim room. Scoring correlates to the child's awake or sleep state. Infants are scored according to response in many areas, including:

- **Habituation**: Ability to diminish response to repeat stimuli
- **Visual and auditory orientation**: Ability to respond to stimuli, fixate, and follow a visual object
- **Motor activity**: Assessment of body tone in various activities
- **Variations**: Changes in color, state, activity, alertness, and excitement during the exam
- **Self-quieting activities**: Frequency and speed of self-calming activities, such as sucking on their hand, putting their hand to mouth, and focusing on objects or sounds
- **Social behaviors**: Ability to cuddle, engage, and enjoy physical contact

Stress Responses

The neonate may exhibit a number of different stress responses:

- **Motoric responses:** Instead of normal and consistent muscle tone, the neonate may exhibit hypotonia with flaccid extremities and jaw. Some may exhibit hypertonicity with extremities hyperextended and/or hyperflexion of extremities. Some neonates may exhibit flailing, twitching, and tremors.
- **Attentional responses:** The neonate may react poorly to auditory, social, and visual stimuli and may exhibit poor sleeping, inability to be consoled, and staring or eye-roving behavior. The neonate may appear stressed and panicked or close eyes and withdraw.
- **Self-regulating/comforting responses:** The neonate may exhibit a number of behaviors to attempt to reduce stress. Motor activities may include grasping hands, moving hands toward the mouth, sucking, grasping blankets and tubing, moving about, and bracing feet against blankets or other barriers. The neonate may cry loudly and rhythmically to reduce stress and induce sleep. These tactics help the neonate to modulate responses to stimuli so that the newborn is not overwhelmed by the stress response.

Autonomic Stress Response

The autonomic nervous system is part of the peripheral nervous system and includes sympathetic nerves. The sympathetic nervous system (T1-L2 or L3) activates in times of stress and is implicated in pain. The nerves innervate deep structures, viscera, and skin. The autonomic nervous system mediates the body's organs and maintains homeostasis. When a neonate is stressed, the neonate typically responds by crying. Other signs of the **autonomic stress response** in the newborn include:

- **Change in skin color**: flushing, pallor, mottling rather than stable pink color
- **Respiratory changes**: when stable, respirations are regular and smooth; with stress, the neonate may exhibit gasping, sighing, apneic periods, and tachypnea
- **Cardiovascular changes**: heart rate and blood pressure increase
- **Visceral/GI response**: hiccups, gagging, coughing, vomiting, sneezing, passing flatus, choking, grunting

The caregiver must recognize the signs of stress, respond to the neonate's needs, and reduce stimuli. For example, a combination of stimuli, such as sound, lights, and touch, may overwhelm a newborn. Additionally, newborns may react to the stress of caregivers.

Stress Related to Light

Light is a necessary component of caring for both sick and healthy neonates in the delivery room and nursery. Adequate lighting is required to evaluate the at-risk neonate, to assess color, to complete procedures such as intubation, or to give medications. Light also discourages the growth of pathogens. However, constant bright light interferes with the development of natural diurnal rhythms because it arouses the central nervous system and stresses the infant. Controlling light helps to stabilize the infant. Some simple methods to protect the neonate from light over-stimulation and to establish a normal sleep cycle include:

- Reducing overhead light levels when direct visualization is not necessary
- Covering incubator hoods to reduce light entering the incubator
- Dimming the lights at night to help establish a natural day/night pattern (circadian rhythm)

Stress Related to Noise

Excessive **noise** causes agitation in all neonates, but especially in preterm neonates. The preterm neonate has less ability to self-calm, and over-stimulation results in decompensation, as demonstrated by increased oxygen requirements and increased apnea and bradycardia episodes. The American Academy of Pediatrics (AAP) recommends noise levels in the nursery and NICU be kept at **≤45 decibels**. A normal speaking voice is between 50-60 decibels. Noise levels above 80 decibels can damage the cochlea and cause hearing loss in adults. To keep noise acceptably low:

- Turn radios/TVs off or down.
- Designate a daily quiet time.
- Close incubator portholes gently, because closing a plastic porthole can spike the decibel level more than 80 dB.
- Whisper and, as much as possible, avoid speaking loudly.
- Remove bubbling water from ventilator tubing.
- Educate parents about the deleterious effects of over-stimulating their infant with loud noises.

Environmental Stressors and "Time Out"

Premature neonates have a very limited ability to deal with **environmental stressors,** but these stressors can affect all neonates. Signs of stress in neonates include:

- Color changes, such as mottling or cyanosis
- Episodes of apnea and bradycardia
- Activity changes, such as tremors, twitches, frantic activity, arching, and gaze-averting
- Flaccid posture (sagging trunk, extremities, and face)
- Easy fatigability

When the infant shows signs of stress, a **time-out** recovery period is indicated:

- Stop the activity causing the stress.
- Reduce unnecessary stimuli (e.g., lower the lights and postpone non-essential manipulation of the neonate).
- Give the neonate a chance to calm down or self-soothe.
- Bundle the neonate and place him/her in a comforting, side-lying position with the shoulders drawn forward and the hands brought to the midline.

Non-Nutritive Sucking

Non-nutritive sucking occurs when an infant sucks on an item such as a pacifier or his/her own fist. Non-nutritive sucking is not associated with nutritional intake, but it is an important method of self-quieting and begins in the uterus at about 29 weeks of gestation. Extremely premature infants often lack basic neurodevelopmental capabilities, and cannot coordinate sucking, swallowing, and breathing simultaneously. Typically, the ability to suck and swallow in a coordinated fashion is not present until 32-34 weeks of gestation. Premature infants should be encouraged to perform non-nutritive sucking during the gavage feeding process if they can accomplish it. Benefits of non-nutritive sucking include:

- Improved digestion of enteral feeds because digestive enzyme release is stimulated
- Facilitated development of coordinated nutritive sucking behavior
- Calming of the distressed infant

Positioning of the Premature Neonate

Correct positioning of the premature neonate minimizes outside stimuli and mimics the enclosed and calming environment of the womb, helping with the transition to extrauterine life:

- Place the neonate in a flexed position, with his hands close to midline and near his face.
- Create a nest of blankets or pillows to:
    - Help block out light and noise.
    - Give him the impression of a closed environment.
    - Minimize abnormal molding of the head from prolonged pressure on one side.
- Cover the incubator to further keep out sound and light.
- Place the neonate in the prone position (on his stomach) to help to stabilize the chest wall, improve ventilation, and increase the amount of time the infant is in quiet sleep. However, infants should be placed supine (on the back) most of the time, to decrease the chance of SIDS.

Clustering Care

The concept of clustering care for the premature neonate centers on allowing the neonate to have prolonged periods of rest or sleep in between required care procedures and manipulations. Long periods of rest and quiet simulate the uninterrupted and fairly constant environment of the womb. Clustering care means performing multiple tasks at the same time, such as feeding, bathing, wound care, drawing laboratory samples, or examining the infant. However, the premature infant may not be able to tolerate multiple manipulations and may show signs of decompensation before all the planned procedures are completed. The premature infant may need a time-out period to recover before performing more stressful procedures. Balance clustering care with observing the infant for cues of stress.

Provision of Sensory Experiences

While sensory interventions are important for neurobehavioral development, preterm neonates or those who are seriously ill may be able to tolerate only one or two types of sensory interventions, so each neonate must be assessed individually and carefully observed for signs of stress. **Sensory experiences** that benefit the neonate can include:

- **Auditory**: Talking to the neonates in a calm and soothing high-pitched tone of voice or providing toys that produce soft or low sounds (such as music) may be used, but loud or sudden noises should be avoided.
- **Tactile**: Gently massaging the neonate, starting from the head down to the extremities, abdomen, and back as the neonate can tolerate is highly beneficial for the neonate; however, light touch should be avoided. Neonatal hand-to-mouth activity should be encouraged.
- **Visual**: Keeping eye contact with the child during all interactions, providing other visual items (mirrors, bright red item, mobiles), and keeping lights low benefits the infant's visual development.
- **Vestibular** (middle ear/brain) **and proprioceptive** (position): Swaddling (legs flexed and hands near mouth), holding, and slowly rocking the neonate back and forth for at least 5 minutes benefits the neonate.

Family Education

Educational Needs of New Mothers

The educational needs of the new mother and family vary depending on age, background, education, experience, and expectations. The needs of the adolescent mother with no experience may be quite different from those of the multiparous mother. Assessing individual needs can be difficult in the short time women are usually hospitalized, so education should cover a wide range of topics. A checklist of topics may be a helpful starting point for the mother to indicate her needs. Because mothers are usually fatigued for the first 24-48 hours, teaching after that time is most effective, but many mothers leave the hospital on the second day. Demonstration with return demonstration is an effective method to ensure that a mother can carry out tasks, but education should anticipate other needs and concerns that may arise. Mothers often have concerns about a variety of issues, such as childcare, contraception, and resuming sexual relations. Pamphlets, website information, or videos that can be sent home with the mother are very helpful.

Safe Positioning for Infants

Infants should be placed on their **backs** for sleeping. Sleeping on the stomach increases the risk of **sudden infant death syndrome (SIDS)**.

- Position the infant on the back when unattended or sleeping, but alternate the direction the head faces to prevent one side of the head from flattening (**positional molding**).
- Provide supervised time each day with the infant lying on the abdomen (only on firm surfaces) to strengthen head and neck muscles and to prevent positional molding.
- Hold the infant, rather than leaving them in a carrier.
- Position baby in side-lying position, alternating from one side to the other, using specially designed supports to maintain the position.

Infant Car Seat

All infants, regardless of age, must be placed properly in an infant car seat during transit. Holding an infant while the car is in motion is not safe. Car seats should be new or in very good condition and fastened according to the manufacturer's guidelines to ensure safety.

- Place the car seat in the back seat and away from any side airbags.
- Always securely buckle the child into the seat.
- Face the infant seat toward the rear of the car.
- Recline the seat so the infant's head does not fall forward.
- Place padding around (not under) the infant if the infant slouches to one side.
- Place blankets over the straps and buckles, not under.

Umbilical Cord Care

Education surrounding the umbilical cord should include the following information:

- Protect the cord from moisture, with top of diaper folded under the cord instead of covering it.
- If the cord becomes soiled, wash with mild soap and water, rinse, and dry. Swabbing with alcohol is no longer recommended and may increase skin irritation.
- Avoid covering the cord stump with clothing, which may cause irritation.
- Give the infant only sponge baths until the cord falls off in about 10-14 days.
- Report signs of infection, such as erythema, swelling, or purulent discharge.

Note: The umbilical cord changes color from grayish-brown to black as it dries and finally falls off.

Fecal Elimination

The first stool (**meconium**) is usually passed within 24 hours and is black and tarry looking. The stool then transitions to greenish as the baby nurses or takes formula, and by the third day, the stool is usually yellow or yellow-green for breastfed babies and yellow or light brown for formula-fed babies. Typically, babies have 2-3 stools daily by day 3 and ≥4 daily by day 5, but this may vary.

- Report abnormalities, such as bloody stools, watery stools, very hard stools, clay-colored or whitish stools, black stools (after meconium has passed), and "currant jelly" stools.
- Cleanse skin thoroughly after defecation with mild soap and water, plain water, or unscented baby wipes.
- Examine skin carefully for irritation.

Urinary Elimination

Urination is estimated according to the number of **wet diapers** in a 24-hour period. Typically, the infant has 1 wet diaper the first day, 2 the next, and so on until urination stabilizes at 6-8 wet diapers by about day 6.

- Check diaper frequently. Infants often urinate during or after feeding.
- Change diapers when wet, gently cleansing skin with mild soap and water, plain water, or unscented baby wipes.

Cradle Cap

Cradle cap may appear as scaly, crusted, or flaky skin on the scalp and other parts of the face. It is not contagious and usually clears by 1 or 2 months. It is not usually a sign of poor hygiene.

- Cleanse scalp or affected areas thoroughly, gently rubbing the area with a terry cloth or brushing to loosen crust or flakes.
- If persistent, try softening the crusts with olive oil. Leave it in for 15 minutes, and then brush or gently comb to loosen crusts or flakes. Finally, wash with baby shampoo.

Diaper Rash

Diaper rash usually results from leaving the infant in soiled/wet diapers and/or not adequately cleansing the skin, although breastfed infants sometimes react to foods the mother has eaten. A rash may also indicate an allergic response to baby wipes or other products, such as lotions or creams. Antibiotics may cause diaper rash. In some cases, a **fungal infection** may occur, usually characterized by red, weepy open areas. Purulent discharge may indicate infection.

- Change diapers as soon as possible when wet or soiled.
- Cleanse skin gently with water.
- Remove diaper and expose skin to air whenever possible.
- Apply barrier cream or ointment especially formulated for diaper rash to prevent or treat diaper rash.
- Contact physician if rash worsens and does not respond to treatment, as antifungals, cortisone, or topical antibiotics may be indicated.

Choking or Gagging in Infant

Education regarding chocking/gagging should include the following:

- Ensure small hazardous items, such as pins and cotton balls or materials, such as baby powder are out of reach.
- DO NOT prop bottle for feeding.
- Burp infant regularly during feedings, whether breast or bottle.
- Keep baby in upright position with head elevated during feedings.
- Check nipple of bottle to ensure it is dripping and not running freely.
- If the infant is choking, secure face down on forearm, tilted downward, and use the heel of the hand to thump on the mid-back. Repeat as necessary. If choking does not resolve with evidence of breathing immediately, call 911 and begin CPR.

Note: Prevention is important, as most **choking and gagging episodes** can be avoided.

Burping the Infant

Both breastfed and bottle-fed babies require **burping** because they swallow air when feeding, although bottle-fed babies tend to require more burping. Infants often show indications (grimacing, squirming, spitting up, and crying) that they are uncomfortable and need to burp.

- Burp the infant routinely after 2 or 3 ounces of formula or after nursing on one breast.
- Position the infant on the shoulder with a burp cloth under the infant's head and gently pat or rub the infant's back.
- Change to a different position if the baby doesn't burp. Try on the opposite shoulder or with the infant sitting on the lap supported by one hand while the other hand pats or rubs the infant's back.

Bathing the Infant

The infant should receive **sponge baths** until the umbilical cord falls off at 10-14 days, and then a bath in an **infant tub** (NOT in an adult tub). Mild soap/shampoo intended for babies or water alone may be used for the bath.

- Make sure the environmental temperature is warm.
- Fill tub with 2-3 inches of water.
- ALWAYS check water temperature to make sure it is warm and NOT hot.
- Set water heaters ≤120 °F to prevent inadvertent scalding.
- Support the baby during the bath with one arm under upper back to support the neck and head while holding the infant under the axillae.
- Pour water over the child with the free hand and use that hand to wash the hair and the body.
- Lift the baby from the tub and wrap in a towel to dry.
- Dry thoroughly, making sure all skin folds and crevices are dry to prevent irritation and rashes.
- Avoid use of lotions or creams.

Fontanels

The infant's fontanels (anterior and posterior) are covered by thick membranous tissue and should feel flat but firm.

- Do not be afraid to touch the fontanels or cleanse the scalp.
- Report **bulging** above the level of the skull, as this may indicate increased intracranial pressure.
- Report a **soft fontanel** that sinks below the level of the skull, as this may indicate dehydration.

Circumcision

Circumcision rates have dropped by 10% over the last 30 years, with about 58% of male infants now being **circumcised** in the United States. The American Academy of Pediatrics has confirmed that the benefits outweigh the risks, though they do not have a formal recommendation for circumcision and instead leave that decision up to the parents. Benefits including decreased risk of prostate cancer, urinary tract infections, and sexually transmitted infections such as HIV. Most parents make their decision based on cultural or religious beliefs or the factor of cost, as some insurance companies and many Medicaid programs do not cover the cost of circumcision. While at one time infants were not thought to experience pain, it is now clear that they do, so circumcision should be done using a local anesthesia or topical EMLA cream.

Post-Circumcision Care

After circumcision, the end of the foreskin is typically swollen and red, and a small amount of bleeding may persist for 24 hours.

- Change the diaper immediately, because urine may cause pain to the open tissue.
- Cleanse the area gently with water and pat dry.
- Apply petroleum jelly gauze to the incision area as directed by the individual physician.
- Avoid using soap or commercial cleansing products, such as baby wipes, until the circumcision heals.
- Report any change, such as increased swelling, redness, temperature, or purulent discharge.

Care of the Uncircumcised Penis

The infant's foreskin is different from that of the adult male. It does not **separate and retract** until the child is around 5 years old.

- Do NOT attempt to retract the foreskin.
- Do NOT use cotton swabs to clean.
- Wash the penis with soap and water or just water during the routine bath.

Shaken Baby Syndrome

Shaken baby syndrome is believed to be the result of vigorous shaking of a neonate, causing acute subdural hematoma with subarachnoid, and retinal hemorrhages. The shaking of the brain may damage vessels and nerves with resultant cerebral edema. Parents should be advised of the importance of always supporting and protecting the neonate's head and avoiding activities that may injure the child, such as throwing and catching a neonate or small child. Parents should be advised that sometimes children may not exhibit obvious neurological symptoms immediately after trauma but have learning disabilities and behavioral disorders that appear in school.

Neonatal CPR

Most cardiac arrests in newborns are associated with respiratory arrest rather than cardiac arrest, so **cardiopulmonary resuscitation** of newborns follows the ABC protocol rather than the compressions only protocol used for adults. The parent should be advised to take a CPR course, especially if the neonate is at risk and if arrest occurs, immediately call 911 for help or ask someone else to call and begin CPR:

- **Airway:** Tilt the head slightly back and lift the chin to open the airway.
- **Breathing:** If the neonate does not begin breathing, administer 2 puffs to ventilate the lungs. For small neonates, place the mouth to cover the neonate's nose and mouth and ventilate each time for approximately one second, observing the chest to ensure it is rising. For the infant with a heart rate ≥60/minute without normal breathing, administer one breath every 2-3 seconds (20-30 breaths per minute).
- **Compressions:** Infants that require chest compressions should receive two breaths per 30 compressions (30:2) for a single rescuer, and two breaths per 15 compressions for two rescuers (15:2). The chest should be depressed approximately 1.5 inches, using two fingers or two thumbs while encircling the hands around the baby's body. The optimum rate of compressions is approximately 100-120 per minute.

Commonly Used Medications

Principles of Drug Administration to Neonates

Dosage and Interval

The half-life of a drug ($t_{½}$) is the time required to reduce serum concentrations by half, and half-life must be considered when determining **dosage and interval** of drugs for neonates. Steady state is usually achieved within 4-5 half-lives. Half-life is a factor of clearance, and small or preterm infants often have reduced clearance because of slow metabolism, resulting in longer half-life. In determining dosage, the infant's weight, gestational age, and post-natal age must be considered.

One major problem with dosing and interval for neonates is that most drugs are not tested on infants, so about 98% are prescribed off-label. There are a number of reference tools available, including software programs, to assist with determining proper dosage and interval for neonatal medications.

Neonatal Tolerance and Weaning

Tolerance and weaning from drugs are often concerns with the administration of opiates. **Tolerance** occurs after repeated administration results in a lessening of effects, requiring an increase in dosage to achieve the same results. When a neonate is weaned from a medication or a dosage is decreased, only one class of medications should be involved. Thus, if the infant is receiving both an opiate and a benzodiazepine, they should not be weaned from both at the same time. The infant should be evaluated for level of pain prior to weaning and reassessed at least every 4 hours during the weaning process. Usually medications are reduced at a rate of 10% per day or 20% every other day. Infants often tolerate an initial reduction in dose better than subsequent reductions, so careful observation for signs of increased pain or withdrawal must be made. Careful control of the environment—temperature, light, and noise—should be done to reduce infant stress during the **weaning process**.

Principles of Neonatal Absorption

Principles of neonatal absorption can be discussed specific to various elements of the process of absorption:

- **GI tract**: Medications may have increased or decreased rates of absorption depending on the rate of gastric emptying, the acidity of the GI tract, the availability of pancreatic or other enzymes, the presence of intestinal bacteria, and GI perfusion as well as disease processes, such as vomiting or diarrhea, and medical procedures, such as GI suctioning.
- **Skin/muscle**: Skin maturation occurs between 23 and 33 weeks of gestation and continues to mature in the weeks after birth. The neonate's skin is thinner and more readily absorbs topical preparations because of increased permeability. Muscle is thinner and generally has less perfusion, so absorption may be slow in the premature or seriously ill neonate, but if perfusion increases, the faster absorption of retained medication may result in overdose.
- **Blood drug levels**: Medications are absorbed immediately but distribution to some organs may vary, and therapeutic levels must be monitored carefully as toxic concentrations may occur if medication administered by IV push or over a short period. Dosage and concentration may be inconsistent because clearance is prolonged.
- **Drug incompatibilities**: Occur when two drugs undergo a reaction when combined that results in the deterioration of one or both of the drugs and can result in inadequate therapeutic effect. Parenteral drugs/solutions may appear cloudy or develop precipitates. The greater the number of drugs administered, the greater the risk of incompatibilities.
- **Drug withdrawal** (therapeutic drugs): Withdrawal protocols vary according to the medication. Some medications, such as some heart medications, must be withdrawn slowly in decreasing doses to avoid a negative response while others can be stopped abruptly. Because clearance may be slowed, the effects of the drug may continue after the medication has been discontinued, so this must be considered when changing medications.
- **Drug resistance**: Ineffectiveness of a drug to treat an infection or condition. For example, some forms of *Staphylococcus* are resistant to vancomycin because of antimicrobial resistance.

Protein Binding in Neonatal Drug Therapy

Protein binding is an important consideration for neonatal drug therapy because when drugs are bound by proteins in the blood, they are not available to be biologically active. The portion of the drug that is **not** bound to a plasma protein is the active portion. **Protein binding** is significant in premature neonates because they typically have:

- Lower levels of plasma proteins, such as albumin.
- Lower binding capacity.
- Susceptibility to competition from endogenous substances like bilirubin, which also attaches to plasma proteins.

Drugs that are normally highly protein bound in the adult have a higher free percentage (activity) in the neonate. Lower than expected dosages may give clinical results. Examples of drugs that are highly protein bound include phenobarbital and indomethacin. If a drug with a high affinity for plasma proteins is administered, it may displace bilirubin from binding sites, increasing the neonate's risk for kernicterus.

Placental Transfer of Drugs

The **placenta** acts as a barrier to protect the fetus, but its main function is to provide oxygen and nutrients for the fetus by linking the maternal and fetal circulation. Virtually all **drugs** cross the barrier to some degree, some by active transport. Some drugs are readily diffused across the placental barrier and can affect the fetus. Drugs that are non-ionized, fat-soluble and have low molecular weight diffuse easily as glucose does. Once a substance crosses the barrier, the lower pH of the fetal blood allows weakly basic drugs, such as local anesthetics and opioids, to cross into fetal circulation where they become ionized and accumulate because they can't pass back into maternal circulation (ion trapping). Giving an intravenous injection during a contraction, when uterine blood flow decreases, reduces the amount of the drug that crosses the placental barrier. A few drugs with large molecules (heparin, insulin) have minimal transfer, and lipid soluble drugs transfer more readily than water-soluble.

Surfactants

Surfactants reduce surface tension to prevent collapse of alveoli. Beractant (Survanta) is derived from bovine lung tissue and calfactant (Infasurf) from calf lung tissue. Surfactant replacement therapy is used to prevent RDS for infants born at 27-30 weeks gestation. It is also used for infants showing signs of worsening lung disease. Surfactant has traditionally been given via the endotracheal tube (ETT) as an inhalant, but with advancing efforts to reduce mechanical ventilation in the context of RDS, other routes of administration are being considered, including minimally invasive surfactant therapy (MIST) through a thin catheter in the trachea while being oxygenated throug noninvasive means, or via nebulizer through a laryngeal mask. Both endoctracheal and MIST approaches have different protocol for determining the need of secondary doses, and facility policy for surfactant therapy should be followed closely.

Steroids

Steroids are commonly administered to mothers to promote fetal lung development for preterm births. These drugs include betamethasone and dexamethasone. Steroids may also be administered to the neonate, but they are associated with significant side effects:

- **Betamethasone** may be used for chronic lung disease (CLD) in the neonate and post-intubation airway edema, but high dose treatment has been associated with cerebral palsy, growth depression, hypertension, hyperglycemia, hypokalemia, and increased risk of infection. Airway edema is treated with 200 mcg/kg orally or IV every 8 hours beginning 4 hours before extubation. Dosages for other treatment vary widely with tapering of doses.
- **Hydrocortisone** may be used for physiologic replacement or acute hypotension. Replacement is begun with 1-2 mg orally every 8 hours and increased to 6-9 mg/m2/day. Hypotension is treated with 2 mg/kg IV loading dose and maintenance of 1 mg/kg IV every 8-12 hours.

VITAMIN K

Vitamin K deficiency in newborns may cause vitamin K deficiency bleeding (VKDB), also called **hemorrhagic disease of the newborn**. Vitamin K is a fat-soluble vitamin produced in the gut. Vitamin K is required by the liver to produce four of the clotting factors—II, VII, IX, and X. At birth, all infants are Vitamin K deficient because of limited transfer of vitamin K across the placenta. Newborns are injected with one intramuscular (IM) dose of vitamin K (AquaMEPHYTON), 0.5-1.0 mg within six hours of birth. The injection quickly raises the infant's vitamin K level to normal and maintains the normal level for several months. Vitamin K should be given prior to circumcision. Infants who do not receive vitamin K prophylaxis at birth will take several weeks (formula-fed) to several months (breastfed) to attain normal vitamin K levels. Formula contains higher levels of vitamin K than human breast milk. VKDB occurs in two forms:

- **Early-onset form** occurs within the first 24 hours after birth and is related to maternal medications that interfere with Vitamin K.
- **Late-onset form** occurs after two weeks of age, because of exclusive breastfeeding, diarrhea, hepatitis, cystic fibrosis, alpha 1-antitrypsin disease, or celiac disease.

NEONATAL ANALGESICS

SUCROSE ANALGESIA

Sucrose analgesia (Sweet-Ease) is used to relieve stress and discomfort in infants before and during medical procedures, such as heel sticks, IV insertion, injections, suctioning, and insertion of NG tubes. Sweet-Ease, a commercially prepared product, is 24% sucrose in an oral solution into which a standard pacifier is dipped and given to the infant, usually 2 minutes before a procedure. The pacifier may be re-dipped every 2 minutes for a total of 4 times. If the infant cannot suck, 0.1 mL of solution is placed on the anterior tongue with a medical syringe with the same frequency. For more painful procedures, such as lumbar puncture and circumcision, sucrose analgesia may be used in conjunction with other forms of analgesia to provide comfort. Contraindications include <32 weeks gestation, hyperglycemia, history of asphyxia or intolerance to feedings, critical illness, paralysis, opioid sedation, and infants NPO for surgery unless cleared by an anesthesiologist.

ACETAMINOPHEN

Acetaminophen (Tylenol) is used both for control of mild to moderate pain and fever. Acetaminophen can be administered orally and rectally, but absorption is less reliable with the rectal route. Acetaminophen has a half-life of 4 hours, is conjugated in the liver, and is excreted through the kidneys. **Oral dosage** is typically 24 mg/kg as a loading dose and 12 mg/kg every four hours (or 8 hours in infants <32 weeks); **rectal dosage** is 36 mg/kg (loading), followed by 24 mg/kg every 8 hours. Serum levels should be checked if treatment is to continue for >24 hours. Serum levels of 12-24 mg/L are required for adequate pain control. Acetaminophen is commonly used for control of pain after **circumcision**, although it is not sufficient for pain control during the procedure.

Fentanyl and Morphine

Fentanyl and morphine are opioid analgesics/narcotics that treat moderate-to-severe pain:

- **Fentanyl** is for painful dressing changes or procedures. Duration of action is 1-2 hours and half-life is 2-4 hours. Dosage is 1-4 mcg/kg every 1-2 hours or by continuous infusion. Rapid tolerance develops, requiring higher doses to create the same relief, and increasing the chance of overdose. Fentanyl is metabolized by the liver and excreted by the kidneys. *Side* effects of fentanyl include respiratory depression, peripheral vasodilatation, inhibition of intestinal peristalsis, and chest wall rigidity at higher doses, which compromises ventilation. Fentanyl is less likely to cause hypotension than morphine.
- **Morphine** is for postoperative pain. Duration of action is 3-4 hours, and half-life is 2-4 hours. Morphine is metabolized by the liver to an inactive metabolite and excreted by the kidneys; 2-12% is excreted unchanged in the urine. Dosage is 0.02-0.10 mg/kg every 1-4 hours or by continuous infusion. Side effects of morphine include respiratory depression, histamine release, and seizures.

Resuscitation and Stabilization

Minimum Neonatal Resuscitation Equipment

The minimal equipment that should be present for neonatal resuscitation includes the following:

- **Temperature**: Thermometer, warmed drying towels, warmed swaddling blankets, radiant warmer, phototherapy equipment.
- **Respiration**: Oxygen tank and hood, flow meter, humidifier, heater, tubing, nasal prongs. Bag and mask set-up (assorted sizes). Laryngoscope with size 0 and 1 blades. Endotracheal tubes, sizes 2.5-4. Bulb syringe, suction catheters (sizes 6, 8, and 10 Fr.), suction canister. Cardiorespiratory monitor, oxygen analyzer.
- **Fluids**: IV needles and tubing, infusion pump, umbilical catheters (sizes 2.5 and 5 Fr.). Blood pressure monitor, pulse oximeter. Isotonic saline, D10W, sodium bicarbonate. If transfusions are done here, blood drainage system, volume expander, and blood warmer.
- **Drugs**: Epinephrine, Naloxone.
- **Procedures**: Various sterile surgical packs, dressings, chest tubes, scalpels, hemostat. Arterial blood gas equipment and portable x-ray machine.

ABCs of Neonatal Resuscitation

The ABCs of resuscitation are a device to help remember in what order to do the steps of the resuscitation process. In this device, the letters stand for the following:

- **Airway**: An airway should be established as the very first thing to tend to. If there is no airway, air cannot be moved during resuscitation attempts. This step includes clearing the mouth and nose of secretions and properly positioning the infant in the "sniff" position.
- **Breathing**: This step involves initiating breathing after the airway has been established. This can be done with stimulation, supplemental oxygen, or through artificial ventilation. Oxygen should be initiated at 21% (up to 30% in preterm neonates) and titrated as needed.
- **Circulation**: Once an airway is open and breathing has been established, then circulation is considered. Chest compressions or the administration of volume expanders may be indicated. Epinephrine is only indicated if the heart rate remains <60 despite warming, ventilation, and chest compressions.

Establishing Airway and Stimulating Respirations

To **establish an airway**, the infant is placed supine with the head slightly extended in the "sniffing" position. A small neck roll may be placed under the shoulders to maintain this position in a very small premature infant. Once the proper position is established, the mouth and nose are suctioned (mouth first, to prevent reflex aspiration of secretions when the nose is suctioned) with a bulb syringe or catheter if necessary. The infant's head can be turned momentarily to the side to allow secretions to pool in the cheek where they can be more easily suctioned and removed to establish the airway. **Stimulating** the newborn is often all that is needed to initiate spontaneous respirations. This tactile stimulation can be accomplished by gently rubbing the infant's back or trunk. Another technique used to provide stimulation is flicking or rubbing the soles of the feet. Slapping neonates as stimulation is no longer practiced and should NOT be used.

Administration of Free-Flow Oxygen

If an infant remains cyanotic in the chest area (central cyanosis) after the initial steps of resuscitation have taken place, administering **free-flow oxygen** is the next step to take. Free-flow oxygen is administered to the neonate by the use of either a mask hooked up to an oxygen source or by the use of the oxygen tubing itself. If the tubing alone is used, the nurse can hold the tube with a cupped hand to help direct and concentrate the oxygen at the infant's airway. Free flow oxygen should be administered at a rate of 5 L/minute, initiated at 21% (up to 30% in preterm neonates). If the infant starts to turn pink, the oxygen can be carefully and slowly removed while continuing to closely monitor the infant for returning cyanosis. If the infant remains centrally cyanotic after the administration of free-flow oxygen, bag and mask ventilation must be considered as the next step.

Bag and Mask Ventilation

Ventilation using a bag and mask is indicated when one or more of the following occurs and has not responded to other resuscitation attempts:

- Apnea that does not respond to tactile stimulation such as rubbing the chest or back or flicking the soles of the feet
- Gasping respirations
- Heart rate of <100 bpm, determined by auscultation at the apex of the heart or palpation of the base of the umbilical cord
- Central cyanosis that persists after administering free-flow oxygen (Acrocyanosis alone is NOT an indication for the need for further oxygenation or ventilation.)

The flowmeter is set at 5-10 L/min, and opening breath pressures of 30-40 cmH_2O are used for full term infants and 20-25 cmH_2O for preterm. Ventilation is done at 40-60 breaths/min with pressure of 15-20 cmH_2O for normal lungs and 20-50 cmH_2O for immature or compromised lungs.

Flow-Inflating Bag and Mask Ventilation

Bag and mask ventilation is indicated for persistent apnea or gasping respirations, bradycardia (<100 bpm), and persistent cyanosis unrelieved by free-flowing oxygen.

Flow-inflating bag and mask (connected to oxygen flow, which inflates bag) equipment includes:

- Oxygen inlet
- Flow control valve
- Pressure manometer attachment
- Patient outlet for mask attachment

Advantages: Flow-inflating bag and mask ventilation has the ability to deliver anywhere from 21% (room air) to 100% oxygen; any pressure desired can be set. This type of bag and mask also has the ability to maintain positive end-expiratory pressure (PEEP) and CPAP.

Disadvantages: Because this bag must be connected to a gas (oxygen) source to inflate, it can only be used where a gas supply exists. It requires some experience to deliver the desired quantity of air with each breath. The high pressures possible with this type of equipment make overinflation of the lungs possible, resulting in pneumothorax. A complete seal is necessary to deliver a tidal volume.

Self-Inflating Bag and Mask Ventilation

Self-inflating bag and mask (does not require gas source) equipment includes:

- Air inlet
- Oxygen inlet
- Patient outlet for mask attachment
- Valve assembly
- Oxygen reservoir
- Pop-off valve
- Pressure manometer attachment

Advantages: Self-inflating bag and mask ventilation is simple to use and does not require much practice or experience to operate. It can be operated anywhere, even if no oxygen source is near, and can easily deliver a tidal volume.

Disadvantages: These bags usually have a pop-off valve that will open at a pressure set by the manufacturer to prevent over inflation of the lungs. This valve popping off can prevent the ability to deliver enough pressure to ventilate very noncompliant lungs. Another disadvantage is that if 90% or higher oxygen delivery is desired, this equipment must have a reservoir attached to deliver this concentration. The inability to deliver PEEP is also a disadvantage to the self-inflating bag and mask.

Gastric Suctioning Following Neonatal Resuscitation

When an infant is resuscitated using a bag and mask, air is inadvertently pumped into the stomach as it is being pumped into the lungs, so **gastric suctioning** is necessary. Once respirations have been stabilized, either spontaneously or with mechanical ventilation, the stomach should be aspirated to remove any air pumped into it. If the air is left in the abdomen, it remains distended, causing an upward pressure on the lungs; this compromises lung capacity and breathing effort. Use this procedure:

1. Select an orogastric catheter or size 8 Fr. feeding tube.
2. Measure the distance from the nose to the earlobe, then to the xiphoid.
3. Mark the tube at this distance.
4. Advance the tube to the mark.
5. Attach a 20 mL syringe to the tube.
6. Aspirate the contents of the stomach.
7. Leave the tube in place, open to air, and taped to the infant's cheek to keep the stomach decompressed.

Chest Compressions

If **chest compressions** are indicated for resuscitation, these steps should be followed.

1. Position the neonate in the "sniffing" position with the neck slightly extended.
2. Make sure there is firm support for the infant's back.
3. Using a two-finger technique, proceed with the compressions on the lower third of the sternum with a depth of one third of the anterior-posterior diameter of the chest. The compression rate is 90 compressions per minute and 30 breaths per minute, equaling 120 "events" per minute. Essentially, one cycle is 3 compressions and 1 breath every 2 seconds.
4. When performing the compressions, the hands should be placed in a circle around the chest to provide support to the infant's back. The ratio of compressions to breaths should be 3:1.
5. Check the heart rate again after 30 seconds of compressions—about 45 compressions total.
6. If the heart rate is less than 60 beats per minute, continue with another round of compressions, but if the rate is 60 beats per minute or higher, stop compressions.

During chest compressions, oxygen should be delivered at a concentration of 100%.

Indications for Stopping or Not Providing Resuscitation to Newborn

The decision to **discontinue or not perform resuscitative efforts** in the newborn (DNR) is very difficult to make. Whenever possible, the decision to withhold or stop resuscitative efforts in the newborn should be made by the attending physician with parental input, especially in situations with variable degrees of morbidity and mortality. Infants born under these conditions associated with certain death should not be resuscitated:

- Extreme prematurity (less than 23 weeks gestation)
- Extremely low birth weight (less than 400 grams)
- Congenital anomalies that are incompatible with life (anencephaly, trisomy 13 or 18)

Discontinue resuscitation of the infant who has not responded to appropriate resuscitation for 10 minutes and shows no signs of life (no heart rate or respiratory effort).

Resuscitation Medications

Epinephrine

Epinephrine is a naturally-occurring hormone produced by the adrenal glands. Epinephrine is used to resuscitate both adults and children. It is a sympathomimetic that supports the circulatory system by:

- Increasing heart rate
- Increasing contraction strength
- Vasoconstricting vessels in the skin, mucosa, and circulation of the gastrointestinal tract, causing a rise in blood pressure

If positive pressure ventilation and chest compressions have not caused the neonate's heart rate to rise above 60 beats per minute during resuscitation, then epinephrine is indicated. The recommended IV dose is 0.01-0.03 mg/kg. The usual concentration of epinephrine is 1:10,000 or 0.1 mg/mL. Endotracheal administration is not widely recommended, but may be used if no IV access is available. Higher doses are required for endotracheal administration (0.05-0.1 mg/kg).

Volume Expanders

Volume expanders used in neonatal resuscitation include:

- Normal saline
- Ringer's Lactate
- O- blood, or blood that has been crossmatched with the mother

Prepare 40 mL in a syringe or IV. Give 10 mL/kg over 5-10 minutes. Repeat if necessary. Rapid infusion of a large volume causes intraventricular hemorrhage. (5% albumin in saline is no longer the solution of choice.) Consider volume expanders in instances where neonatal blood loss is suspected and/or the neonate is showing signs of shock that is not responding to other resuscitative efforts. Blood loss occurs due to trauma of the placenta or umbilical cord, or with neonatal hemolysis. Shock is inadequate perfusion in tissues and organs. Signs and symptoms of shock are pallor, cold extremities, neurological depression, and weak pulse.

Naloxone Hydrochloride

Naloxone hydrochloride, an opiate antagonist, is not used in the routine resuscitation of an infant but is used in one very specific situation following birth. Naloxone is considered the antidote for narcotics administered to the mother of the infant within 4 hours of birth if the infant shows signs of serious respiratory depression from secondary absorption. If the mother of the infant has narcotics in her system as a result of an addiction to narcotics rather than as treatment for labor pain, however, naloxone cannot be given to this infant. If naloxone is given to an infant born to a narcotic-addicted mother, the drug will cause a severe abstinence reaction in the newborn that can result in seizure.

Neonatal Transport

An infant that is severely compromised at birth or <32 weeks gestation often requires **transport** to specialized neonatal care units, usually because of respiratory distress, preterm birth, congenital anomalies, and suspected cardiac abnormalities. The infant should be resuscitated and stabilized prior to transport. Communication with the regional center should be immediate and detailed. The **STABLE program** (**s**ugar, **t**emperature, **a**rtificial breathing, **b**lood pressure, **l**ab work, and **e**motional support) can guide efforts to stabilize the infant. The transport team must take copies of all records and lab reports. Transport teams may include NICU nurses, NNPs, physicians, and respiratory therapists. Adequate supplies (similar to those needed for resuscitation) must be available as well as oxygen, air-blended mixtures, monitors, and transport incubators. The incubator must control temperature while allowing access. Insulating material may be needed for very cold environments.

Maternal Postpartum Complications

Hematologic, Infection, and Diabetes

POSTPARTUM HEMORRHAGE

Postpartum hemorrhage may be early (≤24 hours) or late (≤6 weeks). Normal blood loss with vaginal delivery is about 500 mL and with Cesarean about 1000 mL. ACOG's formal definition of postpartum hemorrhage requires ≥1000 mL of blood loss with signs/symptoms of hypovolemia within the first 24 hours after birth, regardless of the mode of delivery. Blood loss is difficult to estimate because it is mixed with amniotic fluid and mucus, and hemorrhage may be internal and not obvious on examination. Usual indications of hemorrhage, such as increased pulse, decreased blood pressure, and decreased output of urine may be delayed until about 2000 mL of blood loss. A significant drop in hematocrit (10 points) is indicative of hemorrhage. Early hemorrhage poses more risk of mortality than late hemorrhage.

Causes of **early postpartum hemorrhage** include:

- **Uterine atony**: most common with multiple gestations, prolonged labor, labor induction, anesthesia, preeclampsia, and placenta previa; uterine contractions are necessary to occlude blood flow to the placenta
- **Genital lacerations**: may be undetected, or the episiotomy may continue to slowly ooze blood
- **Hematomas**: resulting from trauma to blood vessels, especially with pudendal anesthesia, forceps or vacuum-assisted delivery, macrosomia, and prolonged second stage of labor
- **Inversion of the uterus**: rare but may occur with weak uterine muscles, extended labor, anesthesia, use of magnesium sulfate (for preeclampsia), and manual removal of placenta with excess traction
- **Rupture of uterus**: also rare, but can occur with previous C-section, multiparity, and induction with oxytocin
- **Abnormal implantation of placenta**
- **Coagulopathies**: DIC may occur in response to blood loss or may cause blood loss

Causes of **late postpartum hemorrhage** include:

- **Subinvolution of placental implantation site** (failure of implantation site to shrink and heal) leaves open tissue that may bleed
- **Retained placental tissue**: bleeding occurs when it sloughs from implantation site

Interventions for Postpartum Hemorrhage

Following delivery, the nurse must monitor the woman carefully for increased bleeding, severe pain, tachycardia, and uncontracted uterus, as these signs may indicate **postpartum hemorrhage**. When hemorrhage is suspected, such as with steady flow of lochia rubra, then the woman's vital signs should be checked every 5-15 minutes and perineal pads weighed (1 mL of blood weighs about 1 g). The nurse must massage the fundus and apply firm but gentle fundal pressure only to the contracted uterus to express clots as applying pressure to an uncontracted uterus may result in increased hemorrhage and uterine inversion. The nurse should also relieve a distended bladder, which can prevent uterine contraction. Urinary output <30 mL/hr should be reported to the physician. The patient may need IV oxytocin or bimanual compression of the uterus to control bleeding. If bleeding is caused by trauma, surgical repair is needed. **Balloon tamponade** may be needed to control bleeding. Specially designed catheters have a balloon (usually 500 mL capacity) that is inflated with NS after insertion into the uterus. Many balloon catheters are bi-luminal so that blood can drain and be measured to determine if the pressure applied by the balloon is controlling bleeding. The balloon catheter should control bleeding within 5-15 minutes.

Tranexamic Acid

Tranexamic acid (TXA), a competitive inhibitor of plasminogen activation, inhibits the breakdown of fibrinogen and fibrin clots, thereby decreasing bleeding. TXA is recommended to control postpartum bleeding (>500 mL following vaginal birth or >1000 mL following Cesarean or any bleeding resulting from unstable hemodynamics). According to the World Health Organization (WHO) recommendations (2017), intravenous tranexamic acid should be administered routinely within 3 hours of delivery to women who experience postpartum hemorrhage (regardless of the cause, genital or otherwise) after vaginal delivery or Cesarean or as soon as possible after the onset of bleeding. However, the initial dose should not be administered more than 3 hours after birth. Only intravenous use is recommended at present. If TXA is given intrathecally, it can result in neurotoxicity, with a mortality rate of 50%. **Recommended dosage**:

- First dose: 100 mg/mL IV administered at 1 mL per minute (over a 10-minute period)
- Second dose: 1 g IV if bleeding persists after one-half hour or if bleeding restarts within 24 hours after the first dose is completed

Contraindications include thromboembolism during pregnancy, history of coagulopathy, hypersensitivity to drug, or active intravascular clotting.

Massive Transfusion Protocols

Massive transfusion protocol for postpartum bleeding includes **preparation**:

- Maintain a hemorrhage cart with all necessary supplies, IV equipment, and protocol instructions.
- Assess all patients for hemorrhage risk and measure cumulative loss of blood.
- Administer oxytocin after delivery.
- Carry out performance drills with staff and physicians.
- Institute protocol for cumulative blood loss of >1000 mL (post vaginal birth or Cesarean) and increase surveillance and non-pharmacologic interventions (such as balloon) for 500-1000 mL.

Transfusion protocol (may vary somewhat):

- Stage 1 (blood loss >500 mL vaginal or >1000 mL Cesarean or VS changes >15% [HR ≥110, BP ≤85/45, oxygen saturation <95%]): Ensure IV access (18 gauge); administer oxytocin, methergine; empty bladder.
- Stage 2 bleeding continues with blood loss <1500 mL: Notify blood bank of OB hemorrhage, keep 2 units PRBC at bedside, and administer according to clinical signs (do not wait for results of laboratory tests). Start thawing 2 units of fresh frozen plasma.
- Stage 3 bleeding (>1500 mL) or >2 units PRBCs administered, VS unstable, or indications of DIC: Continue transfusions as needed with whole blood or 1:1 PRBCs and FFP and administer platelets with every fifth unit.

Uterotonic Medications

Uterotonic medications are drugs used to prevent and treat postpartum hemorrhage, most often related to uterine atony:

- **Oxytocin (Pitocin)**: Used to stimulate contractions of the uterus for induction of labor, but also used in the postpartum period to stimulate uterine contractions and prevent atony through rhythmic contractions. Onset is immediate with IV administration. Adverse effects include uterine hyperstimulation, transient hypertension, and water intoxication (rare).
- **Methyl-ergonovine maleate (Methergine)**: A semisynthetic ergot alkaloid used routinely after placental delivery to prevent uterine atony and hemorrhage. Administration may begin after the anterior shoulder is delivered, during the second stage of labor, and causes sustained uterine contractions. Numerous adverse effects include hypertension, dizziness, flushing, tinnitus, nausea, vomiting, palpitations, and chest pain. Overdose or sensitivity reaction may result in vasoconstriction with distal peripheral numbness and tingling, and seizures. It is contraindicated in women with high blood pressure.
- **Ergometrine**: An ergot alkaloid that is used to prevent and control hemorrhage after delivery or abortion. It provides sustained contractions of the uterus. Adverse effects are similar to those of methylergonovine maleate and include hypertension, dizziness, flushing, tinnitus, nausea, vomiting, palpitations, and chest pain. It is contraindicated in women with high blood pressure.
- **Prostaglandins**: Include carboprost tromethamine (Hemabate) and dinoprostone (Prostin). Used for control of refractory postpartum hemorrhage related to uterine atony after other agents have failed to control hemorrhage. Adverse effects include gastrointestinal disorders, headache, flushing, bradycardia, respiratory distress (wheezing, cough, and bronchospasm), chills, and fever. It is contraindicated in women with cardiovascular, kidney, or liver disease or asthma. Women receiving prostaglandins must be monitored carefully for signs of fever or respiratory distress. Antipyretic medications may be needed to control fever/chills.

POSTPARTUM THROMBOPHLEBITIS

Thrombophlebitis may occur in the postpartum period, with indications of **septic thrombophlebitis** typically evident 3-7 days after delivery. **Clot formation** occurs in the vessel walls, leading to occlusion and inflammation. **Fibrinolytic activity** decreases during pregnancy to prevent hemorrhage occurring with delivery; however, this change can promote development of deep vein thrombosis and thrombophlebitis. Additionally, inactivity and bed rest increase risk. Coagulation usually returns to normal within about 3 days after delivery, so later onset often relates to other factors, such as a history of varicose veins. **Superficial thrombophlebitis** is usually evident by observable symptoms and poses less risk of clots breaking free and migrating than deep vein thrombophlebitis.

- **Femoral**: localized pain and swelling with edema of the leg from impaired circulation, often accompanied by fever and chills.
- **Pelvic**: abdominal pain, fever, and chills as well as generalized lethargy and malaise.

Treatment varies, depending on size and type, but may include heat, anticoagulation, compression (stockings), elevation of affected limb, and limitations on activities.

SEPTIC PELVIC THROMBOPHLEBITIS

Postpartum septic pelvic thrombophlebitis (SPT) is an infection that results from venous stasis of the veins that drain the pelvic organs and the presence of bacteria. The infection can extend along the right (most common) and left ovarian veins, resulting in septic thrombosis, which can extend into the vena cava and to the renal vein. This can result in microemboli that migrate through the inferior vena cava to the lungs and other organs. Postpartum SPT is more common after Cesarean than vaginal birth and is associated with postpartum endometriosis/parametritis. Symptoms include chills and fever that is nonresponsive to antibiotics. Patients are otherwise often asymptomatic initially, although some may experience pain in one or both of the lower quadrants or uterine tenderness if endometriosis/parametritis is involved. Diagnosis is per CT or MRI and CBC. Treatment is primarily antimicrobial (typically clindamycin, gentamycin, and ampicillin). Anticoagulation has not been shown to improve outcomes.

POSTPARTUM HEMATOMA

A hematoma may form in the perineal area after delivery, especially if an episiotomy is present. Hematomas may form anywhere from the **vulva** to the **upper vagina** because of trauma. Severe vulvar or vaginal pain that is not relieved by usual analgesia may indicate that a hematoma is forming. Hematomas must be monitored carefully. Those <5 cm may resolve over time. Ice packs may help to reduce discomfort. Vital signs should be monitored carefully for signs of hemorrhage. Larger hematomas require surgical excision of the most dependent portion, followed by drainage. The incision may be closed or left open with drains or packing to prevent recurrence of hematoma. If the hematoma is at the site of the episiotomy, the suture line must be opened to identify the site of bleeding.

Pulmonary Embolus

Because hypercoagulation occurs postpartum, coupled with decreased activity, the risk for **pulmonary embolus** increases, especially in the first 24 hours (but risk may persist for 4-6 weeks). Factors that increase the risk of postpartum DVT include Cesarean section, preterm delivery, hemorrhage, stillbirth, postpartum infection, maternal age ≥35 years, smoking, and medical comorbidities. Up to 70% of patients with pulmonary embolus also have DVT, so a PE should always be suspected with DVT. Symptoms of PE include dyspnea, chest pain, cough, fever, hemoptysis, tachypnea, tachycardia, and anxiety. Massive PE is characterized by hemodynamic instability and can lead to hypotension, PEA, and death. ECG findings of PE may include right axis deviation and inversion of the T-wave. Most patients will exhibit hypoxemia, but normal blood gas values do not preclude PE. Diagnosis is per chest radiograph, D-dimer, and helical CT-angiography, ventilation-perfusion scanning, or bilateral compression ultrasonography. Treatment may include anticoagulation, thrombolysis, or embolectomy, but all increase the risk of postpartum hemorrhage. Vena cava filters may also be inserted to prevent further clots from entering the lungs. $ECMO_2$ may be used to support the patient if respiratory failure occurs.

DIC

Disseminated intravascular coagulation (DIC), or consumption coagulopathy, is a secondary disorder of pregnancy. DIC may be triggered by abruptio placentae, uterine rupture, embolism of amniotic fluid, eclampsia, post-partum hemorrhage, shock (hypovolemic), severe infection with sepsis, and saline/missed abortion. DIC triggers both **coagulation** and **hemorrhage** through a complex series of events that includes trauma causing tissue factor (transmembrane glycoprotein) to enter the circulation and bind with coagulation factors triggering the coagulation cascade. This stimulates thrombin to convert fibrinogen to **fibrin**, causing aggregation and destruction of platelets and forming clots that can be disseminated throughout the intravascular system. These clots increase in size as platelets adhere to the clots, causing blockage of both the microvascular systems and the larger vessels. This can result in **ischemia** and **necrosis**. Clot formation triggers fibrinolysis and plasmin to break down fibrin and fibrinogen, causing destruction of clotting factors, resulting in hemorrhage. Both processes, clotting and hemorrhage, continue at the same time, placing the patient at high risk of death, even with treatment.

Symptoms and Treatment

The onset of symptoms of DIC may be very rapid, or it may be a slower chronic progression. Those who develop the chronic manifestation of the disease usually have fewer acute symptoms and may slowly develop ecchymosis or bleeding wounds.

The **symptoms** of disseminated intravascular coagulation:

- Bleeding from surgical or venous puncture sites
- Evidence of GI bleeding with distension, bloody diarrhea
- Hypotension and acute symptoms of shock
- Petechiae and purpura with extensive bleeding into the tissues
- Laboratory abnormalities:
    - Prolonged prothrombin and partial prothrombin times
    - Decreased platelet counts and fragmented RBCs
    - Decreased fibrinogen

The **treatment** for disseminated intravascular coagulation:

- Identifying and treating underlying cause
- Replacement blood products, such as platelets and fresh frozen plasma, if severe bleeding present
- Anticoagulation therapy (heparin) to increase clotting time if thrombosis is evident
- Cryoprecipitate to increase fibrinogen levels
- Coagulation inhibitors and coagulation factors

DIC Panel Tests

The disseminated intravascular coagulation (DIC) panel includes a number of tests. Generally, test results will show that measurements of materials needed for clotting are decreased and that clotting times are increased. Typical findings that indicate DIC include:

Activated partial thromboplastin time (aPTT)	Increased time
Prothrombin time	Varies from increased time (in 50% of cases) to normal time (25%) to shortened time (25%)
Partial thromboplastin time	Increased time (in 50-60% of cases)
Thrombin time	Increased time
D-dimer (a specific polymer that results when fibrin breaks down, giving a marker to indicate the degree of fibrinolysis)	Increased time (usually more reliable than FSP)
Fibrinogen	Decreased
Platelets	<100,000
Fibrin split products (FSP) or Fibrin degradation product (FDP): occur as more clots form and the further breakdown of fibrinogen and fibrin occur, interfering with blood coagulation by coating platelets and disrupting thrombin, and attaching to fibrinogen so stable clots can't form.	Increased time (in 75-100% of cases)
Clotting factor assays (V, VI, VII, X, XIII)	Decreased time
Antithrombin III	Decreased time (in 90% of cases)

Postpartum Infection

Parametritis

Parametritis (pelvic cellulitis) is inflammation of the connective tissue adjacent to the uterus, particularly in the broad ligament. The infection is rare, but usually occurs postpartum. It may result from bacterial invasion of a cervical laceration or pelvic vein thrombophlebitis. Indications include fever (38-40 °C), chills, lower abdominal pain, uterine subinvolution, local and rebound tenderness, tachycardia, abdominal distension, nausea, and vomiting.

Endometritis

Endometritis is an infection of the lining of the uterus. It occurs more often after Cesarean births than vaginal births. Fever (38-40 °C) occurs about the third day postpartum, accompanied by abdominal pain, malaise, uterine tenderness, tachycardia, and possibly foul-smelling lochia. Risk factors include Cesarean births, prolonged rupture of membranes, protracted labor, repeated vaginal examination, invasive procedures during labor and delivery, excess blood loss and anemia, systemic illnesses, diabetes, kidney infections, and smoking. Historically, it has been the most common cause of maternal death after childbirth. Handwashing is the most effective way to prevent it. Many organisms cause endometritis, reaching the uterus from the lower birth canal. Antibiotics are given parenterally and the infection should respond within 48-72 hours.

Urinary and Wound Infections

Urinary and wound infections in the postpartum period are discussed below:

- **Urinary**
  - May result from birth trauma, urinary retention, and contamination (from a catheter)
  - Indications include dysuria, fever, and urinary retention
- **Wound**
  - May result from contamination of lacerations, episiotomy, and C-section incisions
  - Indications include erythema, local pain, purulent discharge, edema, and (rarely) dehiscence

Postpartum Diabetes Mellitus

Mothers with diabetes mellitus require careful evaluation but should be encouraged to be as independent as possible in monitoring their own blood sugars and taking medications, such as insulin. Insulin requirements usually drop by 50-75% in the 24 hours after delivery because of the drop in hormone levels, so monitoring **glucose levels** and adjusting **insulin dosage** is important to prevent insulin reactions. The insulin needs should be reestablished over the next few days, taking into consideration diet and exercise. Diabetic mothers should be encouraged to breastfeed. Insulin needs are often lower while breastfeeding, even with increased caloric intake, so home glucose monitoring and adjustment of insulin doses must continue after discharge. With gestational diabetes, insulin can usually be discontinued after childbirth with monitoring of glucose levels. Oral medications can be used if necessary, although oral antihyperglycemic medications are contraindicated with breastfeeding.

Mood Disorders

Mood Disorders

Postpartum Depression

Postpartum major mood disorder, commonly referred to as postpartum depression, occurs in about 10-15% of mothers. Onset may occur before or during pregnancy or any time within the first year postpartum, but is most common within the first few months postpartum. Duration varies but is usually 3-14 months. Risk factors include primiparity, history of depression, bipolar disease, or previous postpartum depression, lack of stable and supportive social and family relationships, family history of psychiatric illness, and ambivalence about pregnancy. Symptoms are typical of depression and include sadness, crying, insomnia or excess sleeping, difficulty concentrating or making decisions, phobias, anxiety, lack of interest in activities, and feeling out of control or helpless. The mother may be irritable and hostile, especially toward the child. She may also be suicidal. Treatment may include psychotherapy, antidepressants, antipsychotics, and/or lithium. In some cases, the child may need to be cared for by others until the mother's depression lessens.

Review Video: Peripartum Depression
Visit mometrix.com/academy and enter code: 975380

Postpartum Psychosis

Postpartum psychosis may occur up to 3 months postpartum, but symptoms are usually evident within the first 3 weeks, with sudden onset of **psychotic Criterion A symptoms**, such as delusions, hallucinations, insomnia, anorexia, paranoia, and suicidal or homicidal ideation. In 4% of cases, mothers have committed infanticide, sometimes because of voices urging them to do so, so postpartum psychosis is a **medical emergency** that often requires hospitalization. Mothers should be carefully supervised when caring for their children until symptoms have abated, or children may need to be removed from the mother until the mother stabilizes. While postpartum psychosis is most common in mothers with a history of mental illness (such as schizophrenia or bipolar disease), it can occur in mothers with no such history. The cause is unclear but may be a combination of **hormonal imbalance** and **stress/anxiety**. Treatment includes psychotherapy, mood stabilizers, antipsychotics, and benzodiazepines. Antidepressants may cause mood cycling if psychosis is associated with bipolar disorder.

Newborn Complications

Cardiovascular Complications

Cyanotic and Acyanotic Congenital Cardiac Defects

Congenital heart disease is one of the leading causes of death in children within the first year of life. There are two main types of congenital heart disease: acyanotic and cyanotic. They may also be classified according to hemodynamics related to the blood flow pattern.

Cyanotic defects includes those with decreased pulmonary blood flow or mixed blood flow.

- **Decreased pulmonary blood flow**
  - Tetralogy of Fallot
  - Tricuspid atresia
- **Mixed blood flow**
  - Ebstein anomaly
  - Hypoplastic left heart syndrome
  - Total anomalous pulmonary venous return
  - Transposition of great arteries
  - Truncus arteriosus

Acyanotic defects include those with increased pulmonary blood flow or obstructed ventricular blood flow.

- **Increased pulmonary blood flow**
  - Atrial septal defect
  - Atrioventricular canal defect
  - Patent ductus arteriosus
  - Ventricular septal defect
- **Obstructed ventricular blood flow**
  - Aortic stenosis
  - Coarctation of aorta
  - Pulmonic stenosis

CENTRAL AND PERIPHERAL CYANOSIS

Cyanosis results from lack of oxygen and desaturated hemoglobin level of at least 5 g/dL. The two primary types of cyanosis are central and peripheral:

- **Central cyanosis**: Results from desaturated blood (decrease in oxygen transport from the lungs to the bloodstream), often because of a heart lesion, heart failure, or respiratory disorder. Because the arteries carry insufficient oxygen, cyanosis is apparent in the tongue, conjunctiva, and mucous membranes.
- **Peripheral cyanosis**: Results from peripheral vascular constriction from various causes, including hypothermia, stress, hypovolemia, or from conditions that interfere with blood flow to the extremities, such as cardiogenic shock or sepsis. Because blood supply to the extremities is inadequate, cyanosis becomes evident in the distal hands (fingers, nailbeds) and feet as well as the lips, tip of the nose, perioral areas, periorbital areas, and earlobes. However, PaO_2 levels generally remain normal.

Note that cyanosis may be more difficult to assess in dark-skinned neonates and may appear as a gray "ashy" discoloration rather than blue. **Acrocyanosis** (about mouth and extremities) is often a normal finding in neonates for up to 48 hours.

CARDIAC AND PULMONARY CYANOSIS

Cyanosis can reflect underlying cardiac and pulmonary disease:

- **Cardiac cyanosis:** This generally presents as cyanosis without respiratory distress. Cyanotic heart disease is likely a factor if the neonate's PaO_2 remains <70 mmHg while the neonate breathes 100% oxygen. Typically, with cyanotic heart disease, central cyanosis is a diagnostic factor although the degree of cyanosis at onset may vary. With structural heart defects that result in right-to-left shunting, cyanosis is generally evident, often from birth, and heart murmurs or extra heart sounds are evident. In some cases, such as tetralogy of Fallot, the cyanosis is more noticeable during crying.
- **Pulmonary cyanosis**: The neonate often has obvious signs of respiratory distress, including grunting respirations and sternal retraction, as well as central cyanosis. PaO_2 usually remains >100 mmHg while on 100% oxygen. Pulmonary conditions that may cause cyanosis include pulmonary hypoplasia, pulmonary edema, pneumothorax, pleural effusion, pneumonia, phrenic nerve palsy, hypoventilation, and diaphragmatic hernia.

TETRALOGY OF FALLOT

Tetralogy of Fallot (TOF) is a combination of 4 different defects:

- **Ventricular septal defect** usually with a large opening
- **Pulmonic stenosis** with decreased blood flow to lungs
- **Overriding aorta** (displacement to the right so that it appears to come from both ventricles, usually overriding the ventricular septal defect), resulting in the mixing of oxygenated and deoxygenated blood
- **Right ventricular hypertrophy**

Infants with TOF are often acutely cyanotic immediately after birth, while others with less severe defects may have increasing cyanosis over the first year.

Symptoms include:

- Intolerance to feeding or crying, resulting in increased cyanotic "blue spells" or "tet spells"
- Failure to thrive with poor growth
- Clubbing of fingers may occur over time
- Intolerance to activity as child grows
- Increased risk for emboli, brain attacks, brain abscess, seizures, fainting, or sudden death

Treatment: Total surgical repair at ≤1 year is now the preferred treatment rather than the palliative procedures formerly used.

TRANSPOSITION OF THE GREAT ARTERIES

Transposition of the great arteries is a congenital heart defect in which the aorta is connected to the right ventricle instead of the left ventricle, and the pulmonary artery is connected to the left ventricle instead of the right ventricle. This transposition means that deoxygenated blood is being pumped back to the body and the oxygenated blood returns to the lungs instead of going to the body. Septal defects may also occur, allowing some mixing of blood, and the ductus arteriosus allows mixing until it closes.

Symptoms vary depending upon whether there is mixing of blood but may include:

- Mild-to-severe cyanosis
- Symptoms of congestive heart failure
- Cardiomegaly developing in the weeks after birth
- Heart sounds vary depending upon the severity of the defects

Treatment may include:

- Prostaglandin to keep the ductus arteriosus and foramen ovale open; balloon atrial septostomy to increase size of foramen ovale
- Surgical repair to transpose arteries to the normal position ("arterial switch") as well as to repair septal defects and other abnormalities

Acyanotic Heart Disease

PDA

Patent ductus arteriosus (PDA) is failure of the ductus arteriosus that connects the **pulmonary artery and aorta** to close after birth, resulting in left-to-right shunting of blood from the aorta back to the pulmonary artery. This increases the blood flow to the lungs and causes an increase in pulmonary hypertension that can result in damage to the lung tissue.

While some infants may be essentially asymptomatic, **typical symptoms** include:

- Cyanosis
- Congestive heart failure
- Machinery-like murmur
- Frequent respiratory infections and dyspnea, especially on exertion
- Widened pulse pressure
- Bounding pulse
- Atrial fibrillation/palpitations
- Increased risk for bacterial endocarditis, congestive heart failure, and development of pulmonary vascular obstructive disease

Treatment includes:

- Pharmacologic therapy: Nonselective COX inhibitors such as ibuprofen and indomethacin have proven effective in closing PDA. Ibuprofen has shown to equally effective as the traditional pharmacologic approach of indomethacin, and less-likely to induce necrotizing enterocolitis or renal dysfunction. Both of these options carry a risk for bleeding. For patients with contraindications to nonselective COX inhibitors, acetaminophen is a supported option, but requires high dosages for maximal effect which places the neonate at risk for liver damage.
- Surgical repair can be done with ligation of the patent vessel.

Ventricular Septal Defect

Ventricular septal defect is an abnormal opening in the **septum** between the right and left ventricles. If the opening is small, the child may be asymptomatic, but larger openings can result in a left-to-right shunt because of higher pressure in the left ventricle. This shunting increases in the 6 weeks after birth, with symptoms becoming more evident, but the defect may close within a few years.

Symptoms include:

- Congestive heart failure with peripheral edema
- Tachycardia
- Dyspnea
- Difficulty feeding
- Heart murmur
- Recurrent pulmonary infections
- Increased risk for bacterial endocarditis and pulmonary vascular obstructive disease

Treatment includes:

- Diuretics, such as furosemide (Lasix), may be used for heart failure.
- ACE inhibitor (Captopril) decreases pulmonary hypertension.
- Surgery, including pulmonary banding or cardiopulmonary bypass, can be performed to repair the opening with sutures or a patch, depending upon the size.

Atrial Septal Defect

An atrial septal defect (ASD) is an abnormal opening in the **septum** between the right and left atria. Because the left atrium has higher pressure than the right atrium, some of the oxygenated blood returning from the lungs to the left atrium is shunted back to the right atrium, where it is again returned to the lungs, displacing deoxygenated blood.

Symptoms may be few or even absent depending upon the degree of the defect but can include:

- Congestive heart failure
- Heart murmur
- Increased risk for dysrhythmias and pulmonary vascular obstructive disease over time

Treatment may not be necessary for small defects, but larger defects require closure:

- Open-heart surgical repair
- Heart catheterization and placing of closure device (Amplatz device) across the atrial septal defect

Coarctation of the Aorta

Coarctation of the aorta is a stricture of the aorta, proximal to the ductus arteriosus intersection. The increased blood pressure caused by the heart attempting to pump the blood past the stricture causes the heart to enlarge and also increases blood pressure to the head and upper extremities while decreasing blood pressure to the lower body and extremities. With severe stricture, symptoms may not occur until the ductus arteriosus closes, causing sudden loss of blood supply to the lower body.

Symptoms include:

- Difference in blood pressure between upper and lower extremities
- Congestive heart failure symptoms in infants
- Headaches, dizziness, and nosebleeds in older children
- Increased risk of hypertension, ruptured aorta, aortic aneurysm, bacterial endocarditis, and brain attack

Treatment includes:

- Prostaglandin (alprostadil), such as Prostin VR Pediatric, to reopen the ductus arteriosus for infants
- Balloon angioplasty
- Surgical resection and anastomosis or graft replacement (usually at 3-5 years of age unless condition is severe); infants who have surgery may need later repair

Congestive Heart Failure

Types

Congestive heart failure results from the inability of the heart to adequately pump the blood the body needs. In infants, it is usually secondary to cardiac abnormalities with resultant increased blood volume and blood pressure:

- **Right-sided failure** occurs if the right ventricle cannot effectively contract to pump blood into the pulmonary artery, causing pressure to build in the right atrium and the venous circulation. This venous hypertension causes generalized edema of lower extremities, distended abdomen from ascites, hepatomegaly, and jugular venous distension.
- **Left-sided failure** occurs if the left ventricle cannot effectively pump blood into the aorta and systemic circulation, increasing pressure in the left atrium and the pulmonary veins, with resultant pulmonary edema and increased pulmonary pressure. Symptoms include respiratory distress with tachypnea, grunting respirations, sternal retraction, rales, failure to thrive, and difficulty eating, often leaving the child exhausted and sweaty.

Children often have some combination of right and left-sided failure. Increased pressure in the lungs after birth may delay symptoms for 1-2 weeks.

Management

Management of congestive heart failure (CHF) in infants can be difficult. It is extremely important to establish the etiology and to treat the underlying cause. For infants with structural cardiac abnormalities, surgical repair may be needed to resolve the CHF. There are some medical treatments that can relieve symptoms:

- **Diuretics**, such as furosemide (Lasix), metolazone, or hydrochlorothiazide to reduce pulmonary and peripheral edema
- **Antihypertensives**, such as Captopril or Propranolol to decrease heart workload
- **Cardiac glycosides**, such as Lanoxin, may relieve symptoms if above medicines are not successful
- **High caloric feedings**, either by bottle or nasogastric feeding to provide sufficient nutrients
- **Oxygen** may be useful for some children with weak hearts
- **Restriction of activities** to reduce stress on the heart
- **Dopamine or dobutamine** may be given to increase the contractibility of the heart

Hypotension

Hypotension is a systemic mean arterial blood pressure <2 standard deviations less that average values for gestational age. The lowest reading that is within normal limits for preterm infants is calculated as gestational age plus five. Thus, a 31-week preterm acceptable low BP would be 31-36 mmHg. Hypotension in the neonate most often relates to dysregulation of peripheral vascular tone and/or myocardial dysfunction. Hypotension may also occur as the result of hypocalcemia, hypovolemic, cardiogenic, or distributive shock, so determining the cause of hypotension is critical to planning appropriate intervention. Early signs of hypotension are those of compensated shock and later signs of decompensated shock. Tachycardia, respiratory distress, pallor, lethargy, and cyanosis may be evident. Dopamine (2-20 μg/kg/min) is the most commonly used drug to treat neonatal hypotension as it improves myocardial function and improves peripheral vascular tension without causing vasodilation. Oxygen is administered to combat hypoxia as well as saline bolus (10-20 mL/kg).

Hypertension

Hypertension is a relatively rare finding in the neonate. Signs of elevated blood pressure include lethargy, increased apnea episodes, seizures, irritability, tachypnea, and intracranial hemorrhage. The nurse often discovers elevated blood pressure through a routine check of vital signs. Most **causes of hypertension** in the neonate are **renal** in origin and include:

- **Thrombus formation in the kidneys** from an umbilical artery catheter (the most common cause in the NICU)
- **Other vascular causes**, such as renal vein thrombosis, or renal artery stenosis, or coarctation of the aorta
- **Compression of renal artery** by a mass

Non-renal causes include:

- **Iatrogenesis**, due to administration of dopamine, Aminophylline, or glucocorticoids
- **Neurological**, secondary to seizures or intraventricular hemorrhage
- **Endocrine**, secondary to congenital adrenal hyperplasia or hyperthyroidism
- **Pulmonary**, secondary to pneumothorax or bronchopulmonary dysplasia

Shock

Shock is the result of circulatory failure in which there is inadequate perfusion to meet the metabolic needs of the body. There are a number of different causes, but the **physiologic responses** are essentially the same:

- Hypotension (which may not be present initially because of reactive vasoconstriction)
- Hypoxemia resulting in hypoxic tissue
- Metabolic acidosis

There are essentially **3 stages** in the progression of the shock response:

1. **Compensated shock**: The sympathetic nervous response causes vasoconstriction, which may mask essential underlying hypotension but serves to provide blood flow for vital organ functions, although there may be decreased circulation at the microvascular (small vessel) level.
2. **Decompensated shock**: The cardiovascular system is unable to adequately compensate and microvascular perfusion decreases.
3. **Irreversible/terminal shock**: Damage to internal organs, such as the heart and brain, is so extensive that therapeutic measures cannot reverse eventual death.

Compensated Shock

During compensated shock, the blood pressure may remain normal initially as the compensatory sympathetic nervous response results in vasoconstriction and an increase in the heart rate and contractibility that combine to maintain cardiac output at a level adequate to supply the heart and brain while shifting circulation from other organs:

- **Skin:** Skin cold and clammy
- **Gastrointestinal tract**: Bowel sounds absent or decreased
- **Kidneys**: Urinary output decreased

Because of a decrease in tissue perfusion, lactic acid begins to build up, producing metabolic acidosis. The acidosis results in an increased respiratory rate, which serves to expel excess carbon dioxide. However, this also raises the pH of the blood and may result in respiratory alkalosis. Fluid replacement and medications to increase blood pressure and perfusion of the tissues are critical during this stage.

Decompensated Shock

Decompensated shock occurs as the body can no longer compensate, the blood pressure falls below normal, and all organ systems suffer from hypoperfusion. The heart is overworked and becomes dysfunctional, and chemical changes cause myocardial depression, so that the heart begins to fail. The permeability of the capillaries increases with fluid buildup in the interstitial tissues and decreased venous return to the heart. Multi-system effects occur:

- **Respiratory**: Respirations become rapid and shallow as the hypoxemia causes an inflammatory response and pulmonary edema, with collapse of alveoli and fibrotic changes in the lung tissue.
- **Cardiovascular**: Dysrhythmias and ischemia of the myocardium result in tachycardia. The myocardium is depressed and ventricles may dilate.
- **Neurological**: Hypoperfusion of the brain leads to changes in mental status, including lethargy and loss of consciousness. Pupils may dilate or react sluggishly.
- **Renal**: Acute renal failure occurs with decrease in urinary output, increase in BUN and creatinine, and electrolyte shifts.
- **Hepatic**: The liver loses the ability to filter and metabolize medications and metabolic waste products. Liver enzymes rise, and the skin becomes jaundiced.
- **Gastrointestinal**: Mucosal ulcerations may occur, causing bleeding and bloody diarrhea. Bacterial toxins may invade the lymphatic system where they are carried to the bloodstream, causing infection and increasing adverse cardiovascular responses.
- **Hematologic**: Disseminated vascular coagulation (DIC) may occur with both clotting and bleeding. The skin may show ecchymoses and petechiae. Clotting times are prolonged.

Treatment during this stage is dependent upon the underlying cause but includes intravenous fluids, medications to control blood pressure, cardiac function, infection, and gastrointestinal ulcerations and bleeding. Ventilatory support with oxygen and administration of sodium bicarbonate may be needed to treat metabolic acidosis. The infant must be monitored constantly, including hemodynamic monitoring, blood gases, urinary function, EKG, fluid and electrolytes, blood chemistries, enzyme levels, and neurological status.

Irreversible/Terminal Shock

The irreversible/terminal stage of shock can be difficult to determine because the progression of shock is a continuum rather than clearly defined stages, so the usual strategy is to continue to treat the patient with fluids, vasoactive medications to improve cardiac function, and nutritional support. During this stage hypotension persists, and complete liver and renal failure occurs. As perfusion causes necrosis of tissue, the toxins created result in severe metabolic acidosis. There is also increased lactic acidosis. Adenosine triphosphate (ATP) levels are depleted and there are no mechanisms left to store energy. **Multiple organ dysfunction syndrome (MODS)** occurs. There is no specific treatment that can reverse MODS, so treatment at this point becomes supportive. The mortality rate for MODS ranges from 30-100%, depending upon the number of organ systems that are involved.

Cardiogenic Shock

Cardiogenic shock in infants usually relates to congenital heart disease (usually with systemic to pulmonary shunting), myocarditis, and dysrhythmias, such as AV block and paroxysmal atrial tachycardia. These disorders interfere with the pumping mechanism of the heart, decreasing oxygen perfusion. Cardiogenic shock has 3 **characteristics**:

- Increased preload
- Increased afterload
- Decreased contractibility

Together these result in a decreased cardiac output and an increase in systemic vascular resistance (SVR) to compensate and protect vital organs. This results in an increase of afterload in the left ventricle with increased need for oxygen. As the cardiac output continues to decrease, tissue perfusion decreases, coronary artery perfusion decreases, fluid backs up, and the left ventricle fails to adequately pump the blood, resulting in pulmonary edema and right ventricular failure.

Cardiac Dysrhythmias

Cardiac dysrhythmias (abnormal heart beats), although more common in adults, can occur in infants and are frequently the result of damage to the conduction system during major cardiac surgery.

Bradydysrhythmias are pulse rates that are abnormally slow:

- Complete atrioventricular block (A-V block) may be congenital or a response to surgical trauma.
- Sinus bradycardia may be caused by the autonomic nervous system or a response to hypotension and decrease in oxygenation.
- Junctional/nodal rhythms often occur in post-surgical patients when absence of P wave is noted but heart rate and output usually remain stable, and unless there is compromise, usually no treatment is necessary.

Tachydysrhythmias are pulse rates that are abnormally fast:

- Sinus tachycardia is often caused by illness, such as fever or infection.
- Supraventricular tachycardia (200-300 bpm) may have a sudden onset and result in congestive heart failure.

Conduction irregularities are irregular pulses that often occur post-operatively and are usually not significant. Premature contractions may arise from the atria or ventricles.

Cardioversion Procedures for Arrythmia Types

Cardioversion procedures for arrythmia types are as follows:

- **Stable tachyarrhythmia:** Vagal maneuver to increase parasympathetic input to the heart and slow it. Apply ice to the neonate's face, which triggers the diving response to slow the heart rate. If unsuccessful, try adenosine, digoxin, or propranolol.
- **Unstable arrhythmia with narrow QRS complex:** Synchronized electrical cardioversion is appropriate for atrial flutter or fibrillation, WPW, or PJRT. Set the defibrillator for 0.5-2.0 J/kg. Place two electrode pads on the infant's chest. Wait for the optimum moment in the cardiac cycle. Pass electrical current through the infant's heart.
- **Unstable arrhythmia with wide QRS complex:** Asynchronous cardioversion is appropriate for ventricular tachycardia or fibrillation, SVT with BBB, or antidromic SVT in WPW. Defibrillate because there is no R wave present to time the shock.
- **Stable arrhythmia with wide QRS complex:** Administer amiodarone or procainamide for rate control. If unsuccessful, consider adenosine (0.1 mg/kg, with a maximum of 6 mg, rapid IV push and up to 0.2 mg/kg or 12 mg for a second dose). If pharmacologic interventions are unsuccessful, consider cardioversion at 0.5-1.0 J/kg for the first attempt, and then 2 J/kg if the first attempt is unsuccessful.
- **Bradydysrhythmias:** For 1:1 sinus bradycardia, complete AV block, Wenckebach's phenomenon, and sinus exit block: Check airway, breathing, and circulation. Treat underlying cause. Give oxygen, atropine, and isoproterenol. Start transvenous pacing.

Respiratory Complications

Respiratory Distress Syndrome

Respiratory distress syndrome (RDS) (hyaline membrane disease) occurs in 14% of low-birth-weight infants. RDS is caused by the absence or deficiency of surfactant. Surfactant is a lipoprotein that reduces surface tension in the alveoli. Surfactant causes the lungs to be more compliant (alveoli expand with less effort) and the alveoli do not collapse on end expiration. Surfactant production begins at 22 weeks of gestation, but levels are inadequate until 36 weeks of gestation. Lack of surfactant produces alveolar collapse (atelectasis) and less compliant lungs that cause laborious breathing. Collapsed areas of lung may still receive blood flow, but no exchange of gases occurs (ventilation perfusion mismatch). If RDS is left untreated, hypoxemia and hypercarbia develop, leading to respiratory acidosis. Acidosis and hypoxemia lead to a cycle of increased pulmonary vascular resistance and vasoconstriction, causing increased hypoxemia.

Air Leak Syndromes

Premature infants have more fragile lung tissue and often require respiratory resuscitative measures, such as positive pressure ventilation (PPV), ventilator support, and administration of pulmonary drugs (e.g., surfactant) that make them more susceptible to air leak syndrome. **Air leak syndrome** occurs when an alveolus ruptures and air leaks into a space that it normally does not occupy. Different syndromes occur, depending on the area that air leaks into.

- **Pneumothorax**: Air leakage into the pleural cavity that surrounds the lungs
- **Tension pneumothorax**: One-way air flow into the pleural cavity, with pressure build-up and significant collapse of lung tissue, causing respiratory compromise
- **Pneumomediastinum**: Air traveling along the pulmonary blood vessels that enters the mediastinum
- **Pneumopericardium**: Air in the sac that surrounds the heart
- **Pulmonary interstitial emphysema**: Air trapped in the lung's interstitial spaces

Pneumothorax

Pneumothorax is the most common type of air leak syndrome. In infants, increased air pressure caused by the use of mechanical ventilation is the most common cause, but infants may develop spontaneous pneumothorax. Infants with fragile lung tissue are at especially high risk:

- Infants with lung disease, including hyaline membrane disease (HMD)
- Premature infants
- Infants with meconium aspiration

Symptoms vary according to the type of pneumothorax (spontaneous, traumatic, or tension) but can include:

- Increased respiratory distress with tachypnea and chest wall retractions
- Absence of breath sounds on auscultation
- Paradoxical chest movement in which the chest contracts during inhalation and expands during exhalation
- Shift in maximum intensity sounds of heart
- Bradycardia and cyanosis

Treatment includes:

- Evacuating air with needle aspiration or chest tubes to water seal drainage
- Correction of underlying cause

Review Video: Pneumothorax
Visit mometrix.com/academy and enter code: 186841

Pneumomediastinum

A pneumomediastinum is an air leak in the mediastinum, the area of the chest between the sternum and the spine, and between the lungs. Causes of neonatal **pneumomediastinum** vary. Often, this complication arises after or in conjunction with neonatal respiratory distress, pneumonia, mechanical ventilation use, meconium aspiration, or as a result of birth-related trauma. While pneumomediastinum is often asymptomatic, it can also present with cyanosis, diminished heart sounds or shallow respirations. The condition often resolves spontaneously, but the patient must be monitored closely for complications and may require mechanical ventilation despite this being a common cause of the condition. Diagnosis of pneumomediastinum is through chest x-ray, with ABG's to evaluate the impact of the condition on the newborn's gas exchange and oxygenation.

Apnea of Prematurity

Premature infants (especially those <34 weeks) often exhibit **apnea of prematurity (AOP).** AOP begins at birth and is believed to be caused by immaturity of the nervous system, and improves as the brain matures. It may persist for 4-8 weeks. There are 3 **types of apnea**:

- **Central**: no airflow or effort to breathe
- **Obstructive**: no airflow, but effort to breathe
- **Mixed**: both central and obstructive elements (75% of AOP)

Symptoms include:

- Swallowing during apneic periods
- Apnea >20 seconds
- Apnea <20 seconds with bradycardia 30 beats <normal
- Oxygen saturation <85% persisting ≥5 seconds
- Cyanosis

Treatment includes:

- Tactile stimulation (rubbing limbs or thorax or gently slapping bottoms of feet) or gently lifting the jaw to relieve obstruction
- Oxygen or bag/mask ventilation for bradycardia and decreased oxygen saturation
- Continuous positive airway pressure (CPAP) for mixed or obstructive apnea
- Aminophylline/theophylline or caffeine (for central apnea) may increase contractions of the diaphragm

TTN

Transient tachypnea of the newborn (TTN) occurs when fluid in the lungs is not adequately absorbed after birth. The neonate usually exhibits symptoms within 36 hours of birth, and the condition typically resolves within 3 days. TTN is most common in infants delivered by Cesarean section, but premature birth and having a mother who smokes or has diabetes increases risk to the infant.

Symptoms include:

- Dyspnea (>60/min)
- Sternal retraction (mild)
- Expiratory grunt
- Nasal flaring
- Poor feeding (because of increased respiratory rate)

Laboratory findings include:

- ABGs: hypoxemia
- Chest radiograph: fluid in lungs

Treatment includes:

- Monitor oxygen saturation levels
- Provide supplemental oxygen as indicated
- Provide intravenous fluids or nasogastric feedings if infant is unable to take oral feedings

Meconium Aspiration Syndrome

Meconium aspiration syndrome (MAS) occurs when meconium, expelled in the amniotic fluid (occurring in about 20% of pregnancies), is aspirated by the fetus *in utero* or the neonate at first breath. Blood and amniotic fluids may be aspirated as well. Some infants may present with **symptoms** at birth, but sometimes symptoms are delayed for a number of hours:

- Tachypnea
- Lethargy, depressed state
- Hypoxemia and hypercapnia
- Metabolic acidosis may occur
- Hyperventilation may occur in early stages with hypoventilation in later stages

Symptoms are similar to transient tachypnea of the newborn (TTN) but they are more severe and the infant appears more compromised. Chest x-rays may show infiltrates, atelectasis, and hypoinflated areas as well as hyperinflated areas. Pulmonary hypertension may result. **Treatment** includes:

- Preventive suctioning of the oropharynx as soon as the head is delivered
- Intubation and suctioning of the trachea for infants with respiratory distress (weak respirations, bradycardia, hypotonia)
- Supplemental oxygen and/or mechanical ventilation as indicated

PPHN

Persistent pulmonary hypertension (PPHN) occurs when the high pulmonary vascular pressure that keeps fetal blood from circulating through the lungs fails to reduce after birth, so that blood continues to bypass the lungs, and the foramen ovale and ductus arteriosus are forced by pressure to remain open with venous blood shunting into systemic circulation instead of being oxygenated in the lungs. Infants are usually near or full-term, but present at birth with respiratory distress and cyanosis. PPHN is the cause of about 50% of neonatal deaths. There are 3 **classifications**:

- **Primary** is idiopathic with normal lung tissue but arterial hyperplasia and/or premature constricting of ductus arteriosus *in utero*.
- **Secondary** is precipitated by another disorder, such as meconium aspiration pneumonia (MAP), transient tachypnea of the newborn (TTN) or hyaline membrane disease. This is the most common form.
- **Hypoplastic** is related to pulmonary hypoplasia with anatomic changes in alveoli and vasculature in the lung.

PPHN has been linked to maternal use of SSRIs and NSAIDs.

Symptoms are usually evident within the first 12 hours of birth and progress over the next 24-48 hours:

- Cyanosis with poor cardiac perfusion, tachycardia
- Hypoxemia, persisting even with supplemental oxygen
- Systolic murmur with regurgitation of the tricuspid valve
- Tachypnea and general respiratory distress

Treatment

Treatment for persistent pulmonary hypertension (PPHN) will be specific for the underlying cause, and can include:

- Intubation and mechanical ventilation with HFV especially with parenchymal lung disease
- Central venous lines for administration of solutions, such as calcium gluconate
- Arterial line to monitor arterial blood gas
- Surfactants (beractant) to reduce surface tension in patients without primary PPHN
- High frequency ventilation (HFV) is used with underlying lung disease resulting in low volume
- Extracorporeal membrane oxygenation (ECMO) is used if other forms of support are not successful, and most often if the infant also has congenital diaphragmatic hernia
- Sodium bicarbonate is often used to correct metabolic acidosis in practice, however there is no evidence of short or long-term benefits
- Sedation (fentanyl) to reduce restlessness. Induced paralysis (pancuronium, vecuronium) has been used but is implicated in increased mortality rates, atelectasis, sensory hearing loss, and ventilation-perfusion mismatch
- Inhaled nitrous oxide

Pulmonary Hemorrhage

Pulmonary hemorrhage is bleeding within the alveoli. This usually is the result of some other event, such as intracranial hemorrhage, asphyxia, aspiration, heart disease, or sepsis. This can also be the result of a trauma from over-aggressive suctioning. **Pulmonary hemorrhage** presents as bright red blood from the trachea found with suctioning and as rapid, sudden respiratory deterioration. Pulmonary hemorrhage can cause rapid death if the bleeding is severe and is often only found during an autopsy. A more minor hemorrhage can be managed with blood transfusions and assisted ventilation. Pulmonary hemorrhage may result in hemothorax. In some cases, pneumothorax may also be present, resulting in mediastinal shift that increases the difficulty of identifying and repairing the bleeding vessel. If the infant is stabilized, computed tomography may provide accurate diagnosis to isolate the area of hemorrhage. The underlying cause of the hemorrhage must be discovered and treated.

Surfactant Therapy

Pulmonary hemorrhage is sometimes treated with **surfactant** although there are no adequate randomized studies at this time to show efficacy. However, preliminary reports appear positive. In some cases, pulmonary hemorrhage may be associated with the use of surfactant. The use of surfactant therapy is common in preterm infants to reduce morbidity and mortality related to respiratory distress syndrome. It is also sometimes used for infants receiving prolonged ventilatory support. Surfactant improves lung compliance, decreases pulmonary vascular resistance, and increases flow (right to left) through a patent ductus arteriosus or persistent foramen ovale. However, these very improvements in lung function can result in pulmonary hemorrhage, especially if ventilatory support is not adjusted with respect to the improved pulmonary function, so it's very important that ventilation be monitored carefully after administration of surfactant.

CDH

Congenital diaphragmatic hernias (CDH) may cause severe respiratory distress. The primary CDHs that affect infants are **posterolateral** (Bochdalek hernia).

- **Left-sided** in 85% of cases; includes herniation of the large and small intestine and intra-abdominal organs into the thoracic cavity
- **Right-sided** in 13% of cases; may be asymptomatic or involve only the liver and part of the large intestine herniate

Neonates with left CDH may exhibit **severe respiratory distress** and **cyanosis**. The lungs may be underdeveloped because of pressure exerted from displaced organs during fetal development. There may be a left hemithorax with a mediastinal shift, with the heart pressing on the right lung, which may be hypoplastic. Bowel sounds are heard over the chest area. Pulmonary hypertension and cardiopulmonary failure may occur. **Treatments** include:

- Immediate surgical repair
- HFOV and nitric oxide for pulmonary hypoplasia
- Extracorporeal membrane oxygenation (ECMO) for cardiopulmonary dysfunction

Despite treatment, mortality rates are 50%, and children who survive may have emphysema, with a larger volume but inadequate number of alveoli.

Neurological Complications

Neonatal Neurosensory Capabilities

A neonate is born with the following neurosensory capabilities:

- **Hearing**: The neonate's crying after birth clears middle ear mucus and the eustachian tubes, and hearing becomes acute with hearing thresholds similar to adults and children. Because hearing deficit is one of the most common congenital abnormalities, all infants should be assessed for hearing.
- **Vision**: The neonate's vision is about 10-30 times less acute than that of an adult, but the infant has peripheral vision, can fixate at 8-14 inches, and can accommodate to large objects. The neonate is able to perceive shapes, colors, and faces.
- **Tactile sense**: The neonate has a good sense of touch and reacts emotionally to tactile stimulation.
- **Smell**: The neonate has a strong sense of smell after nasal passages clear and will react to the smell of milk or turn away from strong smells.
- **Pain**: Neonates experience pain, and pain prevention/management should be part of neonatal care.

Birth Asphyxia

Birth asphyxia is the cause of many problems after birth. **Birth asphyxia** is defined as an event that alters the exchange of gas (oxygen and carbon dioxide). This interference with gas exchange leads to a decrease in the amount of oxygen delivered to the fetus along with an increase in the level of carbon dioxide the fetus is exposed to. This gas imbalance causes the fetus to switch from normal aerobic metabolism to anaerobic metabolism. Fetal distress results, which then leads to increased fetal heart rate, release of meconium into the amniotic fluid, and lowered pH. Infants experiencing birth asphyxia will often present at birth with APGAR scores that are less than 5. Symptoms of birth asphyxia include:

- **Mild**
  - Overly alert for the first 45 minutes to one hour following birth (infants are normally sleepy after about 15 minutes following birth)
  - Pupils dilated
  - Respiratory rate and heart rate both slightly increased
  - Newborn reflexes and muscle tone normal
  - Oxygen may be administered
- **Moderate**
  - Hypothermia as evidenced by low body temperature
  - Hypoglycemia as glucose stores are used up trying to supply organs needed energy
  - Pupils are constricted
  - Signs of respiratory distress evident
  - May experience seizure activity at 12-24 hours of age
  - Lethargy (floppy infant)
  - Bradycardia
- **Severe** (Requires close monitoring in a NICU)
  - Pale color related to the inability of the heart to perfuse the body
  - Cerebral edema related to apnea episodes and/or intracranial hemorrhage

Resuscitation will vary according to the infant's condition, but warming the infant, stabilizing the glucose level, and providing oxygen or EMCO (in severe cases) may be indicated.

HIE

Hypoxic-ischemic encephalopathy (HIE) results when oxygen supply to the brain is impaired. A common cause of HIE is perinatal asphyxia. The degree of insult to the neonate depends on the severity of the ischemic event. HIE is typically divided into three categories:

- **Mild HIE**: Characterized by increased muscle tone with brisk deep tendon reflexes. The infant may also exhibit poor feeding, irritability, and excessive sleepiness. These abnormalities generally resolve after 3-4 days.
- **Moderate HIE**: Characterized by significant hypotonia and lethargy with diminished deep tendon reflexes. Moro and grasp reflexes may be absent. Seizures may occur. Full recovery may still occur after 1-2 weeks.
- **Severe HIE**: Generalized hypotonia with depressed deep tendon reflexes and coma. The infant may not respond to physical stimulus. Breathing may be irregular and the infant requires ventilatory support. Basic neonatal reflexes may be absent. Pupils may be dilated and fixed. Generalized seizure activity is present and may be difficult to treat.

Risk Factors and Treatment Options

Neonatal **risk factors** for hypoxic-ischemic encephalopathy include:

- Cardiac arrhythmias
- pH <7.10 (umbilical artery), indicating acidosis during delivery
- Meconium-stained amniotic fluid
- Apgar <7 at 5 minutes after birth or <4 for more than 5 minutes
- Seizures during the first 24 hours
- Neurological dysfunction as demonstrated by coma, lethargy, irritability, hypotonia, and/or altered reflexes
- Symptoms of multiple organ damage: Cardiac damage, indicated by reduced contractility with hypotension; renal damage, indicated by oliguria; and damage to the intestinal tract, indicated by poor peristalsis, delayed gastric emptying, and the development of necrotizing enterocolitis

Identifying infants at risk and instituting treatment may decrease neurological impairment. **Treatment** may include:

- Phenobarbital given in high doses after birth decreases seizures and improves long-term outcome.
- Calcium channel blockers may improve cerebral blood flow during ischemia.
- Mild to moderate hypothermia for 5-72 hours may decrease damage; studies are in progress.
- Allopurinol (40 mg/kg) 4 hours after birth reduces mortality rates.

Subdural and Subarachnoid Cranial Hemorrhages

Subdural hemorrhage between the dura and the cerebrum, usually from tears in the cortical veins of the subdural space, tends to develop more slowly and can result in a subdural hematoma. If the bleeding is acute and develops within minutes or hours of injury, the prognosis is poor. Subacute hematomas that develop more slowly cause varying degrees of injury. Subdural hemorrhage is a common injury related to birth trauma and child abuse, although it can result from coagulopathies or aneurysms. Symptoms of acute injury may occur within 24-48 hours, but subacute bleeding may not be evident for up to 2 weeks after injury. Symptoms may include bradycardia, tachycardia, hypertension, and alterations in consciousness. Subdural taps may suffice for infants, but some infants will require surgical evacuation of the hematoma.

Subarachnoid hemorrhage may result from childbirth (one of the most common causes) or from shaken impact syndrome. The presenting symptom may be seizures, and other symptoms are similar to those of subdural hematoma. Symptoms worsen as ICP rises.

Intraventricular Hemorrhage

Intraventricular hemorrhages (IVH) are common in premature neonates less than 32 weeks estimated gestational age. IVH presents within the first 72 hours of life in 90% of affected neonates, and within the first 24 hours in 50% of cases. Infants less than 35 weeks gestational age or who weigh less than 1500 grams have a 50% incidence rate of IVH; however, this rate is declining due to improvements in obstetrical care and nursing management of fluids and respiration. Depending on the amount and location of bleeding seen on cranial ultrasound, IVH is **graded** as follows:

	Anatomy	**Severity**
Grade I	The hemorrhage is limited to the germinal matrix (subependymal region).	Mild (5% death rate; 5% motor or cognitive impairment)
Grade II	The hemorrhage extends 10-40% into the lateral ventricles on sagittal view, but has not dilated them significantly.	Moderate (10% death rate; 30-40% motor or cognitive impairment)
Grade III	The hemorrhage extends 50% or more into the lateral ventricles with significant ventricular dilation.	Severe (27-50% death rate; 35% motor or cognitive impairment)
Grade IV	The hemorrhage extends into brain tissue.	Periventricular hemorrhagic infarction (80% death rate; 90% motor or cognitive impairment)

Symptoms and Treatment

IVH is also categorized based on **symptoms**:

- **Asymptomatic**: 25-50% of IVH infants are asymptomatic or have only a fall in hematocrit and anemia, but ultrasound shows an IVH.
- **Saltatory**: Infants are pale or ashen and have gradual neurological deterioration (attention, movements, level of consciousness, eye movements).
- **Catastrophic**: Acute onset of decreased level of consciousness, bulging fontanel, cranial nerve abnormalities, decerebrate posturing, and hypotension with drop in hematocrit.

IVH **treatment** must be approached with extreme caution. The pediatrician orders one of the following to suppress CSF production:

- **Indocin** 0.1 mg/kg/dose IV when the baby is 6 hours old, 24 hours old, and 48 hours old

  OR

- **Diamox** 5 mg/kg/dose PO or IV every 6 hours, which is increased by 25 mg/kg/day (with a maximum dosage of 100 mg/kg/day)

Craniosynostosis

Types of craniosynostosis (early fusing of the skull) include the following:

- **Sagittal craniosynostosis** (scaphocephaly) is the fusion of the sagittal suture at the top of the skull, front to back, resulting in a long narrow skull. This typically has little impact on development of the brain but may result in increased intracranial pressure (ICP). This is the most common form. Of craniosynostosis.
- **Coronal craniosynostosis** is the fusion of one or both sutures that extend from each ear to the top of the skull, resulting in a wide, short skull. If both sides fuse (brachycephaly), the forehead may bulge forward. If one size fuses (plagiocephaly), the nose and eye socket on the affected size are affected. May result in vision impairment and increased ICP.
- **Metopic craniosynostosis** (trigonocephaly) is the fusion of the suture from top of nose to anterior fontanel and sagittal suture, causing a triangular forehead and associated with developmental delays and cognitive impairment
- **Lambdoid craniosynostosis** (posterior plagiocephaly) is the fusion of the suture along the back of the head. One side of head may be flat, ears at different levels, and head tilted laterally. This does not typically affect brain development but can cause vision impairment.

Complex craniosynostosis affects multiple sutures and is often part of genetic syndromes, such as Crouzon and Apert. It is associated with increased ICP, cognitive impairment, developmental delays, and other

Periventricular Leukomalacia

Periventricular leukomalacia is necrosis of the brain's white matter (described as "white spots") in the area surrounding the ventricles of the brain, likely due to inadequate oxygenation or blood flow to the area. It occurs most often in preterm infants born before 32 weeks of gestation or in very low birth weight (VLBW) infants. The necrosis can be identified on ultrasound and is associated with poor outcomes. If bilateral occipital cysts are present, this is a reliable predictive factor for cerebral palsy. With VLBW infants, a more diffuse pattern of white spots can be seen on magnetic resonance imaging scans. Additional risk factors include twin-twin transfusion syndrome, hypocarbia, infections (e.g., antenatal and postnatal), intraventricular hemorrhage, and necrotizing enterocolitis. Signs and symptoms vary depending on the severity of the injury but can include motor impairments, developmental delays, visual impairment, cognitive impairment, seizures, and cerebral palsy (typically spastic diplegia). Periventricular hemorrhage is a frequent complication. There is no treatment other than supportive care.

Hydrocephalus

Hydrocephalus occurs when there is an imbalance between production and absorption of cerebrospinal fluid in the ventricles, resulting from impaired absorption or obstruction, which may be congenital or acquired. There are **primarily 2 types** of hydrocephalus that affect infants:

- **Communicating**: CSF flows (communicates) between the ventricles but is not absorbed in the subarachnoid space (arachnoid villi).
- **Noncommunicating**: CSF is obstructed (non-communicating) between the ventricles with obstruction, often stenosis of the aqueduct of Sylvius but it can occur anywhere in the system.

In early infancy, before closure of cranial sutures, head enlargement is the most common presentation while brain damage occurs later as pressure causes damage to the central nervous system. **Early infancy symptoms** include bulging, non-pulsating fontanels (usually anterior) with increasing head circumference, dilated scalp veins, separating sutures, and positive Macewen sign (resonance on tapping near the frontal-temporal-parietal juncture), irritability, seizures, vomiting, and setting-sun sign (the upper eyelids retract and the eyes turn downwards due to pressure on the mesencephalic tegmentum and paralysis of upward gaze).

Causes

Hydrocephalus can be acquired or congenital. Approximately 75% of neonates with intraventricular hemorrhage (IVH) develop hydrocephalus. **Congenital hydrocephalus** is present at birth and can occur due to:

- **Aqueductal stenosis**, the most common cause, when the cerebral aqueduct connecting the third and fourth ventricles is blocked by an infection (toxoplasmosis, mumps, syphilis, or cytomegalovirus), tumor, hemorrhage, or developmental narrowing, and fluid accumulates in the third ventricle
- **Spina bifida**, where 80-90% of infants born with meningocele or myelomeningocele also have hydrocephalus.
- **Arnold-Chiari malformations** in the base of the brain where the spinal column joins the skull, characterized by parts of the cerebellum protruding through the foramen magnum into the spinal canal, which interferes with the normal flow of CSF.

Treatment

Hydrocephalus is diagnosed through CT and MRI, which help to determine the cause. Treatment may vary somewhat depending upon the underlying disorder, which may also require treatment. For example, if obstruction is caused by a tumor, surgical excision to directly remove the obstruction is required. Generally, however, most hydrocephalus is treated with **shunts**:

- **Ventricular-peritoneal shunt**: This procedure is the most common and consists of placement of a ventricular catheter directly into the ventricles (usually lateral) at one end with the other end in the peritoneal area to drain away excess CSF. There is a one-way valve near the proximal end that prevents backflow but opens when pressure rises to drain fluid. In some cases, the distal end drains into the right atrium.
- **Third ventriculostomy**: A small opening is made in the base of the third ventricle so CSF can bypass an obstruction. This procedure is not common and is done with a small endoscope.

Neural Tube Defects

The neural tube is the embryonic structure that eventually forms the brain and spinal cord. **Neural tube defects** (NTD) are a spectrum of congenital disorders involving the meninges covering the spinal cord. Mild forms are asymptomatic. Severe cases are incompatible with life. Diagnosis is often made in pregnancy by ultrasound or by an elevated level of alpha-fetoprotein in the amniotic fluid or in the mother's serum. Causes are multifactorial, with both genetic and environmental components. **Risk factors** for NTD include:

- Poor diet lacking in folic acid
- Family history of a NTD in a parent or sibling
- Maternal obesity with poorly controlled diabetes
- Maternal use of valproic acid or carbamazepine during pregnancy
- Increasing core temperature 3-4 °F (2 °C) through saunas, hot tubs, or fever

Studies have shown that if the mother ingests 400 micrograms of folic acid daily before and during pregnancy, it protects the fetus from developing an NTD.

Types

The neural tube defects, spina bifida and myelomeningocele, are often used interchangeably, but there is a distinction. Spina bifida is a neural tube defect with an incomplete spinal cord and often missing vertebrae that allow the meninges and spinal cord to protrude through the opening. There are **5 basic types**:

- **Spina bifida**: Defect in which the vertebral column is not closed with varying degrees of herniation through the opening.
- **Spina bifida occulta**: Failure of the vertebral column to close but no herniation through the opening, so the defect may not be obvious.
- **Spina bifida cystica**: Defect in closure with external sac-like protrusion with varying degrees of nerve involvement.
- **Meningocele**: Spina bifida cystica with meningeal sac filled with spinal fluid.
- **Myelomeningocele**: Spina bifida cystica with meningeal sac containing spinal fluid and part of the spinal cord and nerves.

Myelomeningocele

Myelomeningocele, which involves spina bifida cystica with a meningeal sac containing spinal fluid and part of the spinal cord and nerves, comprises about 75% of the total cases of spina bifida. There are numerous **physical manifestations**:

- **Exposed sac** poses the danger of infection and cerebrospinal fluid leakage; so surgical repair is usually done within the first 48 hours although it may be delayed for a few days, especially if the sac is intact.
- **Chiari type II malformation** comprises hypoplasia of the cerebellum and displacement of the lower brainstem into the upper cervical area, which impairs the circulation of spinal fluid. It may result in symptoms of cranial nerve dysfunction (dysphonia, dysphagia) and weakness and lack of coordination of upper extremities.
- **Neurogenic bladder** is common and may require the Credé maneuver for infants and later intermittent clean catheterization.
- **Fecal incontinence** is common and is controlled with diet and bowel training as the child gets older.
- **Musculoskeletal abnormalities** depend upon the level of the myelomeningocele and the degree of impairment but often involve the muscle and joints of the lower extremities and sometimes the upper. Dysfunction often increases with the number of shunts. Scoliosis and lumbar lordosis are common. Hip contractures may cause dislocations.
- **Paralysis/paresis** may vary considerably and be spastic or flaccid. Many children require wheelchairs for mobility although some are fitted with braces for assisted ambulation.
- **Seizures** occur in about a quarter of those affected, sometimes related to shunt malfunction.
- **Hydrocephalus** is present in about 25-35% of infants at birth and 60-70% after surgical repair with ventriculoperitoneal shunt. Untreated, the ventricles will dilate and brain damage can occur.
- **Tethered spinal cord** occurs when the distal end of the spinal cord becomes attached to the bone or site of surgical repair and does not move superiorly with growth, causing increased pain, spasticity, and disability and requiring surgical repair.

Anencephaly

Anencephaly is a neural tube defect in which the **embryological neural tube**, which forms the brain and spinal cord, fails to close at the **cephalic (head) end**, resulting in an infant without most of the brain, skull, or scalp, so that the top of the head is open. The eyes bulge forward. Because the forebrain is missing, the child has no cognitive ability or sensation of pain. A rudimentary brain stem may be present, supporting reflexive breathing and cardiac function, but the child's condition is not compatible with life. Most are stillborn, and others live a few hours or days. There is no treatment possible other than supportive care until death. The condition is often diagnosed with ultrasound. An ethical dilemma exists about the use of these infants' organs for donation, with some authorities believing that viable organs should be harvested before brain death.

Encephalocele

Encephalocele is a neural defect that involves a bony defect and herniation of the brain and/or cerebrospinal fluid through part of the skull in a skin-covered sac. In the United States, most commonly the mass is midline in the occipital and occasionally the frontal area. The **encephalocele** may be as large as the skull or may look like a small nasal polyp. In many cases, other abnormalities may exist, so thorough examination, including angiography and MRI, are usually required. Often, the part of the brain that herniates is disorganized, so the condition may be associated with cognitive impairment, although in mild cases the child has normal mentation. Surgical repair to place the herniated mass inside the skull and to repair the bony defect is the standard treatment. If the sac is left in place, the skin can erode, resulting in meningitis.

Neonatal Seizures

Causes

Causes of neonatal seizures are listed below, roughly in order of frequency:

- **Hypoxic-ischemic encephalopathy** after a difficult or traumatic delivery
- **Metabolic abnormality**:
    - Low levels of glucose, calcium, or magnesium
    - Elevated or low levels of sodium
- **Infections**:
    - Bacterial meningitis caused by Group B strep, *E. coli, S. pneumoniae*, or Listeria
    - Viral encephalitis caused by herpes simplex, cytomegalovirus, or enterovirus
- **Cerebrovascular accidents**:
    - Intraventricular hemorrhage
    - Subarachnoid hemorrhage
    - Subdural hematoma
    - Sinus thrombosis
- **Seizure syndromes**:
    - Epileptic encephalopathies (early myoclonic or early infantile)
    - Benign neonatal seizure syndromes, such as benign familial neonatal convulsions, benign idiopathic neonatal seizures, or benign sleep myoclonus

Types

Seizures indicate an abnormality of the central nervous system and are differentiated by their associated abnormal movements:

- **Subtle seizures** are more common in full-term infants, who present with feet pedaling, chewing, apnea, eye movements, or a blank stare.
- **Tonic seizures** are more common in preterm infants, who present with tonic flexion or extension of the limbs, which may be focal (one limb) or generalized.
- **Clonic seizures** occur primarily in full-term infants, indicate a focal cerebral injury, and involve slow, clonic movements (1-3 movements per second), often in one extremity or on one side of the body.
- **Myoclonic seizures** are rare in neonates and may be focal, multi-focal, or generalized, with rapid jerking movements of the extremities.

Treatment depends upon identifying underlying cause but may include glucose (if related to hypoglycemia), phenobarbital (drug of choice), fosphenytoin, and phenytoin.

Review Video: Seizures
Visit mometrix.com/academy and enter code: 977061

Initial Management

Seizures in the neonate require immediate treatment to avoid brain injury from hypoxia and hypoglycemia:

- Glucose (10% solution) if indicated for hypoglycemia with bolus 2 mL/kg and maintenance ≤8 mL/kg.
- Provide supplemental oxygen and ventilation.
- Give a loading dose of phenobarbital (20 mg/kg IV); if the initial loading dose is ineffective, give an additional 10-20 mg/kg IV.
- Draw STAT blood glucose and electrolyte levels.
- Correct electrolyte abnormalities such as low calcium, magnesium, and sodium.
- Give a maintenance dose of 4-6 mg/kg of phenobarbital IV every 12-24 hours.
- Monitor blood pressure and respiratory status frequently, because large doses of phenobarbital cause respiratory and cardiac depression.
- Give fosphenytoin, phenytoin, and lorazepam per order if seizures are uncontrolled.

Jitteriness

Jitteriness (tremor of chin and extremities) occurs in about half of neonates within the first few days of life and may persist intermittently when the child is excited or crying for ≤2 months. Jitteriness may also be present with drug withdrawal, hypoglycemia, hypocalcemia, and encephalopathy. Jitteriness must be differentiated from seizures, which may have a similar appearance. **Characteristics of jitteriness** include:

- There is a lack of ocular deviation or other abnormalities.
- Gentle restraint halts jitteriness.
- Stimulation elicits jitteriness.
- Clonic jerking has both fast and slow elements.
- Autonomic changes involving the heart rate, respirations, and blood pressure are not present.
- EEG is normal.

Jitteriness is distinct from shuddering, a 10-15 second period of fast tremors that may recur ≤100 times daily. Both jitteriness and shuddering are benign conditions that require no treatment.

Monitoring Neonatal Brain Activity Using aEEG

Amplitude-integrated electroencephalography (aEEG) is a continuous method of monitoring brain function and seizure activity in critically ill or preterm neonates, especially those with suspected hypoxic-ischemic encephalopathy. For the aEEG, usually 2–4 electrodes are placed on the scalp to record brain waves. The signals are processed and compressed to emphasize the brain wave amplitude over time. The tracing on the screen is time-compressed so that several hours of brain activity are displayed on a single screen. Abnormal aEEG patterns include:

- Burst suppression: low activity (suppression) with bursts of high activity, representing severe brain injury.
- Continuous low voltage: low amplitude, representing significant brain dysfunction
- Isoelectric: flat tracing, no detectable brain activity
- Repetitive spikes/sharp waves: seizure activity

If an abnormal aEEG pattern develops, then a cEEG (continuous electroencephalography) is often done because it provides more comprehensive information about brain activity. The cEEG is usually done for 24 hours or longer with 19–21 scalp electrodes applied.

Near-Infrared Spectroscopy (NIRS) Monitoring

Near-infrared spectroscopy (NIRS) is a noninvasive device to measure tissue oxygenation and hemodynamics, primarily cerebral, renal, and intestinal oxygenation in neonates. The NIRS device emits near-infrared light that passes through the tissue and is absorbed by different tissues at different wavelengths. Sensors detect the amount of light absorbed and calculate concentrations of oxyhemoglobin and deoxyhemoglobin. NIRS measures oxygen saturation at 2–3 cm below the sensors, so deeper tissues may not be assessed accurately. NIRS is used most commonly to assess cerebral oxygenation but is also used to detect hypoxia and to assess perfusion, such as during cardiac surgery. NIRS can be used to guide interventions for neonates with hypoxic-ischemic encephalopathy. Normal regional oxygen saturation (rSO_2) in cerebral tissue is 55–85%. Lower than normal rSO_2 is associated with hypoxia while higher than normal rSO_2 indicates hyperoxia and risk for retinopathy of prematurity.

Therapeutic Hypothermia

Therapeutic hypothermia for the neonate is used for neuroprotection to prevent neonatal asphyxia leading to severe hypoxic-ischemic encephalopathy. The temperature of deep brain structures is lowered to 33-34 °C through the whole body, hypothermia or head cooling only (CoolCap). **Therapeutic hypothermia** should be initiated within 6 hours after resuscitation for neonates ≥35 weeks with moderate to severe HIE. Other indications include fetal heart disorders, fetal anemia, meconium in amniotic fluid, SGA, LGA, and maternal prenatal hypoxemia. Criteria includes asphyxia as evidenced by Apgar ≤5 after 10 minutes. The goal of hypothermia is to reach the target temperature within 60 minutes. Cooling is typically carried out for about 72 hours followed by 12 hours of rewarming. The neonate must receive sedation and ventilatory support to ensure oxygen levels and ventilation are adequate. The neonate must be monitored carefully (ECG, BP, oxygen saturation, $ETCO_2$). The heart rate normally decreases about 15 bpm per 1 °C decrease, so bradycardia may occur. Temperature must be constantly monitored and temperature alarms set. EEG and neurological monitoring may be necessary because almost half of infants with HIE have seizures during cooling, especially during the first 48 hours. Fluids are limited to 40-60 mL/kg/day.

Birth-Related Nerve Trauma

Cranial Nerve Trauma

Injury to cranial nerves can occur during birth (most commonly the recurrent laryngeal nerve) and is caused by compression of the head against the sacrum during birth or from the use of forceps. Symptoms relate to the specific type of nerve injury but may present as temporary or permanent paralysis. Often asymmetry, drooping of the eye or mouth, or failure of the eyelid to close is noted, especially when the infant cries. Traumatic injury to nerves usually resolves over time, beginning by the end of the first week but symptoms may persist to some degree for months. An open eye must be protected by the use of synthetic tears and patching to prevent damage. Those with injury to the laryngeal nerve may have dyspnea and dysphagia and may require small frequent feedings or enteral feedings until the condition resolves. In most cases, treatment is symptomatic with careful observation so that complications can be treated promptly.

Brachial Plexus Trauma

Trauma to the brachial plexus may cause a full-term infant to hold his or her arm adducted and internally rotated after a delivery complicated by shoulder dystocia. There is movement in the hands. About 1-3 infants per 1,000 live births suffer **trauma to the brachial plexus**. The brachial plexus is a collection of nerve tissue located in the shoulder area that is the pathway for nerves traveling from the spine to the arm and shoulder. These nerves control the movement of the shoulder and arm. Most commonly, the upper portion of this plexus is damaged, leading to weak arm muscles (Erb's palsy). When examined, the infant holds the arm adducted and internally rotated. The startle reflex is abnormal on the affected side, but the grasp reflex is normal. If the lower portion of the plexus is damaged, the hand is paralyzed also, and the grasp reflex is absent (Klumpke's paralysis). Most infants recover fully, but recovery depends on the degree of damage to the brachial plexus (complete tear vs. stretching).

Gastrointestinal Complications

Development of GI Tract

The **gastrointestinal (GI) tract** is anatomically complete by about 24 weeks gestation but functional development continues through 36-38 weeks:

- Fetal swallowing of amniotic fluid begins at about 11 weeks gestation.
- Peristalsis begins at 28-30 weeks. In the preterm infant, it is bidirectional, so milk is not propelled toward the stomach. With normal peristalsis, meconium should pass within 24 hours of birth, but this is delayed in preterm infants.
- The cardiac sphincter and neural control of the stomach are immature at birth, resulting in frequent regurgitation.
- Coordination of sucking and swallowing begins at 33-36 weeks.
- Enzymatic activity and ability to transport nutrients matures by 36-38 weeks.
- Salivary glands are inactive until 3 months.
- Lactase deficiency causes poor carbohydrate digestion, pancreatic lipase deficiency causes poor fat digestion (10-20% excreted), but protein digestion is good.
- Bowel sounds are evident 30-60 minutes after birth. Stomach capacity is 50-60 mL, and emptying time is 2-4 hours.

Short Bowel Syndrome

The neonate's small bowel is approximately 250 cm long. Most absorption of nutrients and vitamins takes place in the first 100-150 cm of the jejunum while the ileum absorbs vitamin B_{12} and bile acids. Infants with less than 100 cm of jejunum after surgical removal have significant malabsorption and require aggressive nutritional support. Infants with **short bowel syndrome** (SBS) have diarrhea, steatorrhea, bloating, anemia, electrolyte imbalances, malnutrition, and poor weight gain secondary to decreased absorption of nutrients and vitamins. The severity and exact nature of their symptoms depend on the amount and type of bowel that has been removed. Removal of significant portions of the ileum results in steatorrhea and poor absorption of fat-soluble vitamins (K, A, D, E) and vitamin B_{12}. Removal of significant portions of the jejunum results in poor absorption of calories, proteins, carbohydrates, and fats. Infants require careful monitoring of serum electrolytes, multivitamins, and a combination of parenteral and enteral nutrition. Over time, the small bowel adapts, increases its absorption, and grows in length.

Sucking and Swallowing Disorders

Sucking and swallowing disorders are very common in the preterm infant because of immaturity (coordination of sucking and swallowing occurs at 33-36 weeks) but may be caused in term infants by a number of conditions, including trisomy 21, FAS, cleft palate, central nervous system disorders (anoxia, hydrocephalus), congenital infection (rubella, cytomegalovirus), respiratory disorders (apnea, pneumonia, RDS), and cardiac or ENT anomalies. Typical characteristics of swallowing disorders include:

- Silent aspiration (not associated with cough or clearing airway)
- Laryngeal penetration (associated with lack of pharyngeal response)
- Nasopharyngeal reflux (especially common in preterm infants and may trigger apnea)

Pneumonia frequently develops in infants with sucking and swallowing disorders, so diagnosing the cause is critical. Observation is not sufficient because of the frequency of silent aspiration. Feeding infants in the upright position can reduce nasopharyngeal reflux. Tests include radiographic (videofluoroscopy) or fiberoptic evaluation of swallowing.

Hirschsprung's Disease

Hirschsprung's disease (congenital aganglionic megacolon) is failure of **ganglion nerve cells** to migrate to part of the bowel, usually the distal colon, so that part of the bowel lacks enervation and peristalsis, causing stool to accumulate, leading to **distension** and **megacolon**. There is a genetic predisposition to the disease that affects more males than females and is associated with trisomy 21 (Down syndrome).

Symptoms include:

- Failure to pass meconium in 24-48 hours
- Poor feeding
- Bilious vomitus
- Abdominal distension

Delayed diagnosis includes:

- Chronic constipation
- Failure to thrive
- Periods of diarrhea and vomiting
- With infection—severe prostration, watery diarrhea, fever, and hypotension

Treatment includes:

- Resection aganglionic section and perform colorectal anastomosis
- There are a number of procedures—Swenson, Duhamel, and Soave—but recently, minimally invasive laparoscopic or transanal approaches have proven successful

Gastroesophageal Reflux

Gastroesophageal reflux (GER) is involuntary regurgitation of stomach contents into the esophagus, usually caused by decreased tone in the lower esophageal sphincter in neonates, especially preterm.

Symptoms include:

- Frequent non-bilious regurgitation (especially after feeding, usually not associated with respiratory distress)
- Some neonates may have colicky symptoms, and some may cough, choke, wheeze or have periods of apnea

Treatment includes:

- **Regulating feeding**: Small, more frequent amounts, thickened with rice cereal. Continuous gavage rather than bolus may reduce reflux.
- **Positioning**: Prone positioning after feeding/eating reduces regurgitation (although some concern remains about SIDS with neonates). Placing the neonate in an upright position (avoiding slumping) after meals or carrying the neonate upright can help, but placing in infant seat position may increase intraabdominal pressure.
- **Medications:** Medications are only recommended in severe cases. Histamine-2 receptor blockers (famotidine) or proton pump inhibitors (omeprazole) may be used short term.
- **Surgery:** Considered for severe or life-threatening symptoms.

Malrotation/Volvulus

During weeks 4-8 of embryonic development, the GI tract is rapidly expanding and the abdominal cavity cannot accommodate it. Therefore, part of the intestinal loop buckles into the yolk stalk area, which will be the future umbilicus. As the intestinal loop buckles out of the abdomen, it begins a normal rotation of the bowel. As it continues to grow and returns to the abdomen during weeks 8-10, there is additional rotation occurring until it is situated into the anatomically correct position. Sometimes this rotation fails, and the result is a malrotation. **Malrotation** is a congenital defect in which the intestines are attached to the back of the abdominal wall by one single attachment, rather than a broad band of attachments across the abdomen, essentially suspending the bowels so they can easily twist, resulting in a **volvulus** (twisted bowel), cutting off blood supply. It may untwist but can lead to **bowel infarction.** Some children with malrotation have no symptoms, but most develop some of these **symptoms** by 1 year:

- Cycles of cramping pain about every 15-30 minutes
- Abdominal distension
- Diarrhea, bloody stools, or no stools
- Vomiting, occurring soon after crying begins, usually indicating small intestine obstruction; later vomiting usually indicative of large intestine blockage
- Tachycardia and tachypnea
- Decreased urinary output
- Fever

Treatment is by surgical repair.

Midgut Volvulus

A midgut volvulus is twisting of the bowel from the second portion of the duodenum to the mid-transverse colon around its mesenteric attachments. Signs depend on the extent of compromised blood flow to the bowel, blockage of lymphatic drainage, and obstruction of intestinal contents. **Signs** include bilious vomiting, gastric distension, rapid clinical deterioration, and shock. Midgut volvulus is usually secondary to congenital malrotation of the intestines. If this is the case, then it often presents during the first week of life, with complete obstruction and severe symptoms. Mortality rates range from 3-15%. The infant's prognosis depends on the amount of ischemic bowel and the length of time that elapsed before the volvulus was diagnosed and treated.

Imperforate Anus

Imperforate anus (anorectal malfunction) is a congenital abnormality in which the **rectum is absent, malformed, or displaced** from normal position. It may include disorders of the urinary tract. Imperforate anus occurs in 1 in 5000 births, more commonly in males than females. Imperforate anus may include stenosis or atresia of the anus. There are 3 main **categories**, classified according to the relationship of the rectum to the puborectalis musculature:

- **Low anomalies:** no external opening, but rectum otherwise in normal position through the puborectalis muscle, with normal function and no connection to the genitourinary tract.
- **Intermediate anomalies:** rectum at or below the level of puborectalis muscle, anal dimple evident, and external sphincter in normal position.
- **High anomalies:** rectum ending above the puborectalis muscles, internal sphincter absent often with a rectourethral fistula in males or a rectovaginal fistula in females, and sometimes fistulas to the bladder or perineum.

Diagnosis, Symptoms, and Treatment

Imperforate anus is **diagnosed** by physical examination, digital or endoscopic examination, and contrast radiography with the infant inverted. An opaque marker at the anal dimple will outline the location of a pouch in relation to the normal position of the anus.

Symptoms include:

- Absence of anal opening, no meconium in 24-48 hours, abdominal distension, and vomiting
- Rectovaginal fistula or rectourethral fistula (may not be evident at first because stool passes through fistula)
- Fistula between the rectum and the bladder with gas or fecal material possibly expelled through the urethra
- Displacement of the anus, with chronic constipation developing over time

Treatment includes:

Surgery performed in most cases, type depending upon extent of abnormality:

- With low anomalies, simple excision of anal opening
- Two- or three-step procedure for higher anomalies; colostomy first, with later reconstruction of the anus in the proper position, involving anoplasty and pull-through procedures
- Manual dilation to treat stenosis

Intestinal Atresia

When a portion of the bowel comes to a stop and then starts back up again forming a discontinuous or segmented bowel, this is called **intestinal atresia.** This condition usually relates to failures during the 5th to 10th week of fetal development, so it is often associated with other anomalies. The most common site for atresia to occur in the neonate is the duodenum. Atresia can also occur in the ileum, jejunum, colon, and even rarely the stomach. An atresia that occurs anywhere in the intestine except the duodenum is not associated with any other disorders. However, an atresia that occurs in the duodenum (the most common type) is usually (30% of the time) associated with other disorders such as trisomy 21, congenital heart disease, and VACTERL association. (VACTERL stands for **v**ertebral defects, **a**nal atresia, **c**ardiac defects, **t**rachea-**e**sophageal fistula, **r**enal anomalies, and **l**imb abnormalities.) The only treatment for intestinal atresia is surgical reconnection of the bowel.

Duodenal Atresia

Duodenal atresia occurs when the duodenum fails to correctly form in the fetus. Often, duodenal atresia is discovered prenatally via ultrasound examination. Neonates with **duodenal atresia** vomit within hours after birth. The vomitus may or may not be bilious, depending on the exact location of the defect. The infant may have a scaphoid abdomen and usually passes meconium. X-rays often show the "double-bubble" sign: The distended stomach is the first bubble and the distended duodenum proximal to the defect is the second bubble. One-third of all patients with duodenal atresia also have Down syndrome. An orogastric tube is immediately placed to relieve the abdominal distension, and IV fluids and TPN nutrition are administered. When IV hydration is delayed, infants with duodenal atresia often develop hypokalemia, hypochloremia, and metabolic alkalosis. Definitive treatment is surgical repair.

Esophageal Atresia and Tracheoesophageal Fistula

Esophageal atresia often occurs with tracheoesophageal fistula (TEF). In esophageal atresia, the esophagus has a blind pouch and does not completely pass to the stomach. In TEF, an abnormal connection is present between the trachea and the esophagus. A congenital tracheoesophageal fistula (TEF) is present in 1 out of every 2,000-4,000 live births. There are 5 different **types of TEF**:

- **Esophageal atresia with distal TEF** (87%) is the most common type. The proximal esophagus ends in a blind pouch and the distal esophagus is connected to the trachea.
- **Isolated esophageal atresia without TEF** (8%), where the proximal esophagus ends in a pouch and there is no connection with the trachea.
- **Isolated TEF** (4%), where the esophagus is patent, traveling to the stomach with a fistula from the esophagus to the trachea. It is also called "H" type because of its resemblance to the letter H.
- **Esophageal atresia with proximal TEF** (1%), where the proximal esophagus connects with the trachea and there is no connection to the distal esophagus.
- **Esophageal atresia with proximal and distal TEF** (1%), where both the proximal and the distal esophagus connect with the trachea.

Infants born with tracheoesophageal fistula (TEF) are often diagnosed prenatally with ultrasound. TEF is often associated with polyhydramnios, as esophageal atresia prevents the fetus from swallowing amniotic fluid. Infants born with TEF have **symptoms** that include:

- Fine, white, frothy bubbles of mucous in the mouth and nose
- Copious secretions, despite suctioning
- Episodes of coughing, choking, and cyanosis that worsen with feeds
- Associated genetic anomalies, such as trisomy 13, 18, or 21
- Other digestive tract problems, heart problems, or kidney and urinary tract problems

Bowel Obstructions

Bowel obstruction occurs when there is a mechanical obstruction of the **passage of intestinal contents** because of constriction of the lumen, occlusion of the lumen, or lack of muscular contractions (paralytic ileus). Obstruction may be caused by congenital or acquired abnormalities/disorders:

Small Bowel Obstructions:

- Duodenal atresia
- Malrotation and volvulus
- Jejunoileal atresia
- Meconium ileus
- Meconium peritonitis

Large Bowel Obstructions:

- Hirschsprung disease
- Anorectal malformations
- Meconium plug syndrome

Symptoms include:

- Abdominal pain, distension, and rigidity
- Vomiting and dehydration
- Diminished or no bowel sounds
- Severe constipation (obstipation)
- Respiratory distress from diaphragm pushing against pleural cavity
- Shock, as plasma volume diminishes and electrolytes enter intestines from bloodstream
- Sepsis, as bacteria proliferate in the bowel and invade the bloodstream

Hypertrophic Pyloric Stenosis

Hypertrophic pyloric stenosis (PS) is obstruction of the pyloric sphincter between the gastric pylorus and small intestine, caused by hypertrophy and hyperplasia of the circular muscle of the pylorus so the enlarged tissue obstructs the sphincter. PS is more common in boys than girls and has a genetic predisposition. Onset of **symptoms** is usually >3weeks:

- Projectile vomiting (1-4 feet) usually shortly after eating but may be delayed for a few hours. Emesis may be blood-tinged but non-bilious
- Infant is hungry and eats readily, but shows weight loss and signs of dehydration
- Upper abdominal distension with palpable mass in epigastrium (to right of umbilicus)
- Visible left to right peristaltic waves

Diagnosis is based on ultrasound. Decreased sodium and potassium levels may not be evident with dehydration.

Treatment includes:

- Intravenous fluids to restore hydration and electrolyte balance
- Surgical pyloromyotomy: longitudinal incisions through the circular muscle fibers down to the submucosa to release the restriction and allow the muscle to expand

Meconium Plug Syndrome

Meconium plug syndrome (also called functional colonic obstruction) occurs when the first stool obstructs the intestinal tract and no other pathology is present. This will be evident in the first 24 to 48 hours of life, when the infant fails to pass the first meconium stool. Meconium plug syndrome usually occurs in full-term infants, infants of diabetic mothers, or infants with hypermagnesemia. The infant may have abdominal distension, poor feeding, and vomiting (often bilious in nature). An x-ray of the abdomen will show dilated loops of bowel. A contrast enema is diagnostic and helps differentiate from other causes of intestinal obstruction. It may also be therapeutic, causing the plug to pass. Infants usually do well after the plug has passed. A small percentage of infants initially identified as having meconium plug syndrome (5 to 10%) have Hirschsprung disease. The cause of meconium plug syndrome is thought to be immaturity of the ganglion cells of the colon.

Meconium Ileus Caused by Cystic Fibrosis

Cystic fibrosis is a congenital disease associated with the collection of thick mucus in the **lungs and intestines**. **Meconium ileus** is obstruction of the ileum with inspissated (thick) mucilaginous meconium that clings to the side of the narrowed lumen of the intestine and forms hard pellets (usually the first clinical sign of cystic fibrosis). The mucus interferes with the absorption of fat, protein, carbohydrates, and other nutrients, leading to malabsorption syndromes. **Diagnosis** is by abdominal x-rays to show air-to-fluid levels and contrast enemas to show obstruction.

Symptoms include:

- **Uncomplicated: abdominal distension, vomiting, no meconium in the first 24-48 hours**
- **Complicated** (may include volvulus, gangrene, perforations, or bowel atresia): pain, fever, erythema, and edema of abdominal wall consistent with peritonitis

Treatment includes:

- Contrast enema with water-soluble contrast (may relieve obstruction by emulsifying fecal material)
- 10-15 mL small volume enemas to flush stool, especially after contrast enema
- Enterotomy, with proximal instillation of wetting agent
- Resection of colon/fecal diversion for perforated or gangrenous bowel
- High protein diet with pancreatic enzyme supplementation

Necrotizing Enterocolitis

Necrotizing enterocolitis (NEC) is the most common gastrointestinal emergency in premature neonates. Seventy-five percent of neonates who develop NEC are less than 37 weeks gestation and weigh less than 2,000 grams. NEC is rare in healthy, full term infants. NEC is an acute necrosis (death of cells) in a bowel segment anywhere from the stomach to the rectum. Inflammation, bacterial invasion, and perforation often occur. NEC is fatal in up to 30% of cases. Risk factors other than prematurity and size should trigger careful observation. These risk factors include:

- **Prenatal**
    - Maternal age >35 years
    - Maternal cocaine use
    - Maternal infection requiring antibiotics
- **Perinatal**
    - Birth asphyxia
    - Respiratory distress syndrome
    - Systemic hypotension
    - Depressed 5-minute Apgar score
- **Postnatal**
    - Congestive heart failure
    - Use of hyperosmolar formula
    - Patent ductus arteriosus
    - Umbilical artery catheterization

The causes of necrotizing enterocolitis (NEC) are not completely understood, but it appears to be related to an ischemic episode, colonization by bacteria, and excess/rapid enteral feedings.

Symptoms include:

- Gastric retention, abdominal distension, and vomiting (bilious)
- Periods of apnea
- Occult or frank blood (25%) in stool
- Pneumatosis intestinalis (gas in intestinal wall) (75%)
- Portal venous gas (10-30%)
- Decrease in urinary output
- Jaundice
- Unstable temperature

Treatment includes:

- Cessation of oral feeding
- NG decompression
- Systemic antibiotics
- Correcting fluid and electrolyte imbalance
- Surgical repair with bowel resection may be necessary

Diastasis of Recti Muscles

Diastasis of the recti muscles is a postnatal maternal condition in which the abdominal muscles, specifically the rectus abdominis muscles (that have separated during pregnancy) remain separated. The pressure of the expanding fetus causes the connective tissue to stretch between the vertically running muscles and often after birth, the tissue slowly heals and the separation closes. When the connective tissue does not heal fully within 6 months, the gap can become permanent. This condition can lead to lower back pain, pain during intercourse, incontinence, or constipation in the mother. Diastasis of the recti muscles can be treated with specific physical therapy. Traditional abdominal crunches are avoided as a treatment because they may worsen the condition by making the muscles tighter in the separated position. Abdominal exercises during pregnancy are recommended as preventative measures. Surgical closure is a treatment option for extreme cases.

Neonatal Umbilical Hernia

Umbilical hernia is a skin-covered herniation of intestine and omentum through an abdominal wall defect near the umbilicus caused by an incomplete closure of the umbilical ring. The herniation may range from 1-5 cm in size and may be obvious on physical examination or felt on palpation. It may appear flat when the infant is supine but protrude when the infant is upright or crying. Approximately 1 in 6 infants are born with umbilical hernias. Symptoms are usually absent unless strangulation of the hernia occurs, and then the infant may cry with pain, feed poorly, vomit, and have an increase in temperature. The abdomen may become distended. In this case, emergency surgical repair must be done. Treatment usually involves just observing the hernia for complications as, in most cases, it will reduce on its own. If the hernia is still present at 3-4 years, a simple surgical repair of the hernia may be done.

Gastroschisis

Gastroschisis is extrusion of the non-rotated midgut through the abdominal wall to the right of umbilicus with no protective membrane covering matted, thickened loops of intestine. The abnormality is usually small, but the stomach and almost all of the small and large intestines can protrude. Because the intestines float without protection in amniotic fluid, there may be severe damage to the intestines with bowel atresia and ischemia. Gastroschisis is usually diagnosed with fetal ultrasound and is obvious at birth. These infants lose body temperature, fluids, and electrolytes and receive intravenous fluids. The exposed organs are covered with sterile plastic film for protection and to prevent fluid loss and a nasogastric feeding tube is inserted. Primary closure is done when the infant stabilizes for small abnormalities. Larger abnormalities may require stages with only part of organs returned to the cavity and the remaining covered with a Silastic pouch until the abdominal cavity grows and surgical repair can be completed.

Omphalocele

Omphalocele is a congenital herniation of intestines or other organs through the base of the umbilicus with a protecting amniotic membrane but no skin. The sac may contain only a loop or most of the bowel and the internal abdominal organs. This sac differentiates gastroschisis from omphalocele. Diagnosis is usually with fetal ultrasound.

Symptoms vary widely. Maintaining integrity of tissues by keeping exposed sac or viscera moist and providing intravenous fluids is important. Small omphaloceles are repaired immediately, but more extensive repair is usually delayed until the infant is stable if sac is intact. Silvadene cream toughens the sac, which is usually covered with a Silastic (plastic) pouch to protect the tissue. The abdomen may be unusually small, making correction difficult, so surgeons may wait 6-12 months while the abdominal cavity grows. Surgical repair may be done in stages over 8-10 days.

Hematologic Complications

ABO Incompatibility

About 20-25% of pregnancies involve ABO incompatibility, usually with the mother type O and the fetus A or B. **Anti-A and anti-B antibodies** occur naturally when a woman is exposed to A and B antigens in foods or bacteria, so these antibodies can cross the placenta and result in **hemolysis of fetal RBC**; however, the antibodies are relatively large and do not enter the fetal circulation easily. If fetal blood leaks into maternal blood (a common occurrence), then smaller antibodies form and these can cross the placenta more easily. There is no difference in effect between the first pregnancy and subsequent pregnancies. There are rarely serious complications for the fetus, although the neonate may develop hyperbilirubinemia, so the infant should be observed carefully. Only in severe cases of hemolysis (rare), does the child require exchange transfusions. Anemia may develop in the weeks after delivery because of increased rate of RBC breakdown, so the neonate should be monitored with blood counts.

Maternal Rh Alloimmunization

Rh incompatibility occurs if the mother is Rh- and the father is Rh+, putting their infant at risk for hemolytic disease of the newborn (HDN) or Rh disease, (erythroblastosis fetalis). **Rh alloimmunization** (formation of antibodies against foreign antigens) can occur during abortion, abruptio placenta, amniocentesis, Cesarean section, chorionic villus sampling, cordocentesis, delivery, ectopic pregnancy, and toxemia. To prevent erythroblastosis fetalis, a woman who is Rh- with an Rh+ mate receives the serum **RhoGAM**, containing anti Rh+ antibodies. The purpose of the antibodies is to agglutinate any fetal red blood cells that pass over into the mother's circulatory system and thus prevent the mother from forming antibodies against them that will attack the infant and sensitize her for future pregnancies. Testing and administration of RhoGAM is as follows:

- Order Rh(D) tests. If the mother is Rh- and the father is Rh+, then their infant is at risk for hemolytic disease of the newborn (HDN).
- Order an antibody screen of the mother's blood to find out if she acquired anti-D antibodies from a previous blood transfusion or pregnancy.
- The mother receives 300 mcg RhoGAM (Rhlg, Rh immunoglobulin) intramuscularly at 26-28 weeks of pregnancy and again within 72 hours after her delivery. Do not inject the infant or father. RhoGAM prevents Rh+ cells from the infant that have crossed over to the mother from causing her to create anti-D antibodies that will attack the infant and sensitize her for future pregnancies.
- Miscarriage, ectopic, abortion: At ≤12 weeks, the mother receives 50 mcg of MICRhoGAM. At ≥13 weeks, the mother receives RhoGAM as for pregnancy.

Blood-Loss Anemia

Blood loss is the most common cause of anemia in the neonate. Anemia is hematocrit or hemoglobin level >2 standard deviations below the mean for age. For a term infant, anemia is a hematocrit <45%. The loss of blood may be internal or external, and may occur in utero, during delivery, or post-delivery. **Treatment** may include packed red blood cell transfusions. Common **causes** of neonatal blood loss include:

Antenatal

- Abruptio placentae or placenta previa
- Fetomaternal transfusion (passage of fetal blood to the mother)
- Twin-to-twin transfusion, resulting in one twin with polycythemia and the donor twin with anemia

Perinatal

- Trauma to the placenta or umbilical cord
- Rupture of anomalous cord vessels
- Fetoplacental transfusion that occurs when the infant is positioned above the level of the placenta after delivery

Postnatal

- Internal hemorrhage, such as intracranial hemorrhage or cephalohematoma
- Damage to internal organs, such as the adrenal gland or liver
- Iatrogenic blood loss secondary to frequent laboratory sampling, a major cause of anemia in premature infants

Anemia of Prematurity

Anemia of prematurity (AOP) represents a pathologic exaggeration of the normal decrease in hematocrit that occurs in every newborn. AOP results from a combination of factors:

- **RBC production** decreases because the premature neonate's response to erythropoietin (EPO) has not matured. EPO is the main stimulus for RBC production. The normal progression of EPO production in the fetus is for the liver to initially be the primary site, with transfer to the kidney as the primary site of production in the full-term neonate. The liver is less responsive to hypoxia and allows for a lower threshold of anemia to progress until EPO production is increased. Lowest Hgb levels are usually at 2-3 months of age.
- **Premature RBCs have a shortened lifespan** when compared to the full-term neonate's because of decreased levels of intracellular ATP and enzyme activity.
- **Frequent blood draws** in premature neonates required for close monitoring deplete the blood supply.

Infants with signs of hypoxemia (poor feeling, tachypnea, tachycardia, pallor) may require transfusions.

Anemia of Red Blood Cell Destruction

Causes of anemia of red blood cell destruction are discussed below:

- **Intrinsic causes**—continued production of abnormal red blood cells that have a decreased survival time because of rare hereditary disorders:
  - **RBC enzyme defects**, such as G6PD deficiency, where hemolytic crisis occurs in response to drugs such as sulfonamide antibiotics, or infections
  - **RBC membrane defects**, such as hereditary spherocytosis, where abnormally-shaped red cells are prone to hemolysis
  - **Hemoglobinopathies**, such as thalassemia, which results in the reduced production of one of the protein chains that make up hemoglobin
- **Extrinsic causes**—temporary RBC destruction caused by some external stimulus:
  - **Immune hemolysis** from transfusion of an incompatible blood product (wrong Rh, ABO, or a minor blood group incompatibility)
  - **Acquired hemolysis** from infection, vitamin E deficiency, or poisoning

Polycythemia

Polycythemia is a hematocrit greater than 65%. An elevated hematocrit means that the blood has less plasma and more cellular elements, increasing the viscosity of the blood. Increased blood viscosity results in slowed blood flow and sludging of red blood cells. Small vessels become occluded with microthrombi, resulting in tissue or organ ischemia. **Clinical signs of polycythemia** include:

- **Dermatologic**: plethora and increased capillary refill time
- **CNS**: lethargy, irritability, abnormal cry, cerebrovascular hemorrhage, and seizures
- **Pulmonary**: respiratory distress, cyanosis, apnea, and the development of persistent pulmonary hypertension
- **Renal**: hematuria, oliguria, and renal vein thrombosis
- **Hematological**: thrombocytopenia secondary to the development of disseminated intravascular coagulation
- **Gastrointestinal**: abdominal distension, poor feeding, bloody stools, and necrotizing enterocolitis
- **Metabolic**: persistent hypoglycemia and hypocalcemia

RISK FACTORS

Polycythemia occurs in 4% of live-born infants. Its **etiologies** are divided into conditions that cause hypoxia and increased RBC production and those that cause abnormal transfer of RBCs to the neonate (hypertransfusion):

- **Hypoxia**
  - Disorders that disrupt normal placental function and decrease oxygen delivery to the fetus include preeclampsia, chronic placental abruption, maternal congenital heart disease, postdate pregnancy, and maternal smoking. Many of these are also associated with a growth-restricted neonate (IUGR).
  - Disorders that cause increased oxygen consumption by the fetus include infants of diabetic mothers and those with Beckwith-Wiedemann syndrome. Polycythemia occurs in 30 to 40% of neonates born to mothers with diabetes.
- **Hypertransfusion**
  - Delay in clamping the umbilical cord during delivery allows for increased blood volume to be transferred to the neonate.
  - Twin-twin transfusion creates one twin who is anemic and the second twin with an increased hematocrit in 10% of monozygotic twin pregnancies.

EXCHANGE TRANSFUSIONS

The infant with polycythemia requires a **partial exchange transfusion** with a plasma substitute in these situations:

- The hematocrit is greater than 65%, and the infant is symptomatic
- The hematocrit is greater than 70%, regardless of symptoms

Aliquots of the neonate's blood are replaced with isotonic saline to lower the hematocrit (Hct) to 50-55%. This formula calculates the volume of blood to be exchanged with an equal volume of saline:

$$\text{Exchange vol (mL)} = \frac{\text{initial Hct} - \text{desired Hct}}{\text{initial Hct}} \times \text{weight(kg)} \times 90\frac{\text{mL}}{\text{kg}}$$

The **procedure** is described below:

1. Withdraw no more than 5 mL of blood at a time from the umbilical artery or vein over 2-3 minutes.
2. Slowly infuse an equal amount of sterile normal saline.
3. Repeat the exchange until the desired volume of fluid is swapped.
4. Monitor the infant closely during the procedure.
5. Measure the hematocrit post procedure.

Thrombocytosis

Thrombocytosis is an increase in the platelet level >450,000/mcL; however, preterm infants often exhibit platelet levels of up to 600,000/mcL at 4-6 weeks. The normal reference range for platelets (thrombocytes) is 150,000-400,000/mcL. Thrombocytosis does not require specific treatment, but the underlying cause should be identified and treated. Neonates rarely have symptoms directly related to increased platelet count, but may experience cerebral ischemia with levels higher than 2,000,000/mcL. Treatment is aimed at the underlying cause. Almost all incidences of thrombocytosis in infants are secondary or reactive. **Common causes of thrombocytosis** in the neonate include:

- Infection
- Trisomy 21 (Down syndrome)
- Iron deficiency (often associated with chronic intrauterine blood loss from bleeding into a twin or GI bleeding)
- Congenital adrenal insufficiency
- Maternal abuse of narcotic drugs

Thrombocytopenia

Thrombocytopenia is a platelet count less than 150,000/mcL, caused either by decreased platelet production, increased platelet destruction, or a combination of both. Hematology labs use **mean platelet volume (MPV)**, a measure of the average platelet size, to differentiate the two. The MPV is normal if the cause is reduced production and elevated if the cause is accelerated destruction. Immature platelets are larger than normal and are released into circulating blood by the bone marrow when mature platelets are being destroyed. The lab may also differentiate the cause by a **retic count** (reticulated platelets are newly-produced platelets). If the retic count is elevated, then platelets are being destroyed, and if it is low, the production of platelets is suppressed. General guidelines for transfusing platelets depend on the clinical stability of the neonate. If the infant is stable, the attending physician considers a transfusion when the count is less than 25,000/mcL. If the infant is unstable, the attending physician considers a transfusion when the count is less than 50,000/mcL.

Fetal Onset, Early Onset, and Late Onset

Causes of **fetal onset** include:

- Alloimmune thrombocytopenia: The mother produces antibodies specific to antigens on the neonate's platelets, which cross the placenta, causing thrombocytopenia.
- Autoimmune thrombocytopenia: Mothers with idiopathic thrombocytopenia purpura or lupus produce antibodies against fetal platelets.
- Congenital infection—mediated: CMV, rubella, toxoplasmosis. Neonates with trisomy 18 or 21.

Causes of **early onset** (<72 hours) include:

- Placental insufficiency occurs in infants who are small for gestational age or with intrauterine growth restriction
- Perinatal asphyxia
- Disseminated intravascular coagulation (DIC)

Causes of **late onset** (>72 hours) include:

- Late onset sepsis
- Necrotizing enterocolitis

Hemophilia

Hemophilia is an inherited disorder in which the infant lacks adequate clotting factors. There are 3 **types**:

- Type A: Lack of clotting factor VII (90% of cases)
- Type B: Lack of clotting factor IX (about 5% of cases)
- Type C: Lack of clotting factor XI (affects both sexes, rarely occurs in the US)

Both Type A and B are usually X-linked disorders, affecting only males. The **severity** of the disease depends on the amount of clotting factor in the blood:

- Mild: >5% factor activity
- Moderate: 1-5% factor activity
- Severe: <1% factor activity

Severe neonatal hemophilia is often discovered when slow clotting is noted after circumcision or venipuncture. Approximately 1 to 2% of hemophiliacs have intracranial hemorrhage. Infants with severe hemophilia have a prolonged PTT, but normal PT values. Diagnosis is confirmed by Factor VIII and Factor IX tests.

Treatment includes:

- Desmopressin to stimulate production of clotting factor (if mild)
- Clotting factor or recombinant clotting factors (genetically-engineered)
- Plasma (Type C)

Neutropenia

Reduced neutrophils (neutropenia) indicate infection or bone marrow suppression. In neonates, the most common reasons for neutropenia are infection or stresses, such as respiratory distress syndrome, although it may be associated with congenital disorders, such as Shwachman-Diamond and Kostmann's syndrome. A segmented neutrophil nucleus (seg) is a mature cell. A banded nucleus (band) is immature. To calculate the absolute neutrophil count (ANC), the percentage of segs is added to the percentage of bands and multiplied by the total white blood cell count. A low ANC is more specific for identifying sepsis than an elevated ANC, but ANC by itself is a poor indicator of sepsis. **Normal neutrophil counts**:

- At birth the lower limit of normal is 1,750 cells/mm^3
- At 12 hours it rises to 7,200 cells/mm^3
- At 72 hours it falls to 1,720 cells/mm^3

The immature to total neutrophil ratio (I:T) is a better indicator of sepsis than ANC. An I:T ratio greater than 0.2 indicates sepsis. The formula for calculating the I:T ratio:

$$\text{I:T} = \frac{\text{immature neutrophils}}{\text{immature neutrophils} + \text{mature neutrophils}}$$

Newborn Complications

Hyperbilirubinemia

Hyperbilirubinemia, excess of bilirubin in the blood, is characterized by jaundice. Hyperbilirubinemia is evaluated according to the levels of direct (conjugated) bilirubin and/or indirect (unconjugated) bilirubin:

- **Direct/conjugated bilirubin** levels increase with blockage of bile ducts, hepatitis, or other liver damage, including drug reaction.
- **Indirect/unconjugated bilirubin** levels increase with anemias (such as hemolytic disorders) and transfusion reactions.

Four basic **types** of hyperbilirubinemia and jaundice:

- **Physiologic**: Common in newborns and usually benign, resulting from immature hepatic function and increased RBC hemolysis. Infants have larger red blood cells with a shorter life than adults, leading to more RBC destruction and resulting in an increased load of serum bilirubin, which the liver of the newborn cannot handle. Premature infants have an even greater physiologic jaundice as their RBCs live even shorter lives than the term infant's. Onset is usually within 24-48 hours, peaking in 72 hours for full-term or 5 days for preterm infants and declining within a week. Phototherapy is the indicated treatment.
- **Hemolytic**: Caused by blood/antigen (Rh) incompatibility with onset in first 24 hours. Preventive treatment is RhoGAM prenatally or post-natal exchange transfusion. This type of hyperbilirubinemia may also result from ABO incompatibility but rarely requires treatment other than phototherapy.
- **Breastfeeding associated**: Relates to inadequate calories during early breastfeeding with onset on 2-3 days. This slows the excretion of stool and allows bilirubin levels to rise. More frequent feeding with caloric supplements is usually sufficient, but phototherapy may be used for bilirubin 18-20 mg/dL.
- **Breast milk jaundice**: May result from human breast milk breaking down bilirubin and its being reabsorbed in the gut. Characterized by less frequent stools and onset in 4-5 days, jaundice peaks in 10-15 days but may persist for a number of weeks. Treatment involves discontinuing breastfeeding for 24 hours.

Kernicterus

Kernicterus (also called bilirubin encephalopathy) occurs when elevated serum bilirubin levels cause damage to the brain. The exact serum bilirubin level at which damage occurs is unknown. Premature infants are more susceptible to the development of kernicterus at lower serum bilirubin levels because of the immaturity of their blood-brain barrier, causing it to be more permeable to bilirubin than in full term infants. Disease processes, such as acidosis or meningitis, further lessen the competency of the blood-brain barrier. **Early signs of kernicterus** are divided into three phases:

- **Phase I:** Occurs during the first few days of life and is characterized by decreased alertness, hypotonia, and poor feeding.
- **Phase II:** The onset and duration of this phase is variable. Hypertonia of the extensor muscles develops. Infants may display opisthotonos (extreme hyperextension or arching of the back) and/or retrocollis (extreme arching of the neck).
- **Phase III:** This occurs generally after one week with the recurrence of hypotonia.

Review Video: Jaundice Icterus
Visit mometrix.com/academy and enter code: 339680

PHOTOTHERAPY AND EXCHANGE TRANSFUSION

Hyperbilirubinemia is often treated with **phototherapy** to prevent the need for exchange transfusion. For phototherapy, the infant is placed under lights to decrease bilirubin levels in the blood. The lights usually consist of a single tungsten halogen lamp or 4-8 white or blue fluorescent lights and a Plexiglas shield. The infant is placed under these lights with a protective mask covering the eyes to prevent retinal toxicity. The lights should be 15-20 cm above the infant. The lights convert bilirubin into a water-soluble compound that can be excreted by the liver into bile and eventually into the infant's stool. The success of phototherapy is directly related to the quantity of body surface area that is exposed to the lights, so the infant is clad only in a diaper to expose the most skin to the light as possible. Indications:

Weight	Serum Bilirubin Level
500-750 g	5-8 mg/dL
750-1000 g	6-10 mg/dL
1000-1250 g	8-10 mg/dL
1250-1500 g	10-12 mg/dL

Exchange transfusions may be used for hyperbilirubinemia. Blood <72 hours old is used to maintain potassium levels. Indications include:

Weight	Serum Bilirubin Level
500-750 g	12-15 mg/dL
750-1000 g	>15 mg/dL
1000-1250 g	15-18 mg/dL
1250-1500 g	17-20 mg/dL

There are many risks associated with exchange transfusions, including vascular complications, such as emboli or thrombosis, often related to umbilical catheters. Cardiac complications include dysrhythmias and overload, leading to arrest. Clotting disorders may result from over-heparinization (reversed with protamine sulfate). Electrolyte and glucose abnormalities as well as infection may occur.

BLOOD COMPONENT THERAPY

Blood component therapy is described below:

- **Whole blood** has red blood cells (RBCs), white blood cells (WBCs), and platelets in their normal ratios. Whole blood is not a common neonatal blood transfusion product unless there is massive hemorrhage from trauma. Usually, its components are given individually to treat a specific condition.
- **Packed RBCs** are prepared by removing most of the plasma from blood, leaving a hematocrit of 70-90%. Use packed cells to treat anemia.
- **Leukocyte-poor RBCs** have more than 70% of WBCs removed by centrifuging, washing, or filtration. Much of the RBC mass is also lost. Leukocyte-poor blood products have less chance of passing on CMV infection or triggering a febrile reaction.
- **Washed RBCs** are cleaned with 0.9% sodium chloride to remove more than 95% of the nonviable RBCs and 80-90% of the WBCs. Washing is one method of producing leukocyte-poor RBCs.
- **Fresh frozen plasma** is comprised of 90-92% water, clotting factors, immunoglobulins, albumin, electrolytes, and enzymes and is used to add volume.

Blood Product Administration

In the NICU, **blood transfusions** are common, especially packed red blood cells. Blood should always be warmed to prevent hypothermia. Small volumes may be warmed passively by exposing to room temperature or heated isolette for 30 minutes prior to administration. Transfusions are given through peripheral IVs rather than umbilical lines except in extreme emergency. A filtered line should always be used for blood administration. During the transfusion, vital signs should be monitored and recorded every 15 minutes and the neonate carefully watched for any signs of a transfusion reaction. **Irradiated blood cells** are recommended for neonates <1200 mg and for those who are immunocompromised or receiving transfusions of granulocytes or exchange transfusions. Whole blood is not a common neonatal blood transfusion product unless there is massive hemorrhage from trauma. **Platelets** used for neonates to prevent cerebral hemorrhage with thrombocytopenia are collected from one donor instead of from pooled donations, suspended in plasma, and leukocyte depleted. Usual dose is 10-15 mL/kg given over 60-90 minutes.

Infectious Disease

Immunity

Infants (especially preterm) have **increased susceptibility to infection** when compared to older children and adults because of immaturity or deficiencies in their immune systems:

- **Cellular immunity**: Neutrophils and macrophages in the neonate are deficient in chemotaxis and not as effective in killing invading bacteria. Reserves of neutrophils are easily depleted in neonates.
- **Humoral immunity**: Some passage of immunoglobulin G (IgG) occurs from the mother to the fetus, but mostly during the third trimester. In general, immunoglobulin levels are low. The neonate does not produce IgA until 2-5 weeks after birth. Complement activity is also immature in newborns, leaving them especially susceptible to Gram-negative organisms.
- **Barrier function**: The skin and mucous membranes, which normally act as barriers, are less effective in newborns. Prolonged invasive instrumentation (central lines or endotracheal tubes) associated with infants who are premature or those with complex congenital deformities are other routes for infection.

Humoral Immunity

Humoral immunity in neonates is mainly mediated by maternal transfer of **Immunoglobulin G (IgG)** that greatly increases after 32 weeks of gestation. Infants born prior to 32 weeks have a significantly lower immunoglobulin level than term infants. Endogenous production of immunoglobulins does not begin until 24 weeks after birth, allowing serum immunoglobulin levels to trough until production begins. This trough further lowers the premature infant's ability to fight infections. The lower the infant's gestational age, the higher the incidence of neonatal sepsis. The risk of neonatal sepsis is 10 times higher in infants who weigh less than 2,500 grams, when compared to full term infants. Boost the premature infant's immunoglobulin level with intravenous IgG (IVIG) to prevent the acquisition of nosocomial infections or as adjunctive therapy in neonates with early onset sepsis. (Studies have shown mixed results with only minimal benefits.)

Sources of Neonatal Infection

For the neonate there are three main categories of sources of infection:

- **Transplacental (Intrauterine)** infection is a direct infection from the mother to the fetus prior to birth. Infections such as AIDS, Cytomegalovirus, Rubella, Syphilis and Toxoplasmosis are the most common types in this category.
- **Perinatal acquisition** during labor and delivery occurs at the time of birth rather than *in utero* and is a direct result of contact with a pathogen present on the mother at birth. Infections in this category include Chlamydia, Enterovirus, Group B *Streptococcus*, Hepatitis B and Herpes.
- **Hospital acquisition** in the neonatal period is the third category. This is an infection that the infant did not have at birth but acquired from hospital personnel, equipment, the mother, or visitors.

Nosocomial Infections in Neonatal Unit

A nosocomial infection is acquired while in the hospital and is often responsible for late onset sepsis in neonates. The immature or compromised immune systems of premature neonates, combined with the frequent use of invasive ventilators, catheters, ventricular shunts, chest tubes, and IVs make neonates susceptible to nosocomial infections:

- **Peripheral IVs** are very common in neonates and often require restarting because of their small and fragile veins. Appropriate aseptic technique is essential to lessen infections associated with peripheral IVs.
- **Percutaneously inserted central catheters**, most commonly used in the NICU as they are more permanent than peripheral IVs, are also associated with nosocomial infections and should not be left in place longer than 21 days.

Pathogens commonly involved in nosocomial infections include coagulase-negative staphylococci (CoNS), *Klebsiella*, *Serratia*, *Enterobacter*, *Pseudomonas*, and *Candida*. Viral infections, such as respiratory syncytial virus (RSV), are usually introduced by parents and visitors. Frequent use of antibiotics contributes to the development of opportunistic bacteria and drug-resistant infections, such as Vancomycin-resistant *Enterococci* and methicillin-resistant *Staphylococcus aureus*.

Gram-Positive and Gram-Negative Pathogens in the Nursery

The Gram stain is a rapid lab test that divides bacteria into two classes (gram-positive or gram-negative) depending on their staining characteristics. Gram staining narrows the range of likely pathogens so the doctor can choose an antibiotic, pending a culture and sensitivity, which requires several days.

- **Gram-positive**
  - Group B *Streptococcus* (most common)
  - *Staphylococcus aureus* and *S. epidermidis*
  - *Listeria monocytogenes*
- **Gram-negative**
  - *Escherichia coli* (most common)
  - *Klebsiella pneumoniae*
  - *Pseudomonas aeruginosa*
  - *Haemophilus influenzae*
  - *Enterobacter aerogenes*

Antibiotic resistance is increasing among gram-negative bacilli such as *Klebsiella pneumoniae*, *P. aeruginosa*, and *Enterobacter* spp. Organisms that are deemed significant may vary from one department to another, so that organisms that might prove fatal in the neonatal unit may pose less of a threat to adults.

Candidiasis

Candida albicans is a fungus that can cause late onset sepsis and oral thrush in the neonate. Invasive **candidiasis** is a serious infection and has a mortality rate of 25-30%. The source of infection may be from the mother or from colonized health care workers. It is estimated that up to 30% of health care workers are colonized with *candida*. Immunocompromised patients, such as mothers with AIDS, are especially vulnerable to thrush. **Risk factors for the development** of candidiasis include:

- Birth weight less than 1,500 grams
- Prolonged use of broad-spectrum antibiotics
- TPN with infusion of lipids
- Prolonged urinary catheterization
- History of cutaneous or mucous membrane colonization or infection (thrush or candidal diaper rash)

Amphotericin B is the drug of choice for the treatment of candidiasis. Central lines and catheters may have to be removed.

Enterovirus

Enteroviruses include coxsackievirus, echovirus, and poliovirus (essentially eradicated in the United States). Most **enterovirus infections** (90%) in adults are asymptomatic or non-specific febrile illness with flu-like symptoms. There is no consensus regarding neonatal infections, but most researchers believe they are not acquired transplacentally but that infection occurs perineally (during delivery) or after birth (≥ 2 weeks) from exposure to a mother with the virus or another infected infant. Neonates are at increased risk of developing sepsis-like conditions, such as aseptic meningitis, myocarditis, and hepatitis. It may be difficult to differentiate enterovirus infection from bacterial sepsis. Because of lack of immune response, neonates <10 days are at increased risk from non-polio enteroviruses. Neonates may be lethargic, feverish, and exhibit signs of hypoperfusion (mottled skin, delay in capillary refill time, and cyanosis) and jaundice. They often feed poorly and cry inconsolably.

Bacterial Infections Affecting Newborns

Escherichia Coli

Newborns who are preterm or low birth weight or whose mothers experienced prolonged labor or fever are at increased risk of ***Escherichia coli (E. coli)* infection**. Early recognition of **symptoms** and alerting the physician is critical. Contact precautions must be utilized.

- **GI infection:** Symptoms include green, watery, and bloody diarrhea, fever, and dehydration.
- **UTI:** Symptoms, such as fever pyuria, poor feeding, and irritability, usually occur in the 2nd to 3rd week but may be earlier in preterm neonates or secondary to bacteremia, so urine and blood cultures are usually done and antibiotics administered.
- **Neonatal sepsis:** Infection usually obtained intrapartum with symptoms within 6 hours of delivery. Symptoms include Low APGAR score, poor sucking, apnea, bradycardia, unstable temperature, vomiting, diarrhea, and dyspnea. Mortality rates are higher in low-birth weight and preterm neonates. Treatment is with antibiotics and supportive therapy.
- **Neonatal meningitis:** May progress from diarrhea or UTI. Onset after 48 hours usually includes neurological impairment, stupor, irritability, seizures, posturing, anterior fontanel bulging, and nuchal rigidity. Treatment is with antibiotics and supportive therapy.

Staphylococcus

Neonates may be exposed to *Staphylococcus* through contact with medical personnel or from contaminated equipment, such as ventilators. Risk factors include preterm birth, VLBW (<1500 g), prolonged hospitalization, and invasive procedures such as insertion of venous catheters. Indications of infection may include fever or hypothermia, cardiac changes (tachycardia, bradycardia), vomiting, lethargy, and skin rash or lesions. If the infection enters the bloodstream, the neonate may develop sepsis, which can progress to meningitis and to neurological compromise or death. *Staphylococcus aureus* is one of the most common infective agents and may be either methicillin-susceptible or methicillin resistant (MRSA), which is much more difficult to treat. *Staphylococcus epidermidis*, which is found on skin and mucosa, and coagulase-negative staphylococci both tend to colonize invasive devices, such as catheters, forming biofilms that lead to sepsis and are naturally resistant to antibiotics. Coagulase-negative staphylococci infections may also occur in preterm neonates receiving TPN.

Bacterial Meningitis

Bacterial meningitis is caused by a wide range of pathogenic organisms, varying with the infant's age:

- ≤1 month: *E.coli,* Group B *Streptococci*, *Listeria monocytogenes*, and *Neisseria meningitidis*
- 1-2 months: Group B *Streptococci*

Bacterial infections usually arise from the spread of distant infections but can enter the CNS from surgical wounds, invasive devices, or nasal colonization. The infective process includes inflammation, exudates, white blood cell accumulation, and tissue damage with the brain showing evidence of hyperemia and edema. Purulent exudate covers the brain and invades and blocks the ventricles, obstructing CSF and leading to increased intracranial pressure. Since antibodies specific to bacteria don't cross the blood-brain barrier, the body's ability to fight the infection is very poor.

Diagnosis

Diagnosis of bacterial meningitis is based on examination of cerebrospinal fluid and symptoms. **Symptoms** may be very non-specific, such as hypo- or hyperthermia, jaundice, irritability, lethargy, irregular respirations with periods of apnea, difficulty feeding with loss of suck reflex, hypotonia, weak cry, seizures, and bulging fontanels (late sign). Nuchal rigidity does not usually occur with neonates. Meningitis is often difficult to diagnose in the neonate because it has early nonspecific clinical findings of irritability, lethargy, poor feeding, temperature instability, and hypotension. The more specific neurological symptoms of seizures or bulging fontanels are seen in late onset infection. Antibiotics given to the mother prior to delivery or to the neonate prior to performing a lumbar puncture inhibit bacterial growth in cerebrospinal fluid (CSF), making the diagnosis dependent on other CSF parameters. **CSF findings** suggestive of bacterial meningitis include:

- Decreased glucose
- Elevated protein
- White blood cells values in CSR greater than 100 WBC/dL

A polymerase chain reaction assay test for Group B strep antigen in CSF is available. Values may be more difficult to interpret in the premature neonate, as their blood brain barrier is more permeable.

Hospital-Acquired Pneumonia

Klebsiella Pneumoniae

Klebsiella pneumoniae is a common cause of hospital-acquired infections of the urinary tract, surgical sites, and lower respiratory tract. *K. pneumoniae* is a gram-negative member of the Enterobacteriaceae family and is part of the normal body flora. It can infect children of all ages but is most common in infants who are premature and/or in neonatal intensive care. Infants with invasive devices, such as those with mechanical ventilation, are at increased risk. There have been a number of outbreaks in neonatal units, especially with multi-drugs resistant forms, with the hands of health staff and the gastrointestinal tract of the infants providing reservoirs of bacteria.

When the infection attacks the lungs, the **symptoms** include inflammatory changes that result in necrosis and hemorrhage, clogging the lungs with thick puro-sanguineous exudate. The disease spreads rapidly, with high fever and dyspnea. Mortality rates are high.

Treatment includes antibiotic therapy (such as 3rd generation cephalosporins or quinolones) based on cultures and sensitivities.

Pseudomonas Aeruginosa

Hospital-acquired pneumonias (HAP) are far more lethal than community-acquired pneumonias (CAP), with HAP death rates of 20-40% and up to 90% if the infant is on mechanical ventilation, with ***Pseudomonas aeruginosa*** one of the most lethal (40-60% mortality) because it can invade blood vessels, resulting in hemorrhage. Most infections are spread by contact with contaminated hands of healthcare staff or from invasive devices, such as endotracheal tubes and mechanical ventilators.

Symptoms include fever, cough, bradycardia, and elevated WBC counts.

Treatment includes:

- Antibiotic therapy: Usually combinations of 2 antibiotics are given, such as piperacillin or ceftazidime and gentamicin or ciprofloxacin (based on cultures). Vancomycin is generally avoided because of the rise of vancomycin-resistant organisms.
- Preventive measures include maintaining ventilated patients in 30° upright positions, universal precautions, and changing ventilator circuits as per protocol.

Early-Onset Sepsis

Early-onset bacterial sepsis usually occurs in the first 24 hours after birth, but may occur any time up to day 6 of life. Infants born prematurely have an increased rate of early-onset sepsis and more rapid onset of symptoms. In early onset sepsis, the source of infection is from the mother, either transplacentally, or a microorganism that colonized the mother's birth canal. Pathogens that most commonly cause early-onset sepsis are Group B *Streptococcus*, *E. coli*, *Haemophilus influenzae*, coagulase-negative staphylococci, and *Listeria monocytogenes*. **Risk factors** for the development of early onset sepsis include:

- Premature, preterm, or prolonged rupture of membranes
- Maternal colonization with Group B *Streptococcus*
- Fever in the mother greater than 38 °C during delivery
- Premature birth or low birth weight (<2500 g)

- Maternal urinary tract infection
- Chorioamnionitis
- APGAR score less than 6 at 1 minute or 5 minutes
- Delivery with birth asphyxia or meconium staining

Clinical Manifestations and Diagnosis

The clinical manifestations for **early-onset sepsis** are often vague and nonspecific making it a particular challenge to diagnose early. Sometimes the only noticeable sign is that the mother or nurse will note that the infant just doesn't seem well—nothing that can be specified but general symptoms perhaps starting with a poor feeding or other seemingly minor event. Infection may localize or cause bacteremia and sometimes meningitis. Some **manifestations** that should be noted include:

- The inability of the infant to maintain a normal body temperature
- Apnea, tachypnea
- Vomiting
- Cyanosis
- Lethargy
- Jaundice
- Seizures
- Purpura

If sepsis is suspected, CSF examination is done to evaluate for possible meningitis, a frequent complication of sepsis, especially if the infant is exhibiting symptoms of sepsis, GBS sepsis, or late onset of infection.

Late-Onset Sepsis

Late-onset sepsis occurs after day 6 of life and is more common in preterm infants and those with medical or surgical conditions. The infection is acquired from the environment after birth, rather than from the mother. Infants with indwelling catheters, nasal cannulas, continuous positive airway pressure (CPAP), intubation, ventricular taps, and any other type of prolonged instrumentation are at increased risk. Late onset sepsis generally has a more gradual onset than early onset sepsis, and the site of primary infection relates to the cause. For example, ventilation-associated infection results in pneumonia. **Likely organisms involved in late onset sepsis** include:

- Gram-positive organisms like *Staphylococcus aureus* and Group B *Streptococcus* in 2/3 of cases
- Gram-negative organisms such as *E coli*, *Klebsiella pneumoniae*, *Pseudomonas aeruginosa*, *Serratia*, *Enterobacter*, and *Acinetobacter*
- *Candida*

Treatment of Sepsis/Meningitis

Neonatal sepsis and meningitis are treated with **intravenous antibiotics**. Usually if sepsis is suspected, treatment with broad-spectrum antibiotics (IV aminoglycoside and penicillin) will be started while awaiting the culture results. Once culture results are obtained any adjustment to a more effective medication to treat the now identified organism may be made. Using antibiotics too liberally when not indicated by a confirmed bacterial infection can have serious consequences for the neonate, such as the development of antibiotic resistant strains of bacteria and the killing of the normal flora of organisms that inhabit the intestinal tract leading to digestive problems. These problems must be weighed with the need to quickly treat a suspected sepsis when cultures have not been completed as many of these take days to finish growing. If hydrocephalus occurs with meningitis, then a ventroperitoneal shunt may be inserted surgically. Enteral or parenteral feedings may be necessary to provide adequate nutrition during treatment. Radiant warmers or incubators may be needed for thermoregulation.

RANGE OF SEVERE INFECTIONS

There are a number of terms used to refer to the range of severe infections and often used interchangeably, but they are part of a continuum:

- **Bacteremia** is the presence of bacteria in the blood but without systemic infection.
- **Septicemia** is a systemic infection caused by pathogens (usually bacteria or fungi) present in the blood.
- **Systemic inflammatory response syndrome (SIRS)**, a generalized inflammatory response affecting many organ systems, may be caused by infectious or non-infectious agents, such as trauma, adrenal insufficiency, pulmonary embolism, and drug overdose. If an infectious agent is identified or suspected, SIRS is an aspect of sepsis. Infective agents for infants include a wide range of bacteria and fungi, including *Streptococcus pneumoniae* and *Staphylococcus aureus.* SIRS includes 2 of the following:
    - Elevated (>38 °C) or subnormal rectal temperature (<36 °C)
    - Tachypnea >60 for infants or $PaCO_2$ <32 mmHg
    - Tachycardia >160 for infants
    - Leukocytosis (>12,000) or leukopenia (<4000)
- **Sepsis** is the presence of infection either locally or systemically in which there is a generalized life-threatening inflammatory response (SIRS). It includes all the indications for SIRS as well as one of the following:
    - Hypoxemia (<72 mmHg) without pulmonary disease
    - Elevation in plasma lactate
    - Decreased urinary output <5 mL/kg/hr for ≥1 hour
- **Severe sepsis** includes both indications of SIRS and sepsis as well as indications of increasing organ dysfunction with inadequate perfusion and/or hypotension.
- **Septic shock** is a progression from severe sepsis in which refractory hypotension occurs despite treatment. There may be indications of lactic acidosis.
- **Multi-organ dysfunction syndrome** (MODS) is the most common cause of sepsis-related death. Cardiac function becomes depressed, acute respiratory distress syndrome (ARDS) may develop, and renal failure may follow acute tubular necrosis or cortical necrosis. Thrombocytopenia appears in about 30% of those affected and may result in disseminated intravascular coagulation (DIC). Liver damage and bowel necrosis may occur.

Genetic, Endocrine, and Metabolic Complications

Autosomal Inheritance Patterns

Autosomal inheritance patterns involve genetic **abnormalities in chromosome pairs 1-22**:

- **Autosomal recessive***:* This occurs when two parents (without active disease) each have a copy of the same abnormal recessive gene, and both pass the abnormal copy to offspring. The **recurrence risk** (the chance to have affected offspring) for two carrier parents with the same abnormal gene mutation is 25% for each pregnancy and 50% chance the child will become a carrier. Autosomal recessive disorders, such as cystic fibrosis, Tay Sachs, and sickle cell anemia, are seen more frequently among certain ethnic groups and in offspring of related parents.
- **Autosomal dominant***:* This means that only one abnormal dominant gene needs to be inherited to cause the condition. Autosomal dominant diseases include Huntington's disease and Marfan syndrome. The recurrence risk for an affected parent to pass the disease to a child is 50% with each pregnancy, but there is no carrier state.

Sex-Linked Inheritance

Sex-linked inheritance involves the sex chromosomes (**chromosome 23**). Y-linked disorders such as Klinefelter syndrome are rare, but they will be passed from the father to all male children. X-linked diseases, such as hemophilia and Duchenne muscular dystrophy, usually occur in males because males have only one X chromosome, so a single recessive gene on that X chromosome causes the disease. Females have two X chromosomes, so the normal gene on an unaffected X chromosome can usually compensate. Although the Y chromosome is the other half of the XY chromosome pair in the male, the Y chromosome is much smaller than the X chromosome and doesn't contain most of the genes of the X chromosome—it's not a complete match—so there is no compensating gene to protect the male. Thus, females carry the disease and males inherit the disease. A man with an X-linked recessive disorder will not pass the disease to his sons (because they don't inherit his X chromosome), but his daughters will inherit the mutated gene, so they have one abnormal X (from the father) and one normal (from the mother). These daughters then have a 50% chance of having sons who are affected and a 50% chance of having daughters who carry one copy of the mutated gene. X-linked dominant inheritance also differs depending upon whether the mother or father carries the defective gene. There is no carrier state with X-linked dominant disorders. If the father has the disease, such as Rett's syndrome, all daughters will inherit. If the mother has the disease, each child, regardless of gender, has a 50% chance of inheriting.

Multifactorial Inheritance

Complex or multifactorial inheritance relates to an interaction of many different genes, as well as the environment and lifestyle choices. Thus, a genetic disorder may depend upon genes inherited from both parents as well as unidentified environmental factors (smoking, drug use, diet) interacting in such a way as to produce an abnormality. This type of inheritance pattern is much less predictable than the others. Neural tube defects, for example, are caused by multifactorial inheritance. In some cases, an infant may inherit only a tendency toward a disease, such as diabetes type 2, but development of the disease may depend up weight, diet, smoking, and other factors as the child matures. Complex diseases include such things as asthma, heart disease, and osteoarthritis. Multifactorial traits often run in families, with risk 50% in first-degree relatives (parents), 25% in second-degree (grandparents, aunts, uncles), and 12.5% in third-degree (cousins).

Newborn Screening

Screening of the newborn to detect genetic diseases varies somewhat from one state to another. Because about 1 in 200 newborns has chromosomal abnormalities, screening is an important tool, although many birth defects, such as defects caused by maternal alcohol abuse or vitamin deficiency, are not genetic in origin. Screening tests for these genetic diseases are available:

- Biotinidase deficiency (autosomal recessive)
- Congenital adrenal hyperplasia (autosomal recessive)
- Congenital hearing loss (autosomal recessive, autosomal dominant, or mitochondrial)
- Congenital hypothyroidism (autosomal recessive or autosomal dominant)
- Cystic fibrosis (autosomal recessive)
- Galactosemia (autosomal recessive)
- Homocystinuria (autosomal recessive)
- Maple syrup urine disease (autosomal recessive)
- Medium-chain Acyl-CoA dehydrogenase (autosomal recessive)
- Phenylketonuria (autosomal recessive)
- Sickle cell disease (autosomal recessive)
- Tyrosinemia (Two types are autosomal recessive; a third type is unclear)

Cystic Fibrosis

Cystic fibrosis (mucoviscidosis or CF) is a progressive congenital disease that particularly affects the pancreas and lungs, causing digestive and respiratory problems. It is caused by a genetic defect that affects sodium chloride movement in cells, including mucosal cells that line the lungs, causing the production of thick mucus that clogs the lungs and provides a rich medium for bacteria. While most patients with cystic fibrosis at one time died in childhood, the life expectancy is now about 30 years. About 15-20% of neonates with CF have meconium ileus (obstruction of small intestine with meconium) at birth. Other infants have no symptoms at first but show failure to thrive in the first 4-6 weeks and may develop a cough and wheezing. Cystic fibrosis patients usually suffer from recurrent respiratory infections of the lower respiratory tract. The most common infective agents are *Pseudomonas aeruginosa* and *Burkholderia cepacia* complex. The screening test for CF is IRT/DNA. If the IRT/DNA is positive, the infant is scheduled for a sweat test and buccal swab.

G6PD Deficiency

Glucose-6-phosphate dehydrogenase (G6PD) deficiency is an X-linked recessive disease and can often present as, or similar to, hyperbilirubinemia. Because female infants inherit two X chromosomes, it's rare that both are defective, and the normal chromosome compensates, so X-linked recessive disorders affect primarily male children (who get the X chromosome from the mother, not the father) but are passed on by the mother. G6PD is an enzyme utilized to process carbohydrates and to protect red blood cells. G6PD results in premature destruction of red blood cells and hemolytic anemia, which can be triggered by infection, some medications (antimalarial drugs, sulfa, ASAS, NSAIDS, quinidine, quinine, and nitrofurantoin), and eating or inhaling the pollen of fava beans (favism). Infants may be asymptomatic, although some may exhibit increased jaundice. In the United States, G6PD is most common in African American males (1 out of 10) and those with Middle Eastern heritage. Treatment includes avoiding triggers, treating infections, and transfusions if necessary.

Chromosome Abnormalities

Trisomy 13

Trisomy 13 (Patau syndrome) may occur with complete trisomy, mosaicism, or partial trisomy, so symptoms may vary depending upon the amount of extra genetic material in **chromosome 13**. Diagnosis can be made prenatally with amniocentesis. This disorder occurs in 1 of every 20,000 live births in both males and females. **Indications** include:

- Cleft lip/palate
- Polydactyly and clenched fists
- Microcephaly, abnormal brain structure, profound intellectual disability, seizures
- Small or absent close-set eyes (may be fused into one eye), vision impairment
- Coloboma (split or hole in iris)
- Low-set ears and deafness
- Umbilical/inguinal hernias
- Cardiac abnormalities with heart on right side of chest and congestive heart disease (80%)
- Rocker-bottom feet
- Micrognathia
- Multiple system disorders

Treatment is supportive and symptomatic, but despite interventions, about 80% die ≤1 month. Infants may have profound dyspnea, seizures, and difficulty feeding.

Trisomy 18

Trisomy 18 occurs when the infant has **three number 18 chromosomes**, instead of the normal two. Trisomy 18 is an aneuploidy second only to Down syndrome (trisomy 21) for frequency. Trisomy 18 occurs in 1 of every 6,000-8,000 live births, and is associated with severe malformations and high infant mortality. Only 5-10% of affected children survive beyond the first year of life. **Malformations** include:

- **Neurological**: Microcephaly, anencephaly, hydrocephaly, Arnold-Chiari malformation, hypoplasia of the corpus callosum, wide occipitoparietal skull diameter with narrow frontal diameter, called "strawberry sign" because of its appearance on ultrasound.
- **Facial**: Epicanthal folds, short palpebral fissures, cataracts, short nose with upturned nares, micrognathia, narrow palate, cleft palate, and low-set ears.
- **Skeletal**: Clenched fists, radial hypoplasia, rocker-bottom feet, hypoplastic nails, and short neck with excessive skin folds.
- **Cardiac**: Ventricular septal defect is most common, but some heart problem is present over 90% of the time.
- **Other**: Pulmonary hypoplasia, omphalocele, esophageal atresia, multicystic kidneys, cryptorchidism, and intrauterine growth restriction.

TRISOMY 21

Trisomy 21 (**Down syndrome**) occurs in 1 out of every 800 live births. Trisomy 21 is the most common chromosomal disorder in humans. Advanced maternal age is a risk factor. The definitive diagnosis is made by cytogenetic examination of the infant's DNA from amniocentesis or chorionic villi sampling. Common **physical characteristics** of infants born with Down syndrome are listed below in decreasing order of incidence:

- Low birth weight
- Brachycephaly (head is short in diameter from front to back and disproportionately broad)
- Upslanting palpebral fissures (openings between the eyelids)
- Wide gap between first and second toes
- Small, low set ears
- Hypotonia
- Epicanthic skin folds (redundant skin folds in the upper eyelid from the nose to the inner side of the eyebrow)
- Brushfield's spots (small white or gray spots on the periphery of the iris)
- Short, wide hands
- Single transverse palmar crease
- Heart disease (40-50%); murmur may be heard on physical exam

DIGEORGE SYNDROME

DiGeorge syndrome is a series of congenital defects that results from a deletion of part of the long arm of **chromosome 22**. This same area of the chromosome is also missing in infants with velo-cardio-facial syndrome and conotruncal anomalies face syndrome, so use the preferred name **22q11 deletion syndrome** to describe all three syndromes. The basic **defects** in 22q11 deletion syndrome are:

- Conotruncal heart defects: Tetralogy of Fallot, ventricular septal defect, or interrupted aortic arch (80%)
- Cleft lip or palate (70%)
- Hypocalcemia secondary to hypoparathyroidism (20-60%), which causes seizures
  - Note: Hypocalcemia is often temporary; many children do not require calcium supplementation after their first year of life
- Microcephaly, small ears, hooded eyelids, small mouth, and small chin
- Mild to borderline intellectual disability, with IQs in the 70-90 range (40%)
- Hypoplastic or absent thymus, resulting in T-cell dysfunction, recurrent infections secondary to immune deficiencies, and rarely, severe immune deficiency

Turner Syndrome

Turner syndrome is one of the most common chromosomal abnormalities, occurring in approximately 1 in 2,000 live female births (male fetuses die). **Turner syndrome** is caused by the absence of a set of genes that form the short arm of one of the X chromosomes. Most infants are missing the entire second chromosome (45X). Most pregnancies in which the infant has Turner syndrome end in spontaneous abortions. **Clinical signs** present at birth include:

- Webbed neck from fetal lymphedema; after the swelling resolves, loose folds of skin are still present on the neck
- Broad chest with wide spaced nipples (shield chest)
- Swollen hands and feet
- Short 4th or 5th metacarpals or metatarsals
- Increased incidence of congenital hip dislocation
- Increased incidence of coarctation of the aorta and bicuspid aortic valve

The **diagnosis** of Turner syndrome is confirmed by a karyotype. All infants with Turner syndrome must have their hearts evaluated.

Beckwith-Wiedemann Syndrome

Beckwith-Wiedemann syndrome is a congenital imprinting disorder (80% caused by defect of chromosome 11) of infants that exhibit overgrowth, affecting multiple body systems. Most cases are sporadic, although 10–15% are autosomal dominant transmission. Characteristics may include the following:

- Preterm delivery of LGA infants
- Macrosomia
- Height and weight >95% for age
- Hemihyperplasia
- Macroglossia
- Forehead ridge
- Increased risk of Wilms tumors, adrenal carcinoma, and liver tumors
- Nevus flammeus (erythema of the eyelids and forehead)
- Seizures
- Cryptorchidism
- Abdominal wall defects with enlarged organs (kidneys, adrenal glands, spleen, liver, and pancreas)
- Omphalocele or umbilical hernia, often needing surgical intervention
- Hypoglycemia
- Hemihypertrophy (overgrowth of only one side of body)
- Cardiac abnormalities.
- Hypoglycemia after birth, which can cause seizures
- Ear anomalies, sometimes result in hearing loss

Treatment includes surgical repair of abnormalities (such as abdominal wall defects) and removal of tumors (such as Wilms tumors), with chemotherapy as needed and control of hypoglycemia. Tongue reduction surgery and orthopedic repair may be done. Children who survive infancy have a good prognosis. Intelligence is usually normal although some may have slight cognitive impairment. Children must be monitored for tumor development.

Potter Sequence

Potter sequence or syndrome is a congenital disorder related to oligohydramnios or anhydramnios resulting from renal disease, such as bilateral renal agenesis (BRA), other urinary obstruction, or premature amniotic sac rupture. There are five different classifications of Potter syndrome:

- Classic: BRA present
- Type I: autosomal recessive polycystic kidney disease
- Type II: one kidney missing and the other abnormal
- Type III: autosomal dominant polycystic kidney disease
- Type IV: hydronephrosis from obstruction (rarely causes death)

The lack of amniotic fluid causes the fetus to be compressed by the uterus, resulting in a number of physical manifestations, including the following:

- Potter's facies: parrot-beak nose, micrognathia, low-set ears, flattened nose, wide-set eyes, and skin fold from edge of eye across cheek
- Clubfeet, tibial bowing, or fused legs (sirenomelia)
- Genitourinary and gynecological abnormalities (small bladder, absence or abnormality of reproductive organs)
- Pulmonary abnormalities (underdeveloped alveoli), resulting in severe respiratory distress at birth
- Diaphragmatic hernia
- Genitourinary anomalies, including absent or malformed kidneys

Treatment is supportive and symptomatic, but survival is extremely rare for most types. At birth, immediate respiratory support is needed, including intubation and ventilation or ECMO.

VATER Syndrome (VACTERL Association)

VATER syndrome is a subset of VACTERL association with fewer abnormalities. VATER/VACTERL is an acronym for several different birth defects that often occur together. The letters in the acronym stand for:

- **V** - Vertebral defects (70%): usually consist of smaller than normal vertebrae that may predispose the infant to develop scoliosis
- **A** - Anal atresia or imperforate anus (55%): often requires surgical correction at birth
- **C** – Cardiovascular defects (75%): common heart defects include ventral septal defect, atrial septal defect, and tetralogy of Fallot
- **T** – Tracheoesophageal fistula (70%)
- **E** – Esophageal atresia (70%)
- **R** – Renal anomalies (50%): anomalies can be severe, including incomplete formation of the kidneys or obstruction of urine outflow
- **L** - Limb anomalies (70%): defects include absent or displaced thumbs, extra digits, fusion of digits, and forearm defects

For VACTERL diagnosis, the infant must have 3 of the 7 malformations. An infant with any one of these birth defects must also be evaluated for other defects in the association. For VATER diagnosis, the infant must have 3 of 5 malformations.

CHARGE Syndrome

CHARGE syndrome is a multi-organ autosomal dominant (or new mutation) disorder. The CHARGE acronym represents common features of the syndrome, although abnormalities may vary in different neonates:

- **C**olomba: a hole or gap in eye structures that can affect the iris, retina, optic disc or choroid and can result in impairment of vision or blindness; eyes may be small and underdeveloped
- **H**eart defects: may include tetralogy of Fallot, VSD, ASD, or PDA
- **A**tresia, choanal: one or both nasal passages may be blocked; since neonates are obligate nasal breathers, this can lead to difficulty breathing in the neonate
- **R**etardation of growth/development: delay in meeting milestones
- **G**enitourinary anomalies: hypogonadism and reduced hormone production may result in males with micropenis and cryptorchidism although female external genitalia usually appear normal; puberty may be delayed in both genders
- **E**ar abnormalities/hearing loss: abnormalities in the middle and inner ear, abnormalities of the external ear, and varying decrease of hearing loss

A square-shaped face is common. Other less common disorders associated with the syndrome include cranial nerve abnormalities, impaired sense of smell, difficulty swallowing, tracheoesophageal fistula, renal abnormalities, scoliosis, kyphosis, polydactyly, oligodactyly, club foot, and long-bone abnormalities.

Skeletal Dysplasia

Skeletal dysplasias are a large group (450+) of genetic disorders affecting the bones and cartilage, one bone, or a group of bones, and the mode of inheritance can vary. Some disorders may result from spontaneous mutations or exposure to toxins. For example, X-linked disorders may affect males and not females. Often parents have mild symptoms but the child has a more severe disorder. Some of these disorders, such as osteogenesis imperfecta, may be diagnosed in the fetus by screening or ultrasound during the first trimester, but others may not be diagnosed until the third trimester or birth of the infant. Common dysplasias include thanatophoric, campomelic, achondroplasia, and achondrogenesis. About half of infants with skeletal dysplasias are stillborn or die within a few weeks of birth. If the dysplasia is lethal, then the neonate is provided comfort care, but if the dysplasia is consistent with life, then the infant must be stabilized, consultation with genetic specialists conducted, and non-skeletal complications assessed.

Osteogenesis Imperfecta

Osteogenesis imperfecta (OI) is a genetic disorder of collagen synthesis that results in brittle, easily fractured bones. OI occurs in 1 in 20,000 live births. Collagen is a major component of bone that gives it both strength and flexibility. Infants with OI either produce defective collagen or deficient amounts of collagen. Four different types of OI have been identified, with symptoms ranging from very mild to lethality in the neonatal period. **Common features** of OI include:

- Brittle bones that fracture easily (fractures may be present at birth)
- Bowing of long bones
- Shortened limbs
- Discolored, brittle teeth
- Blue sclera
- Skeletal deformities, including scoliosis
- Respiratory difficulties
- Weak muscles

Generally, OI is inherited in a dominant fashion, but a new mutation may cause the disorder in approximately 25% of cases. Parents of children diagnosed with OI must be instructed on correct methods of handling and bathing their child and placing the child in the crib to minimize trauma and the development of fractures.

Osteopenia of Prematurity

Osteopenia of prematurity (OOP) is a disorder of decreased bone mineralization seen in premature infants. Infants born extremely premature are at greatest risk for developing OOP. During the last trimester of pregnancy, large amounts of calcium and phosphorus are provided to the developing fetus to aid in bone mineralization. Clinical findings that may not be apparent until 2 to 4 months of age are craniotabes and impaired linear growth. Pediatricians diagnose rickets (vitamin D deficiency) when the preterm infant shows thickening of wrists and ankles, rachitic rosaries, and cupping of bone metaphysics in x-rays, and elevated alkaline phosphatase in blood serum. **Risk factors** for the development of OOP include:

- Preterm (less than 34 weeks of gestation)
- Weight less than 1,500 grams
- Delayed onset of enteral feeds
- Chronic use of steroids or diuretics by the mother or infant, which increase excretion of minerals
- Feeding unfortified human milk or full term formulas to preterm infants

Treatment includes supplementing calcium, phosphorus, and vitamin D.

Hypothyroidism

Hypothyroidism is caused by a deficiency in production of the thyroid hormones (TH) T_4 and T_3. All newborns are screened for congenital hypothyroidism because of the severe consequences associated with lack of treatment and the ease of treatment with exogenous thyroid hormone. It may be congenital or acquired. **Congenital hypothyroidism** (formerly called cretinism) may manifest at birth or be delayed for years, but severe early onset can result in profound neurological deficit and intellectual disability if undiagnosed and treated:

- **Neonates***:* Widened posterior fontanel, hypothermia ≤95 °F, edema, respiratory distress, feeding difficulties, lethargy, delayed passage of meconium, prolonged physiologic jaundice, and vomiting
- **≤3 months of age**: Umbilical hernia, dry skin, constipation, enlarged tongue, lethargy, and minimal crying

Treatment includes oral TH replacement therapy. Prompt initiation of therapy is critical for congenital hypothyroidism in order to prevent developmental abnormalities. If symptoms of hypothyroidism are severe, therapy to reach appropriate levels of TH is initially given gradually over 3-4 weeks to avoid hyperthyroidism.

Hyperthyroidism

Hyperthyroidism is caused by excess production of T3 and T4 thyroid hormones. Suppression of TSH may be present in neonates born to thyrotoxic mothers or those with genetic disorders, such as McCune-Albright syndrome. Hyperthyroidism may develop during the fetal stage, resulting in IUGR, fetal hydrops (non-immune), and fetal death. **Symptoms** of neonates include:

- Hyperkinesis
- Diarrhea
- Vomiting
- Failure to thrive or gain weight
- Tachycardia with increased pulse pressure
- Hypertension (systemic and pulmonary)
- Hepatosplenomegaly
- Thrombocytopenia
- Hyperviscosity syndrome
- Ophthalmic abnormalities
- Craniosynostosis

Treatment includes the use of antithyroid medications, such as Propacil or Tapazole, β-adrenergic blockers, and iodine. Digoxin may be necessary as well as glucocorticoids. Remission usually occurs in 20-48 weeks. In rare cases, thyroid ablation (thyroidectomy) may be necessary.

Inborn Errors of Metabolism

Inborn errors of metabolism comprise a wide range of genetic metabolic disorders, usually related to defects in gene coding for enzymes, resulting in toxic accumulations that interfere with metabolism. Disorders are classified according to the type of metabolic disorder and include:

- **Carbohydrates** (glycogen storage disease, fructose intolerance)
- **Proteins** (clotting defects, sickle cell, thalassemia, osteogenesis imperfecta, Marfan's)
- **Amino acids** (phenylketonuria, hyperammonemia)
- **Organic acid** (alcaptonuria)
- **Cholesterol/lipoprotein** (hyperlipoproteinemias, hypoproteinemias)
- **Mitochondrial** (Kearns-Sayre syndrome)
- **Porphyrin** (porphyria)
- **Defective DNA repair** (xeroderma pigmentosum)

Symptoms relate to the specific defect. Some symptoms are present in the neonate but others appear in childhood or adulthood, with some diseases life-threatening and others slowly progressive. Symptoms common to many disorders may include:

- Encephalopathy with poor feeding, lethargy, tachypnea
- Metabolic acidosis and/or hyperammonemia
- Hypoglycemia, hepatic dysfunctions with jaundice
- Dysmorphism (structural anomalies)
- Abnormal body odor or urine odor

Phenylketonuria

Phenylketonuria (PKU) is an inborn error of metabolism that results from a deficiency of the liver enzyme that changes phenylalanine to tyrosine (phenylalanine is a product that results when protein is digested). These infants are unable to digest protein. The symptoms of this disorder will show up sometime before 3 months if not caught in a screening. The first symptoms will be vomiting, poor feeding effort, and irritability. Later, if not treated, the infant will develop eczema and will have urine that smells musty. Once this condition is diagnosed, the infant must be put on a strict diet that restricts phenylalanine. Extensive family training must take place to educate the family about the diet. If the infant does not follow this diet restriction, intellectual disability will result. PKU screening within 7 days of birth is required in all 50 states.

Galactosemia

Galactosemia, an autosomal recessive disorder, is the most common inborn error of metabolism. In this disorder, the infant is lacking the enzyme that converts galactose to glucose. Because lactose is made up of galactose and glucose, the infant who cannot convert the galactose in lactose to glucose cannot tolerate lactose. Usually, the neonate is asymptomatic but develops symptoms rapidly. The clinical manifestations seen with galactosemia include jaundice, vomiting, diarrhea, inability to gain weight, and hypoglycemia. An infant with this condition that does not receive treatment can contract a serious gram-negative infection related to damage to the intestinal lining, and death may occur at 1-2 weeks. This condition must be treated by removing all lactose products and replacing the formula with soy or lactose-free formula. If left untreated, severe intellectual disability can result.

Adrenal Disorders of the Neonate

Congenital Adrenal Hyperplasia

Congenital adrenal hyperplasia (CAH) is an autosomal recessive defect that results in a cortisol deficiency, and is often accompanied by an aldosterone deficiency. 90 to 95% of CAH cases are due to a deficiency in 21-hydroxylase, the enzyme responsible for catalyzing two reactions in the adrenal glands:

- 17-Hydroxyprogestorne → 11-deoxycortisol → cortisol
- Progesterone → deoxycorticosterone → aldosterone

The cortisol deficiency results in shock, hypoglycemia, and circulatory collapse. The infant becomes dehydrated when CAH is accompanied by aldosterone deficiency (salt wasting), because of excessive loss of urinary sodium. Symptoms do not usually occur until the infant is 2 to 4 weeks old. Metabolic abnormalities of hyperkalemia, hyponatremia, hypoglycemia, and metabolic acidosis are present shortly after birth. Some infants have milder forms of CAH and are not diagnosed until later in life. Elevated levels of ACTH cause hypertrophy of the adrenal glands and increased production of androgens. Elevated androgens *in utero* virilize the female infant, so she has ovaries and uterus but external genitalia are often ambiguous.

Adrenal Insufficiency and Adrenal Hemorrhage

Adrenal disorders common to the neonate include the following:

- **Adrenal insufficiency** is the inadequate production of adrenal hormones (cortisol, aldosterone) because of adrenal or pituitary gland dysfunction. Clinical findings may be nonspecific but the condition is characterized by poor feeding, dehydration, hypoglycemia, hyponatremia, hyperkalemia, metabolic acidosis, hyperpigmentation, and hypotension. Treatment includes hormone replacement.
- **Adrenal hemorrhage** is associated with birth trauma, asphyxia, or sepsis. This may be asymptomatic or includes signs of adrenal insufficiency if 90% or more of the adrenal glands are destroyed, including electrolyte imbalances. Some neonates may present with anemia or late onset jaundice. An abdominal mass may be evident if bleeding is significant.

Ambiguous Genitalia

Ambiguous genitalia in the neonate can accompany the following conditions:

- **Congenital adrenal hyperplasia** (female): The adrenal glands are unable to produce glucocorticoids and mineralocorticoids (cortisol and aldosterone) but produce androgen, which is a male hormone. This results in virilization and an enlarged clitoris, which may resemble a small penis. The labia may be partially or completely fused, resembling a scrotum, and the vaginal orifice may be very small or obscured by the labia. Treatment with female hormones may aid in development of secondary sexual characteristics, but the brain was imprinted as male during development, typically leading to gender dysphoria.
- **5-alpha-reductase 2 deficiency:** This autosomal recessive disorder results in genetic males with the inability to convert testosterone to dihydrotestosterone (DHT), which is necessary for masculinization during fetal development, resulting in ambiguous or female-appearing external genitalia (micropenis, bifid scrotum, hypospadias), although internal reproductive organs are male.

- **Ovotestis** (formerly hermaphrodite): Both male and female reproductive organs are present in this condition, although there is considerable variation possible. A vagina may be present but is usually abnormal, penile length can vary but hypospadias is common, and the labia and scrotum vary widely. Most individuals with ovotestis will develop breasts at puberty.
- **Clitoromegaly** is a benign difference in the appearance of the clitoris, which is often enlarged and appearing to be a small penis. This may occur with neurofibromatosis, which should be ruled out.
- **Androgen insensitivity syndrome** is when genetically male neonates have a defect in androgen receptors that prevents response to testosterone and other androgens. External genitalia may appear as typical male or typical female, depending on the type:
    - Complete (CAIS): phenotype is female but no uterus or ovaries, vagina is short, testes are labial or inguinal.
    - Partial (PAIS-1): phenotype is primarily female with clitoromegaly, fused labia, urethra and vaginal openings or urogenital sinus
    - Partial (PAIS-2): phenotype is ambiguous with microphallus (<1 cm), bifid labia (appear scrotal), testes (descended or undescended), urogenital sinus or perineoscrotal hypospadias
    - Partial (PAIS-3: phenotype is primarily male with small or micropenis with perineal hypospadias, bifid scrotum, and testes (descended or undescended)
    - Mild (MAIS): phenotype is male but undervirilized with normal appearing genitalia but impaired spermatogenesis and virilization at puberty

Hypoglycemia

Hypoglycemia is low blood sugar of 30 mg/dL or less during the first day after birth, or below 45 mg/dL thereafter. One neonate in every 25,000 experiences persistent **hypoglycemia**. Half of hypoglycemic neonates develop brain damage. The hypoglycemic patient may be asymptomatic or may have these symptoms: apnea, tachypnea, respiratory distress, vomiting, diminished oral intake, tachycardia, bradycardia, jitteriness, lethargy, brisk Moro reflex, seizures, coma, and temperature instability. Suspect hypoglycemia in these circumstances:

- Elevated insulin levels in the infant with a brittle diabetic mother
- Premature or SGA baby
- KATP-HI diffuse or focal disease, GDH-HI, or GK-HI genetic disorders
- Septic shock
- Hyperthyroidism
- Inadequate glucose stores in malnourished infants and poor feeders
- Hypoxemia or ischemia
- Ingestion of alcohol, beta blockers, or salicylates

Treatment is 5-20 mg/kg/day oral diazoxide, 2-3 times per day. The doctor may also order hydrochlorothiazide, nifedipine, octreotide, and glucagon. Partial pancreatectomy is required if drugs are ineffective.

Causes and Risk Factors

Causes and risk factors for hypoglycemia include the following:

- **Decreased glucose availability**—Risk factors include preterm birth, glycogen storage diseases, intrauterine growth restriction, and prolonged fasting.
- **Increased glucose utilization**—Risk factors include cold stress and hypothermia, sepsis, labored breathing, perinatal asphyxia, Rh incompatibility, persistent neonatal hyperinsulinism, and maternal tocolytic drugs.
- **An umbilical artery catheter placed with the tip right above the pancreas**—delivers glucose directly to the pancreas and can stimulate too much insulin production.
- **Elevated insulin levels**—Risk factors include infant of diabetic mother (elevated glucose levels trigger increased insulin production), islet cell hyperplasia, abrupt cessation of IV glucose, exchange transfusion, and Beckwith-Wiedemann syndrome.

Acute Hypoglycemia/Hyperinsulinism

Acute hypoglycemia/hyperinsulinism can cause damage to the central nervous and cardiopulmonary systems, interfering with development of the brain and causing neurological impairment. **Causes** may include:

- Persistent hyperinsulinemic hypoglycemia of infancy (PHHI) in infants of diabetic mothers, usually apparent in the first 3 months
- Genetic defects in chromosome 11 (short arm)
- Severe infections, such as Gram-negative sepsis and endotoxic shock
- Maternal tocolytic administration

Symptoms in infants include:

- Blood glucose <40 mg/dL
- Central nervous system: seizures, altered consciousness, lethargy, and poor feeding with vomiting, myoclonus, respiratory distress, diaphoresis, hypothermia, and cyanosis

Treatment includes:

- Glucose/Glucagon administration to elevate blood glucose levels.
- Diazoxide (Hyperstat) inhibits release of insulin.
- Somatostatin (Sandostatin) to suppress insulin production.
- Nifedipine.
- Careful monitoring. Surgical removal of 85-90% of pancreas may be needed for infants to reduce insulin but poses risk of diabetes.

Hypoglycemia Secondary to Glycogen Storage Disease

Glycogen storage diseases (GSD) are inherited enzyme deficiencies that prevent/inhibit glycogenolysis and release of glycogen. There are 10 different types, but I, III, and IV are most common. All are autosomal recessive defects. Glycogen is stored in the liver and muscles but cannot be accessed and builds up, eventually resulting in cirrhosis of muscles and organs (heart, liver, kidney). Infants present with hypoglycemia that does not respond to the administration of glucagon, enlarged liver, and failure to thrive. GSD infants require almost continuous enteral feeds to maintain their blood glucose levels. They are susceptible to episodes of damaging hypoglycemia that can cause seizures, apnea, hypothermia, hypotonia, and cyanosis. Some types can be treated with diet, monitoring of symptoms, and medications, but others have no effective treatment. Uric acid may accumulate, so medications to lower uric acid levels may be needed.

Hyperglycemia

Hyperglycemia is a value greater than 100 mg/dL glucose in the newborn and is often iatrogenic (caused by glucose infusion). Premature and very low birth rate infants receiving IV glucose are at greatest risk for developing **hyperglycemia** because these infants often have decreased insulin production or decreased insulin insensitivity. Congenital diabetes mellitus is rare and may either be transient or permanent in nature. One of the main dangers of hyperglycemia is dehydration from osmotic diuresis. The neonate's urine will contain glucose (glucosuria). Intracranial hemorrhage is associated with hyperglycemia. Decreasing the amount of IV glucose usually resolves hyperglycemia. Dehydration must be corrected with IV fluids, if necessary. Enteral feeds stimulate insulin production by the pancreas, so exogenous insulin is rarely required to control the infant's elevated blood sugar levels.

Excess IV Glucose

If excessive IV glucose is administered to a newborn, it will cause hyperglycemia to develop. Newborns utilize glucose at a rate of 4-8 mg/kg/min. Premature infants have a lower glucose tolerance, so start them at 4 mg/kg/min. Full term infants are started at 8 mg/kg/min. At levels greater than 150-180 mg/dL, osmotic diuresis occurs (glucose in the urine). The infant develops dehydration. Dextrose is the d isomer of glucose (d-glucose). In order to supply a 2-kg infant with 7 mg/kg/min of glucose using a solution of D10 (10% dextrose solution, 100 mg dextrose per mL) the following calculations are used:

$$\text{Required dextrose} = \left(7\frac{\text{mg}}{\text{kg}\cdot\text{min}}\right) \times (2\ \text{kg}) = 14\frac{\text{mg}}{\text{min}}$$

$$14\frac{\text{mg}}{\text{min}} \times \frac{1\ \text{mL}}{100\ \text{mg}} = 0.14\frac{\text{mL}}{\text{min}}$$

$$0.14\frac{\text{mL}}{\text{min}} \times \frac{60\ \text{min}}{1\ \text{hr}} = 8.4\frac{\text{mL}}{\text{hr}}$$

IDM

Infants of diabetic mother (IDM) are exposed to elevated levels of glucose during their intrauterine development, as glucose freely crosses the placenta; the blood glucose level of the developing fetus mirrors that of the mother. The fetus increases production of insulin at around 20 weeks of gestation in response to the mother's elevated blood glucose. When the umbilical cord is cut, it abruptly disrupts the neonate's supply of glucose. The infant's greatest risk for hypoglycemia occurs 30-90 minutes after delivery. Because insulin levels are elevated in the fetus, the newborn may have an increased glucose need for several days to prevent hypoglycemia—as high as 10-15 mg/kg/min. Glucose is given as a continuous infusion to prevent the newborn from developing rebound hypoglycemia after a bolus of glucose. IDM infants show fewer symptoms of hypoglycemia when compared to other neonates and may also suffer from hypocalcemia, hypomagnesemia, and hyperbilirubinemia. Hypoglycemia is an easily treatable condition that, when left untreated, causes long-term neurological damage.

Infants of diabetic mother (IDM) often **present** with:

- Birth trauma secondary to cephalopelvic disproportion, including shoulder dislocation
- Hypoglycemia from sudden withdrawal of maternal glucose and elevated insulin in the infant
- Respiratory distress syndrome because elevated insulin inhibits surfactant production
- Polycythemia (excessive red blood cell production) and hyperviscosity because of elevated insulin and glucose increase the metabolic rate and oxygen consumption
- Iron deficiency because polycythemia leaches iron from the heart and brain
- Hyperbilirubinemia because of increased red blood cell destruction after birth
- Cardiovascular malformations, such as intraventricular hypertrophy with outflow tract obstruction, transposition of the great arteries, ventral septal defects, and coarctation of the aorta
- Congenital malformations, such as anencephaly, spina bifida, renal agenesis, and duodenal atresia
- Electrolyte abnormalities, including hypocalcemia and hypomagnesemia

COMPLICATIONS

There are several complications resulting from IDM, including:

- **Seizure activity** can occur in some of these infants due to the lack of sufficient fuel for the brain when the infant becomes hypoglycemic. Glucose is the fuel the brain needs to function properly, and when it is in short supply, the brain is essentially starved.
- **Shoulder dystocia** is a condition that is directly related to an infant that is large for gestational age (LGA) because of diabetes. Large babies will often experience shoulder dislocation at birth as they try to fit through the birth canal.
- **Thrombosis** sometimes forms in the kidneys (venous or arterial) as a result of a high hematocrit and increased viscosity of blood.
- **Increased diabetic risk**—2% of female and 6% of male IDMs will go on to develop juvenile type 1 diabetes.

Magnesium-Related Disorders of the Neonate

Hypomagnesemia in the neonate can result from prematurity, IUGR, and placental insufficiency as well as low maternal levels of magnesium. Hypomagnesemia may also result from increased magnesium loss associated with renal tubular acidosis, short bowel syndrome, and diarrhea, as well as insufficient magnesium in parenteral nutrition.

- Normal values: 1.6–2.6 mEq/L
- Hypomagnesemia: <1.6 mEq/L; critical value: <1.2 mg/dL

Signs and symptoms include irritability, tremors, hyperreflexia, seizure, cardiac arrhythmias, poor feeding, and apnea. Treatment is supportive and oral or IV magnesium according to severity.

Hypermagnesemia can result from maternal magnesium treatment, renal insufficiency, and excess magnesium intake (such as in parenteral nutrition).

- Hypermagnesemia: >2.6 mEq/L; critical value: >4.9 mg/dL

Signs and symptoms include respiration depression/apnea, bradycardia, hypotension, lethargy, poor sucking, flaccidity, hypotonia, decreased reflexes, GI hypomotility, and abdominal distention. Infants born to mothers receiving magnesium may require resuscitation at birth. Treatment includes adequate hydration, furosemide, and calcium gluconate to counteract effects and increased excretion.

Phosphorus-Related Disorders of the Neonate

Hypophosphatemia may occur in preterm and VLBW neonates because of inadequate storage, and this can result in metabolic bone disease with onset generally between 6 and 16 weeks because of bone demineralization. Other causes of hypophosphatemia include insufficient phosphorous in formula, maternal malnutrition, increased loss because of renal tubular disorders, refeeding syndrome, and some medications. Signs and symptoms include poor feeding, irritability, muscle weakness, and hypotonia. Treatment includes phosphate supplementation.

- Normal value: 0-5 days is 4.6–8.0 mg/dL
- Hypophosphatemia: <4.0–5.5 mg/dL

Hyperphosphatemia may result from renal insufficiency, over-supplementation, hypoparathyroidism (congenital or transient), and maternal hyperphosphatemia. Signs and symptoms include tetany (due to associated hypocalcemia), seizures, renal damage, calcium-phosphate precipitation in soft tissues, and oliguria. Treatment includes phosphate binders, limiting phosphate intake, hydration, diuretics, and calcium supplementation.

- Hyperphosphatemia: >6.5–8 mg/dL

Maternal Newborn Nurse Practice Test #1

Want to take this practice test in an online interactive format?
Check out the bonus page, which includes interactive practice questions and much more: **mometrix.com/bonus948/matnewnurse**

1. Correct statements about breastfeeding and formula-feeding include which of the following?

a. there is a faster return to pre-pregnancy weight in mothers of formula-fed infants
b. there is a lower incidence of milk-protein allergy in formula-fed infants
c. there is an improved immunity in breastfed infants

2. The dark red uterine discharge expelled in the first 2-3 days postpartum is

a. lochia rubra
b. lochia serosa
c. lochia alba

3. The fetal/neonatal lung substance that improves pulmonary compliance by decreasing alveolar surface tension is

a. meconium
b. prostaglandin
c. surfactant

4. Obesity during pregnancy is associated with an increased risk of

a. fetuses that are small-for-gestational age
b. cesarean birth
c. rapid postpartum weight loss

5. Immediately after an uncomplicated delivery without meconium, a full-term newborn is warmed, dried, suctioned, and positioned appropriately but has a heart rate of 80 beats/min. According to neonatal resuscitation guidelines, the next step in managing this infant is

a. positive-pressure ventilation
b. chest compression
c. epinephrine administration

6. Clinical practice that is consistent with established recommendations or standards is best characterized by

a. standards that are used primarily to minimize providers' legal liability
b. recommendations that are used to standardize patient care based on evidence-based guidelines
c. standards that are based on methods that have proven effective over a substantial period of time

7. All of the following are elements of the postpartum breast assessment EXCEPT:

a. firmness, tenderness, and redness
b. engorgement and nipple soreness/cracking
c. lumps indicating possible cancerous growths

8. Vitamin K is administered to newborn infants to prevent

a. bleeding
b. neonatal jaundice
c. gonococcal conjunctivitis

9. Perineal pain in the first 4-6 hours after vaginal delivery are initially managed with

a. oral analgesic medications
b. ice packs to the perineum
c. frequent perineal pad changes

10. The biophysical profile evaluates fetal wellbeing by combining fetal heart rate monitoring with

a. ultrasonographic examination of established fetal parameters
b. fetal movement counting ("kick counts")
c. external monitoring of uterine contractions

11. The least expensive type of infant formula is

a. formula concentrate
b. ready-to-feed formula
c. powdered formula

12. Six to twelve hours after the vaginal delivery of a single infant and placenta, the uterine fundus should be palpable at or below the level of the

a. pubic symphysis
b. umbilicus
c. epigastrium

13. Infants delivered by elective cesarean section are at increased risk for

a. neonatal jaundice
b. low birth weight
c. neonatal respiratory distress

14. In caring for a family who has experienced a perinatal fetal death, it is helpful to

a. share personal stories of recovery that have been witnessed in the past
b. maximize consistency in assigned nursing staff
c. guide the family to a bereavement room as soon as possible, to allow privacy in mourning

15. Ineffective or shallow infant latch with breastfeeding may lead to increased

a. reflux in the infant
b. milk let-down
c. nipple pain

16. Reddish-orange crystals noted in the urine of a 48-hour-old newborn are

a. a sign of congenital renal disease
b. a sign of vitamin K deficiency
c. a normal finding

17. Which of the following statements about the nurse's medical record documentation is correct?

a. it provides an accurate account of patient status and response to care
b. it consists of both objective and subjective notes regarding the patient and care provided
c. the physician's medical record documentation is more important than the nurse's medical record documentation in legal proceeding

18. Breastfeeding in the immediate postpartum period can improve uterine contractions because of the release of

a. prolactin
b. oxytocin
c. human chorionic gonadotropin

19. Gas exchange in utero in the fetus is performed by the

a. fetal heart
b. fetal lungs
c. placenta

20. An early sign of magnesium sulfate toxicity is

a. seizure activity
b. loss of deep tendon reflexes
c. flushed skin and nausea

21. Breastfeeding is usually contraindicated if the mother has

a. a history of treated breast cancer
b. human immunodeficiency virus
c. latent tuberculosis

22. A method of heat production unique to newborn infants is the metabolism of

a. bilirubin
b. brown fat
c. prostaglandin

23. If the postpartum uterine fundus is boggy on palpation, the nurse does which of the following?

a. notifies the physician immediately
b. massages the uterus until it feels firm
c. re-examines the fundus in 15-20 minutes

24. A sign of impaired attachment between the postpartum mother and her infant is

a. decreasing maternal interaction with the infant over time
b. maternal request to rest and refuse visitors
c. maternal encouragement for family members to hold the infant

25. An Rh-negative mother who has given birth to an Rh-positive infant and has no evidence of sensitization (i.e., maternal indirect Coombs test negative) should be administered

a. Rh immune globulin (Rhogam) within 72 hours of delivery
b. no additional medication
c. cross-matched packed red blood cells within 4 hours of delivery

26. A common complication in the newborn infant of a diabetic mother is

a. hyperglycemia
b. anemia
c. hypoglycemia

27. Hindmilk (milk that flows later in a feeding) has a higher concentration of which of the following substances than foremilk?

a. fat
b. protein
c. colostrum

28. The postpartum patient who has undergone a forceps-assisted vaginal delivery is at increased risk for

a. postpartum hemorrhage
b. eclampsia
c. postpartum depression

29. Early decelerations with a normal fetal heart rate variability during labor have which of the following indications?

a. they often indicate fetal congenital heart disease
b. they do not indicate fetal hypoxia
c. they may indicate fetal acidemia

30. A cephalohematoma in the newborn infant has which of the following characteristics?

a. it does not cross suture lines
b. it typically resolves within 12 hours of birth
c. it is more common after a cesarean birth

31. Infectious mastitis in the breastfeeding mother has which of the following characteristics?

a. it is treated by cessation of breastfeeding
b. it usually occurs within 48 hours of delivery
c. it can often be prevented with proper breastfeeding technique

32. Neonatal jaundice that is present in the first 24 hours of life is considered

a. physiologic
b. pathologic
c. unconjugated

33. A common cause of neonatal sepsis is

a. *neisseria gonorrhoeae*
b. group B *Streptococcus*
c. *Gardnerella vaginalis*

34. All of the following clinical features would be expected with "postpartum blues" (adjustment reaction with depressed mood) EXCEPT

a. frequent tearfulness
b. irritability
c. suicidal ideation

35. The newborn's sensory capacity to attend to and fixate on a visual stimulus (e.g., caregiver's face) is known as

a. habituation
b. orientation
c. self-quieting

36. To prevent contamination and encourage drying of the umbilical cord stump, caregivers should be advised to

a. give the newborn daily tub baths
b. pull on the cord stump daily
c. fold diapers down to avoid covering the cord stump

37. Compared to infants delivered in occiput anterior vertex presentation, infants delivered vaginally in a breech presentation have which of the following risks?

a. a higher risk of birth trauma
b. a lower risk of fetal asphyxia
c. a lower risk of umbilical cord prolapse

38. Treatment of engorgement in the breastfeeding mother includes

a. application of warm compresses before breastfeeding
b. less frequent breastfeeding
c. antibiotics and cold therapy

39. Pregnancy in the breastfeeding postpartum mother is at the lowest likelihood

a. within one month of delivery
b. throughout the duration of breastfeeding
c. when menstruation resumes

40. The sign most concerning for congenital heart disease in the newborn infant is

a. fever
b. central cyanosis
c. acrocyanosis

41. The expected physiologic weight loss in the term newborn's first week of life is

a. up to 20% of birth weight
b. no weight loss
c. up to 10% of birth weight

42. A mother who gives birth by cesarean delivery is encouraged to

a. ambulate as soon as possible after delivery
b. delay seeing her infant until she is no longer requiring pain medications
c. take shallow, purse-lip breaths to minimize pain

43. In a patient with preeclampsia, the development of eclampsia is characterized by

a. elevated liver enzymes
b. hypertension
c. seizures

44. A gestational age assessment in the preterm newborn is likely to demonstrate

a. hyperflexion of the upper and lower extremities in the infant's resting posture
b. minimal breast bud tissue
c. highly developed ear cartilage

45. The drug-exposed infant is most likely to have symptoms of withdrawal in the newborn period after chronic intrauterine exposure to

a. caffeine
b. marijuana
c. oxycodone

46. In caring for a newborn male's recently circumcised penis (non-Plastibell technique), the infant's caregivers are advised to

a. apply a small amount of petroleum ointment to the glans with diaper changes
b. avoid cleaning the penis with warm water
c. pull off the thin, yellowish film that forms on the glans

47. A respiratory pattern characterized by 10-15 seconds of shallow rapid breathing followed by a 5-10 second respiratory pause with spontaneous return of breathing and no associated distress or color change is called

a. periodic breathing
b. central apnea
c. transient tachypnea of the newborn

48. Sticky, greenish black stool is considered characteristic of

a. a newborn infant
b. a breastfed infant
c. a formula fed infant

49. A newborn infant opens her mouth and turns her head to the right when her right cheek is touched, which is consistent with which of the following reflexes?

a. rooting reflex
b. moro reflex
c. tonic neck reflex ("fencing" reflex)

50. Parents of newborn infants are instructed to place infants on their back to sleep to decrease the risk of

a. gastroesophageal reflux (GERD)
b. sudden infant death syndrome (SIDS)
c. bronchiolitis

51. Characteristics of jitteriness include

a. ocular deviations
b. clonic jerking with fast and slow elements
c. increased heart rate

52. After using a breast pump, the woman should

a. rinse removable parts in cold water, then wash with warm soapy water
b. immediately sterilize the removable parts in boiling water
c. wash removable parts in very hot soapy water

53. The most common neonatal bacterial infection is

a. *Staphylococcus aureus*
b. *Pseudomonas aeruginosa*
c. Group B *Streptococcus*

54. The neonate usually passes meconium within

a. 6 to 8 hours
b. 8 to 24 hours
c. 48 to 72 hours

55. A few weeks after delivery, if a woman complains that she cannot sleep, has little appetite and has begun having anxiety attacks and fears that she cannot take adequate care of her neonate, the most likely cause is

a. postpartum depression
b. postpartum blues
c. postpartum psychosis

56. If a neonate's hemoglobin is 19.3 shortly after birth, a typical value at 7 days is

a. 22.4 g/dL
b. 19.3 g/dL
c. 17.4 g/dL

57. HELLP syndrome is characterized by (H) hemolysis, (EL) elevated liver enzymes, and (LP)

a. lateral pain
b. low (blood) pressure
c. low platelet count

58. The vaccination that should be routinely administered to all newborns within 24 hours of birth is

a. hepatitis A.
b. hepatitis B.
c. rotavirus.

59. If a quad screen shows high AFP, and normal hCG, uE3 and INH-A, this indicates

a. neural tube defect
b. trisomy 21
c. multiple gestation

60. The infantile form of Tay-Sachs disease is classified as a

a. chromosomal abnormality
b. blood disorder
c. metabolic defect

61. The nutritional supplement given to women to prevent neural tube defects is

a. folic acid
b. magnesium
c. iron

62. If a woman complains that she is exhausted because the neonate nurses so frequently during the night that the woman cannot get any sleep, the nurse should advise the woman to

a. give bottle feedings during the night so the neonate will sleep longer
b. nurse the infant on a strict 3- to 4-hour schedule
c. sleep when the baby sleeps, day and night

63. The CARE principles applied to the care of a pregnant woman refer to (C) communication, (A) advocate, (R) respect, and (E)

a. enable
b. educate
c. engage

64. The recreational drug that most increases the risk of spontaneous abortion is

a. marijuana
b. methamphetamine
c. MDMA

65. By about the sixth day after birth, over a 24-hour period, most infants urinate approximately

a. 12 to 14 times
b. 8 to 12 times
c. 6 to 8 times

66. The neural tube defect that is most likely to result in hydrocephalus is

a. spina bifida occulta
b. myelomeningocele
c. meningocele

67. When using the BUBBLE-HE mnemonic to remember the steps to a comprehensive postpartal assessment, the initial BUB refers to

a. breasts, uterus, bladder
b. bowels, urine, and breasts
c. bowels, uterus, and bonding

68. Human milk can be kept frozen in the freezer section of a side-by-side refrigerator-freezer for

a. 2 weeks
b. 3 to 4 months
c. 6 months

69. If a pregnant woman at 38-weeks of gestation complains of dizziness when lying flat, the most likely cause is

a. hyperventilation and shortness of breath
b. nutritional imbalance
c. supine hypotensive syndrome

70. If a woman's pregnancy classification is G4, T2, P1, A1, L3, the number of total pregnancies is

a. 3
b. 4
c. 6

71. If the fundal height is halfway between the woman's symphysis pubic and umbilicus, the approximate weeks of gestation are

a. 8
b. 12
c. 16

72. The cell free fetal DNA test assesses for

a. chromosomal disorders
b. neural tube defects
c. fetal alcohol syndrome

73. How much weight is a woman with a pre-pregnancy BMI of 22.0 is expected to gain during pregnancy?

a. 15 to 20 pounds
b. 25 to 35 pounds
c. 28 to 40 pounds

74. The presence of bilirubin in amniotic fluid usually indicates

a. chromosomal abnormalities
b. infection
c. Rh-sensitized pregnancy

75. Severe post-dural puncture (spinal) headache is best treated with

a. epidural blood patch
b. opioid analgesia
c. caffeinated beverages

76. If bottle-feeding a neonate with cleft lip and cleft palate, the nipple should be

a. shorter than normal size
b. normal size for gestation
c. longer than normal size

77. Ultrasonography can be used to estimate fetal age with crown-rump length (CRL) at approximately

a. 6 to 8 weeks
b. 7 to 12 weeks
c. 13 to 14 weeks

78. When palpating the uterus after delivery, it is necessary to

a. support the lower uterine segment
b. support the upper uterine segment
c. press down firmly with both hands

79. Asymmetric intrauterine growth restriction is caused by problems that occur during the

a. first trimester
b. second trimester
c. third trimester

80. If a woman in labor is receiving a benzodiazepine to relieve anxiety, nausea, and pain, the medication that should also be available on the unit is

a. flumazenil
b. naloxone
c. N-acetylcysteine

81. A patient who experienced placenta previa is at increased risk of hemorrhage during the postpartal period because

a. the placenta was smaller than normal
b. the area of implantation does not contract effectively
c. the placenta implanted very high in the uterus

82. Following spontaneous rupture of the membranes during labor, if the fetal heart rate becomes markedly bradycardic with variable decelerations, this likely indicates

a. cord prolapse
b. placenta previa
c. fetal head compression

83. During the process of lactation, the breasts usually begin filling and feel firm and warm by the

a. first day
b. second day
c. third day

84. The most common cause of subinvolution is

a. uterine atony
b. retained placental fragments
c. hematoma

85. If shoulder dystocia occurred during delivery, the newborn should be examined for

a. fractured clavicle and Erb's palsy
b. skull fracture and cerebral palsy
c. spinal cord injury and paralysis

86. Labor and delivery is defined as precipitate if labor lasts less than

a. one hour
b. three hours
c. five hours

87. Ensuring that a woman has given informed consent and understands her rights and all of the risks and benefits of a procedure or treatment supports the ethical principal of

a. beneficence
b. nonmaleficence
c. autonomy

88. If a woman complains of persistent constipation in the postpartal period, the best treatment approach is usually a(n)

a. increase in fluid intake
b. high fiber diet
c. stool softener

89. When conducting a review of the literature as part of evidence-based research, the level of evidence that is based on a quasi-experimental study, such as a matched case-control study, would be categorized as

a. Level I
b. Level II
c. Level III

90. In the postpartal period, the uterine fundus should no longer be palpable after

a. 14 days
b. 10 days
c. 7 days

91. The antibiotic agent that should be avoided for long-term use while a woman is breastfeeding is

a. tetracyclines
b. erythromycin
c. cephalosporins

92. If a nurse administers the wrong drug to a patient but the patient suffers no ill effects, the elements of malpractice that are missing are

a. Duty to use care and breach of duty
b. Duty to use care and damages
c. Damages and causation

93. Necrotizing enterocolitis in a preterm infant is usually caused by

a. ischemic bowel
b. severe constipation
c. generalized infection

94. If, on palpating the uterus in the postpartal period, the nurse finds the fundus is displaced superior to the umbilicus and to the right, the nurse should suspect that the cause is

a. uterine atony
b. bladder distension
c. uterine hemorrhage

95. Methylergonovine (Methergine®) may be administered to a woman after delivery in order to

a. promote uterine contractions
b. relieve pain and discomfort
c. reduce maternal hypertension

96. A woman who is breastfeeding and needs to take smoking cessation medication in order to stop smoking should avoid

a. nicotine patches
b. nicotine gum
c. varenicline

97. A woman who has taken methadone during pregnancy and wants to breastfeed should

a. take the lowest dose of methadone
b. continue the same dose of methadone
c. stop taking methadone

98. If a neonate's skin is dry and peeling with no vernix and loss of subcutaneous fat, the likely gestational age is

a. 42 to 44 weeks
b. 35 to 40 weeks
c. 24 to 26 weeks

99. In the immediate postpartal period, a woman's gastric motility is generally

a. within normal limits
b. increased
c. decreased

100. If a woman's white blood cell count was 20,000 after delivery and increased to 40,000 by the second day, this likely indicates

a. normal postpartal elevation
b. acute infection
c. chronic infection

101. If testing after birth shows that a neonate has inherited galactosemia, an inborn error of metabolism, the neonate should be fed

a. human milk
b. whey-based formula
c. soy-based formula

102. If a breastfeeding woman shows a nonimmune rubella titer prior to discharge, the woman should be

a. given the MMR vaccine and continue breastfeeding
b. given the MMR vaccine and stop breastfeeding for a few days
c. told to take the MMR vaccine in 3 to 6 months

103. The breastfeeding position that is good to relieve plugged milk ducts and engorged breasts is

a. cradle hold
b. football hold
c. side-lying hold

104. When assisting with the lumbar puncture of a preterm neonate, the correct position for the neonate is

a. lateral with trunk flexed
b. lateral with trunk in neutral position
c. sitting with head supported

105. If a new mother presents with irritation of the nipple and verbalizes discomfort during breastfeeding, it is most likely that the infant is

a. latching to both the nipple and the areola
b. latching only to the nipple, with the nipple ending at the infant's soft palate
c. latching only to the nipple, with the nipple ending at the infant's hard palate

106. If a neonate exhibits neck rigidity after birth, this may indicate injury to the

a. sternocleidomastoid muscle
b. levator scapula muscle
c. platysma muscle

107. B. A demarcated unraised red-purple lesion caused by capillaries below the skin on a child's face is a

a. nevus vasculosus (strawberry mark)
b. nevus flammeus (port-wine stain)
c. erythema toxicum

108. If a woman with flat nipples has started using a nipple shield while breastfeeding but the infant is not gaining adequate weight, the nurse should advise the woman to

a. provide supplemental bottle feedings
b. use the nipple shield for only 1 or 2 minutes
c. stop breastfeeding

109. If a nursing neonate has a 5:1 suck/swallow ratio, this indicates

a. non-nutritive suckling
b. fast but adequate suckling
c. normal suckling

110. If a new mother asks about bottle-feeding human milk so the father can experience feeding the infant, she should be advised to wait for at least

a. 24 to 48 hours
b. one week
c. 4 weeks

111. Until a neonate regains body weight, the neonate should be nursed at least every

a. 2 hours
b. 3 hours
c. 4 hours

112. A normal percentage of weight loss for a neonate in the first few days of life is

a. 5%
b. 8%
c. 10%

113. When expressing milk from the breast, a woman should

a. alternate between the C and the U hold in fixed positions
b. start with the C hold but move about the breast clockwise
c. use the C hold and hold the hand in a fixed position

114. Women may experience exacerbation of autoimmune disorders, such as lupus erythematosus, after labor and delivery because

a. the woman's immune system is no longer suppressed
b. the woman is in a weakened condition
c. the woman is experiencing increased stress and anxiety

115. If, on the first post-partum day, the woman's fundus is firm and lochia appears normal but the woman complains of perineal discomfort and BP falls to 88/50 and pulse increases to 112, the nurse should suspect a(n)

a. uterine hemorrhage
b. vaginal laceration
c. hematoma

116. If a neonate's cardiac status appeared normal at birth but 48 hours later the neonate experiences a precipitous drop in circulation to the lower body, the likely congenital heart defect is

a. ventricular septal defect
b. aortic stenosis
c. coarctation of the aorta

117. Following delivery, if the fundus feels contracted and in the right position but free flow of bright red blood is evident vaginally, this is likely due to

a. vaginal or cervical laceration
b. normal post-delivery lochia
c. uterine hemorrhage

118. The hormone that stimulates the alveoli to produce milk is

a. oxytocin
b. estrogen
c. prolactin

119. If a woman reports that her neonate cries frantically when hungry, this likely means that

a. there is the possibility of an underlying disease process that must be investigated
b. the woman is missing signs of hunger
c. the woman is not breastfeeding correctly

120. Following an unmedicated delivery, a neonate should ideally begin breastfeeding during the first

a. 10 to 20 minutes
b. 1 to 2 hours
c. 3 to 4 hours

121. A woman who develops postpartal DVT should be carefully monitored for signs of

a. pulmonary embolus
b. infection
c. hemorrhage

122. During stage two of milk production (the postpartum period), hormonal changes include

a. increased progesterone and decreased prolactin
b. increased progesterone and decreased estrogen
c. decreased progesterone and increased prolactin

123. In order to prevent post-dural puncture (spinal) headache, the woman should

a. be administered ibuprofen
b. lie flat for several hours
c. increase hydration

124. During the "claiming" part of parent-neonate attachment, the parent usually first compares the child to other family members by noticing how the neonate is

a. similar
b. unique
c. different

125. After delivery, a woman is likely to exhibit signs and symptoms of hypovolemic shock with blood loss greater than

a. 500 mL
b. 1000 mL
c. 1500 mL

126. The phase of maternal role transition during which the woman begins to feel like a mother is

a. taking in
b. taking hold
c. letting go

127. If a neonate's chest circumference is 34 cm, the head circumference would normally be about

a. 32 cm
b. 36 cm
c. 38 cm

128. An indication that the woman may not be bonding with her neonate is when the mother

a. exhibits disgust when the infant urinates and refuses to change the diaper
b. points out that the neonate looks like a paternal grandparent
c. asks that the infant be placed in the nursery during the night

129. Paternal-neonate bonding includes three stages: Commitment, attachment, and

a. knowledge
b. preparation
c. acceptance

130. If a woman admitted in labor plans to relinquish her infant for adoption, the nurse should

a. avoid any mention of adoption
b. acknowledge the adoption plans
c. ask the woman if she has changed her mind

131. To prevent contamination, reconstituted formula for bottle feeding should not be stored in the refrigerator for more than

a. 6 hours
b. 12 hours
c. 24 hours

132. To facilitate bonding between the woman and her neonate if the woman chooses to bottle feed, the nurse should encourage the woman to

a. maintain eye contact with the neonate
b. hold the infant with the head higher than the body
c. swaddle the infant tightly in a blanket

133. The neonate of a diabetic mother whose blood glucose levels were elevated above 145 mg/dL during labor is likely to experience

a. hyperglycemia and hypercalcemia
b. hypoglycemia and hypocalcemia
c. hypoglycemia and hypercalcemia

134. The primary risk factor for metritis (uterine infection) is

a. hematoma
b. vaginal birth
c. Cesarean birth

135. A woman with gestational diabetes is at risk of delivering a neonate with

a. microsomia
b. macrosomia
c. congenital defects

136. If a woman with a history of bipolar disease develops marked hyperactivity about two weeks after delivery with signs of postpartum psychosis, including confusion and anger toward the infant, the first intervention should be to

a. remove the neonate from the home
b. urge the woman to seek treatment
c. immediately refer services to help the mother care for the infant during this period

137. If a neonate is born with gastroschisis, the exposed organs should be

a. pushed back into place and covered with dry dressing
b. irrigated and covered with wet dressings
c. covered with moist gauze and wrapped in plastic

138. Following delivery, the best preventive measure to reduce the risk of developing deep vein thrombosis (DVT) is

a. ASA prophylaxis
b. early ambulation
c. adequate hydration

139. A first-line treatment for gestational hypertensive disorders is

a. nifedipine
b. hydrochlorothiazide
c. furosemide

140. A woman should be encouraged to room-in with her neonate during hospitalization in order to

a. reduce maternal anxiety
b. initiate maternal responsibility
c. facilitate bonding

141. On the day of delivery, a diabetic woman who has been receiving insulin for type 1 diabetes will probably require

a. the same dosage
b. a higher dosage
c. a lower dosage

142. If a neonate has a hematocrit of 67%, this likely indicates

a. polycythemia
b. anemia
c. hypovolemia

143. If a Haitian woman states she does not want to name her baby girl, the nurse should assume

a. the woman is not bonding with the neonate
b. delayed naming is a cultural norm
c. the woman is unhappy with the child's gender

144. Following delivery, postpartum blues typically subsides within about

a. 4 days
b. 10 days
c. 16 days

145. X-linked disorders affect

a. male offspring primarily
b. female offspring primarily
c. male and female offspring equally

146. If a woman expresses concern that her 3-year-old child does not seem to love the neonate, the nurse should advise the woman that

a. the child may need professional help to develop a bond
b. the mother should pay less attention to the neonate
c. young children develop affection over time

147. A woman who is nursing her neonate usually needs to increase fluid intake by about

a. 500 mL day
b. 1000 mL day
c. 2000 mL day

148. An antidepressant that is generally considered reasonably safe to continue during pregnancy for women with a history of severe depression is

a. paroxetine (Paxil®)
b. tranylcypromine (Parnate®)
c. citalopram (Celexa®)

149. A neonate exposed to or infected with herpes simplex is treated with

a. cephalosporin
b. acyclovir
c. corticosteroid

150. Conditions associated with oligohydramnios include

a. urinary tract anomalies
b. chromosomal abnormalities, such as trisomy 21
c. obstructional lesions of GI tract

151. Laboratory abnormalities associated with disseminated intravascular coagulation include

a. increased platelet counts
b. increased fibrinogen
c. prolonged prothrombin

152. When assisting a patient to take a sitz bath to relieve swelling and discomfort of hemorrhoids, the nurse should assure that the water temperature does not exceed

a. 100 °F (38 °C)
b. 105 °F (41 °C)
c. 110 °F (43 °C)

153. If a normal speaking voice is 50 to 60 decibels, the noise levels in the nursery and NICU should be maintained at

a. ≤45 decibels
b. ≤50 decibels
c. ≤60 decibels

154. With kangaroo care, the neonate in minimal clothing is placed

a. in a swaddling blanket and held
b. between the mother's bare breasts
c. in a sling across the mother's breasts

155. If a neonate has a patent ductus arteriosus, the usual initial treatment is

a. captopril
b. prostaglandin
c. indomethacin

156. In the neonate, the nurse should immediately report any periods of apnea that last for more than

a. 10 seconds
b. 20 seconds
c. 30 seconds

157. The wet neonate's temperature falls rapidly after birth if not promptly dried and warmed because of

a. evaporation
b. convection
c. radiation

158. Following birth, damage to the neonate's upper brachial plexus (C5 to C7) is likely to result in

a. Ipsilateral Horner syndrome
b. Klumpke's palsy
c. Erb's palsy

159. The purpose of administering vitamin K to a neonate is to

a. facilitate clotting
b. prevent clotting
c. treat anemia

160. According to Safe Sleep guidelines, parents should be taught to place a neonate on the back

a. when the neonate is sleeping and unattended
b. during the night
c. during the first two weeks

161. Starting immediately after hospital discharge, the neonate should have "tummy time"

a. 2 to 3 times a day
b. whenever the neonate is awake
c. 4 to 6 times a day

162. The normal position for the neonate's ears is with the insertion point of the top of the ear parallel to the

a. eyebrow
b. outer canthus of the eye
c. nostrils

163. When placing a newborn in a safety car seat, the seat should be rear-facing and

a. reclined 30-45 degrees
b. upright
c. flat

164. If a neonate must undergo a medical procedure, sucrose analgesia (SweetEase™) should be given to the infant

a. when the procedure starts
b. 10 minutes before the procedure
c. 2 minutes before the procedure

165. According to the Silverman-Anderson Index, a neonate exhibiting see-saw movement of the chest/abdomen, pronounced intercostal and xiphoid retraction, nasal flaring, and audible grunt would receive a score of

a. 2
b. 6
c. 10

166. The neonatal hearing test that measures the integrity of the middle and inner ear and the outer hair cells of the cochlea is the

a. auditory brainstem response
b. otoacoustic emissions test
c. bone-conduction test

167. The eye prophylaxis for neonates that is generally the drug of choice is

a. erythromycin
b. silver nitrate
c. tetracycline

168. If air becomes trapped in the alveoli because of meconium aspiration during labor and delivery, the neonate is at risk for

a. pulmonary embolism
b. air embolism
c. pneumothorax

169. ABO incompatibility can occur if

a. the mother is B and the fetus is A
b. the mother is O and the fetus is B
c. the mother is A and the fetus is O

170. If a neonate with Down syndrome has skin that appears mottled at times (pale in some areas and flushed in others), especially if the neonate is exposed to cool air, the most likely cause is

a. acrocyanosis
b. erythema toxicum
c. cutis marmorata

171. In order for a child to be born with cystic fibrosis, an autosomal recessive disorder,

a. both parents must carry the defective gene
b. either parent must carry the defective gene
c. the mother must carry the defective gene

172. If a neonate is born to an HIV infected mother, the neonate should begin antiretroviral medications within

a. 6 weeks
b. 24 to 48 hours
c. 6 to 12 hours

173. In order to prevent intracranial hemorrhage, a neonate with thrombocytopenia generally requires a platelet count of at least

a. 100,000
b. 50,000
c. 30,000

174. If a neonate's mother was addicted to methamphetamine use during her pregnancy, the neonate in withdrawal will likely exhibit

a. hyporeflexia
b. high-pitched crying
c. inability to sleep

175. Neonates who are bottle fed need to be burped

a. every 2 to 3 ounces
b. if they appear uncomfortable
c. at the end of feeding, regardless of volume

Answer Key and Explanations

1. C: Whenever possible, breastfeeding is the nutritional method of choice for the newborn infant and has many advantages for both the infant and the postpartum mother. The nutritional composition of human milk is ideal for the newborn infant and cannot be entirely replicated in formula. Breastfed infants have improved immunity relative to formula-fed infants, including a decreased risk for respiratory and gastrointestinal infections, serious bacterial infections, and allergic disease, including milk-protein allergy. Advantages for the breastfeeding mother include faster postpartum weight loss and a lower risk of breast and ovarian cancer later in life.

2. A: The uterine discharge expelled in the postpartum period is called lochia and consists of blood cells, epithelial cells, uterine debris, and the superficial layer of the endometrial decidua basalis. Lochia rubra is expelled in the first 2-3 days of the postpartum period; it is dark red in color and may include expulsion of small clots, usually as a result of pooling of the lochia rubra in the upper vagina. Lochia serosa is a pink-colored discharge and is expelled on days 4-10 postpartum. Lochia alba is a white-yellow discharge that is seen for 1-2 weeks following the lochia serosa. Variations in volume and duration are common, but the overall trend with lochia should be a lighter color and volume as time elapses. Assessment of lochia volume and character is important in the postpartum period to monitor for excessive postpartum bleeding.

3. C: Surfactant is a lipoprotein that is produced in the lung alveoli beginning at 24 weeks' gestation. Surfactant reduces the surface tension of the alveoli by coating their inner surface. This results in a decreased tendency for the alveoli to collapse. Surfactant deficiency leads to progressive respiratory distress as a result of impaired lung compliance, ultimately leading to hypoxia, respiratory failure, and metabolic acidosis, all of which further impair surfactant production. Respiratory distress due to surfactant deficiency is called respiratory distress syndrome (RDS) and is most commonly seen in preterm infants. The morbidity and mortality of RDS are markedly reduced with the early assessment of fetal lung maturity, identification of high-risk infants, and the endotracheal administration of surfactant replacement therapy.

4. B: Maternal nutritional status is an important determinant of both maternal and fetal wellbeing. Women with a normal body mass index whose pregnancy weight gain is within the recommended range have the lowest risk for complications in pregnancy and delivery. Poor weight gain during pregnancy is associated with an increased risk of preterm delivery and low birth weight. Obesity and pregnancy weight gain above the recommended range are associated with an increased risk of gestational diabetes, cesarean delivery, fetal macrosomia, fetal demise, postpartum hemorrhage, fetal neural tube defects, and difficulty with postpartum weight loss.

5. A: Neonatal resuscitation guidelines allow for all care providers managing newborn infants to proceed along a standardized algorithm to stabilize the infant as soon as possible after delivery. Initial steps may vary with deliveries involving meconium-stained amniotic fluid in an attempt to avoid worsening meconium aspiration. In the newborn without meconium-stained amniotic fluid, the infant is warmed, dried, suctioned (if necessary), and placed in a position that allows for unobstructed breathing. Heart rate, respiratory effort, and color are then evaluated. If the infant has poor respiratory effort or rate or the heart rate is lower than 100 beats/min, positive-pressure ventilation is provided. If positive-pressure ventilation does not improve the heart rate to 100 beats/min, then chest compression and epinephrine administration are indicated.

6. B: Medical care providers need to stay up-to-date with current recommendations and care guidelines to ensure that they are providing quality, evidence-based care to patients, while protecting themselves from allegations of medical mismanagement. While methods that have proven effective over a substantial period of time may continue to do so, it is important that clinical practice incorporate recent research and best practices into their standardized methods. When situations arise in clinical practice that require deviation from established standards of practice, thorough documentation in the medical record, detailing the provider's medical decision-making process is particularly important. Medical care that is consistent with established guidelines can minimize a provider's legal liability. The primary purpose of following professionally established standards, however, is providing safe, high-quality, evidence-based care to the patient.

7. C: Assessment of the breasts is an important component of the comprehensive nurse assessment in the postpartum period. During pregnancy, elevated estrogen and progesterone levels cause the breasts to enlarge and become more glandular. The postpartum patient should have her breasts assessed for firmness, tenderness, redness, and engorgement in addition to nipple soreness or cracking. In the breastfeeding patient, a crucial part of the nurse assessment is evaluation of infant latch and removal from the breast. In the non-breastfeeding patient, techniques for lactation suppression and pain management can be reviewed and demonstrated. The postpartum mother should be reminded of the importance of self-breast examinations for lumps indicative of malignancy, but the immediate postpartum period will prove difficult to identify lumps upon assessment due to the number of changes the breasts are going through at this time.

8. A: Newborns are vitamin K-deficient as a result of poor transfer of vitamin K across the placenta and low capability of the liver to store vitamin K in the newborn period. Several clotting factors depend on the presence of adequate vitamin K for proper function. As a result, vitamin K deficiency leads to an increased risk of serious bleeding. Newborns at increased risk for vitamin K deficiency include breastfed infants, as there are low levels of vitamin K in human milk, and infants born to mothers taking anticonvulsant medication. Bleeding as a result of a vitamin K deficiency often presents as bleeding of the umbilicus, gastrointestinal tract, circumcision or venipuncture sites, or (rarely) intracranium. Vitamin K administered routinely after delivery prevents most cases of bleeding in the neonate that results from a vitamin K deficiency.

9. B: Perineal pain is present in virtually all postpartum patients after vaginal delivery. Ice pack application, sitz baths, and careful cleaning after voiding (e.g., using a "peri-bottle" to squirt water onto the perineum) are helpful supportive care measures to reduce and manage postpartum perineal pain. Topical anesthetics or soothing agents (e.g., witch hazel) may also be applied. Analgesics are not typically first line treatment for perineal pain. Changing the "peri-pad" frequently can reduce the risk of contamination of perineal wounds but is not typically helpful for reducing pain. Perineal lacerations need to be monitored for signs of poor healing or infection, such as erythema, marked swelling, and discharge or wound dehiscence.

10. A: There are multiple methods for the evaluation and monitoring of fetal wellbeing. In high-risk pregnancies (e.g., maternal hypertension, multiple gestation) or in cases where there are other concerns for fetal wellbeing (e.g., decreased fetal movement, previous fetal demise), antepartum fetal monitoring is generally indicated. Fetal movement counting (e.g., maternal perception of fetal movement) is considered normal if the mother perceives ten distinct movements over a 2-hour period (after 32-34 weeks' gestation). The nonstress test involves fetal heart rate (FHR) monitoring and is considered reassuring ("reactive") if there are at least two fetal heart rate accelerations (>15 beats/min above baseline, lasting >15 seconds) in a 20-minute period. The biophysical profile combines FHR monitoring with ultrasonographic evaluation of fetal tone, fetal movement, amniotic fluid volume, and fetal respiratory movements.

11. C: Powdered formula is the least expensive form of commercially available infant formula, but it must be reconstituted, using water. Proper mixing (60 mL water for each scoop of powdered formula) is crucial to avoid medical complications in the infant because of inappropriately concentrated or dilute formula. Among the three forms available, powdered formula preparation has the highest risk for contamination. Formula concentrate is mixed with water to its appropriate concentration, while ready-to-feed formula is given without any mixing required. Although ready-to-feed formula is the easiest to use, its cost is significant. Whichever type of formula is used, proper mixing and storage guidelines must be reviewed with postpartum families.

12. B: Immediately after vaginal delivery of the placenta, the normal uterus contracts to grapefruit-size, and the fundus is palpable between the umbilicus and the pubic symphysis. During the first 6-12 hours after delivery, the ligaments and muscles supporting the uterus relax somewhat, and the fundus is palpable at or below the umbilicus. Beginning approximately 24 hours after delivery, the shrinking uterus descends about 1 cm/d into the pelvis, reaching pre-pregnancy size and location by 6 weeks' postpartum. Excessive blood loss, infection, and retained placental fragments can lead to an interruption of the normal postpartum uterine contractions, leading to uterine atony. A common cause of uterine atony and displacement of the uterine fundus after delivery is bladder distension.

13. C: Approximately one-third of infants in the United States are delivered by cesarean section. Cesarean delivery may be performed for maternal indications, fetal indications, or both. Examples of common indications for cesarean birth include placenta previa, breech presentation, placental abruption, congenital anomalies, fetal distress, maternal infection, and previous delivery by cesarean section. Women who deliver by cesarean section are at increased risk for infection, thromboembolic events, and anesthesia complications. Infants delivered by cesarean section are at increased risk for respiratory complications, physical injury (e.g., laceration, fracture), early breastfeeding difficulties, and admission to a neonatal intensive care unit.

14. B: Facilitating and assisting with the family's grief process after a perinatal death is an important nursing intervention and is best accomplished with consistency in the nursing staff. This allows for establishment of a therapeutic relationship between the nurse and the grieving family. Ideally, the nurse assists the family in expressing their feelings about the loss, participating in decision-making about the birth and postpartum period (including seeing the deceased infant), and becoming aware of the resources available for ongoing support during the journey through the grieving process. Sharing personal stories may appear as an effort to normalize an extremely unique and private experience for the family, and should be avoided. Although not all parents choose to see or spend time with the deceased infant, it can be very helpful in assisting the family to accept the loss of the infant, therefore utilizing a bereavement room should not be rushed.

15. C: Establishing successful and satisfying breastfeeding for both the mother and infant depends on proper teaching of multiple factors, including signs of infant hunger, ways to wake the sleepy infant, breast and nipple care, proper positioning of mother and infant, and proper infant latch on the breast. The infant's mouth should be attached not just to the nipple but far back onto the areola. A shallow latch on the nipple is painful for the mother, and milk let-down is often inhibited. The infant's lower lip should be out and the infant's nose should be close to (but not compressed against) the breast. Establishing the proper latch can be time-consuming and frustrating initially, but most infants and mothers ultimately accomplish the proper latch with teaching and support.

16. C: Uric acid crystals appear reddish-orange in color ("brick dust") and are often mistaken for blood in the infant's diaper. Urate crystals form most commonly when an infant is dehydrated and are, therefore, quite common in the neonatal period, particularly in the breastfed infant. The crystals themselves are not harmful or dangerous and require no further intervention aside from an assessment of the infant's hydration status. True hematuria in the neonatal period is not a normal finding and requires further evaluation of the genitourinary tract.

17. A: Timely and accurate medical record documentation is a critical skill of all patient care providers. The bedside nurse is the care provider who most often assesses the patient, and his or her documentation is often the best representation of the patient's clinical status. Although the nurse's priority is providing excellent direct patient care, thorough documentation is important. The maternal/newborn nurse's documentation should include objective data about maternal/fetal status (e.g., vital signs, fetal heart rate monitoring); recognition of problems or complications; nursing actions in response to changes in the patient's status; communication with other providers, including their responses; communication with the patient and family members; and details of the patient's response to interventions. In legal cases alleging medical mismanagement, the medical record is often the most critical document available to a provider who must defend his or her actions.

18. B: Breast stimulation from infant sucking or a breast pump leads to prolactin release from the anterior pituitary and oxytocin release from the posterior pituitary. Milk production is stimulated by prolactin release, while milk secretion is stimulated by oxytocin release. Oxytocin also stimulates uterine contractions. Initiation of breastfeeding in the postpartum period can, therefore, lead to improved uterine contractions and a decreased risk of postpartum hemorrhage as a result of uterine atony. Human chorionic gonadotropin is an important hormone of early pregnancy for maintenance of the corpus luteum.

19. C: One of the most critical physiologic adaptations of the newborn infant is the use of the lungs as the primary organs of gas exchange. In utero, oxygen from maternal blood flows through the placenta into the umbilical vein. From the umbilical vein, it travels to the right side of the fetal heart and is then diverted across the foramen ovale or ductus arteriosus to the fetal body. In the fetal circulation, pulmonary vascular resistance is high, and there is relatively little pulmonary blood flow. Fetal waste and carbon dioxide flow through the umbilical arteries into the placenta and are eliminated through the maternal circulation. When the newborn infant takes a breath after birth, the inhaled oxygen stimulates dilation of the pulmonary vessels, and blood flow to the lungs increases as pulmonary vascular resistance falls. This process is crucial for a smooth transition to extrauterine life.

20. B: Magnesium sulfate is administered in the obstetrical setting for the treatment of preterm labor because it relaxes smooth muscle and for the treatment of preeclampsia and eclampsia because it depresses the central nervous system. Magnesium sulfate is usually administered as a continuous intravenous drip, and side effects are dose-related. Common side effects include nausea, generalized weakness, lethargy, flushing, headache, and blurry vision. Patients need to be monitored closely for signs of magnesium sulfate toxicity to avoid life-threatening complications of magnesium administration. Loss of deep tendon reflexes (typically assessed with the patellar tendon reflex) is often the first sign of toxicity. Other signs of toxicity include a significantly depressed level of consciousness, hypotension, and respiratory depression. If magnesium sulfate toxicity is not recognized and promptly treated, the patient may experience total respiratory or cardiovascular collapse. Calcium gluconate is the antidote for magnesium sulfate toxicity and should be readily available for patients receiving magnesium sulfate.

21. B: Human milk and breastfeeding provide such great benefit to both the breastfeeding mother and infant that true contraindications to breastfeeding are relatively few and should be evaluated on a case-by-case basis. Generally accepted contraindications to breastfeeding (in most cases) include HIV infection, human T-lymphotropic virus 1 infection, active tuberculosis, active herpes breast lesions, illicit substance abuse or dependence, and chemotherapy or radiation therapy in the breastfeeding mother. Galactosemia in the infant is also a contraindication to breastfeeding. Recently diagnosed breast cancer may interfere with breastfeeding so that the mother can initiate treatment, but treated breast cancer is not a contraindication. Similarly, treated or latent tuberculosis is not a contraindication to breastfeeding, in contrast to active, untreated tuberculosis.

22. B: Newborn infants are at risk for significant heat loss because of their large skin surface area relative to body mass, small amount of subcutaneous fat, and limited ability to shiver as a means of generating heat. Brown fat is produced from 26 weeks gestation until 1 month after birth and is metabolized in response to cold stress. Metabolism of brown fat requires oxygen and glucose and produces acids as a byproduct of the process. Brown fat metabolism ("nonshivering thermogenesis") is one of the few means by which the newborn infant produces heat. Cold stress in the newborn infant can lead to hypoglycemia, metabolic acidosis, and increased caloric requirements. Environmental interventions, such as use of a radiant warmer, drying, hats, and blankets, are crucial to prevent cold stress in the newborn infant.

23. B: Periodic assessment of the uterine fundus is a crucial part of postpartum care. The postpartum fundus should feel firm to palpation once the placenta has been delivered. A boggy fundus is a sign of uterine atony or relaxed uterine muscles. Uterine atony is a common cause of postpartum hemorrhage and should be recognized and treated promptly. Many postpartum patients can lose a large amount of blood within the uterine cavity before becoming symptomatic of serious blood loss. The first step in treating uterine atony is external fundal massage to stimulate the uterine muscles to contract. Bladder distension may lead to uterine atony and results in the fundus being displaced laterally. If bladder distension is suspected, the patient is encouraged to void. Should these interventions not be effective, the physician should be notified.

24. A: The postpartum nurse is in an excellent position to observe and support early attachment between the postpartum patient and her infant. Early opportunities for the mother to hold, interact with, and feed the infant as soon as possible after delivery can encourage mother-infant bonding. Important components to assess include the frequency and type of contact between the mother and infant (e.g., eye contact, close touch/hold), sensitivity to the infant's needs, responsiveness to the infant's needs, and the mother's interpretation of the infant's behaviors. Decreasing maternal interaction with the infant over time indicates impaired attachment, while maternal requests for rest or for family members to hold the infant are healthy and supported actions. Factors that may interfere with mother-infant bonding include maternal or infant medical complications, inadequate postpartum pain management, negative past pregnancy or postpartum experiences, and inadequate family or partner support. All patients, but particularly the first-time mother, benefit from education and positive reinforcement for appropriate infant care behaviors in the postpartum period.

25. A: If an Rh-negative woman is pregnant with an Rh-positive fetus and fetal red blood cells enter the maternal circulation, Rh antibodies form in the maternal circulation. This process is referred to as "sensitization." A subsequent pregnancy with an Rh-positive fetus in the sensitized Rh-negative mother leads to hemolysis of fetal red blood cells as maternal anti-Rh antibodies cross the placenta, leading to severe fetal anemia. Rh immune globulin (Rhogam) confers passive antibody protection against Rh antigens, preventing maternal Rh-antigen antibody protection. The indirect Coombs test detects Rh-positive antibodies in the maternal circulation and is, therefore, the test of choice for maternal sensitization screening. If an Rh-negative mother delivers an Rh-positive infant and there is no evidence of maternal sensitization, Rhogam is administered within 72 hours of delivery. Rhogam is also administered after abortion, antepartum hemorrhage, amniocentesis, chorionic villus sampling, trauma, or any procedure or incident where there is a reasonable likelihood of maternal exposure to Rh-positive fetal blood.

26. C: Infants born to a diabetic mother (IDM) are at increased risk for multiple complications in the newborn period. Maternal hyperglycemia causes fetal hyperglycemia as glucose freely crosses the placenta. Fetal hyperglycemia leads to increased fetal insulin production, which exerts a growth hormone-like effect (causing macrosomia). After birth (when the infant is no longer exposed to maternal hyperglycemia), the newborn's elevated insulin level causes a rapid fall in serum glucose, typically within 1-6 hours after birth. Symptoms of neonatal hypoglycemia include temperature instability, tremors, and poor feeding. Other complications in the newborn period of the IDM include hyperbilirubinemia, birth trauma, polycythemia, and respiratory distress syndrome.

27. A: The composition of mature human milk varies significantly as a single feeding progresses. The milk that flows at the beginning of a feeding is called foremilk. The milk that flows beginning at let-down (milk-ejection reflex) is called hindmilk. Foremilk is high in protein and low in fat, while hindmilk is high in fat (and calories) but with a low protein content. The let-down reflex typically occurs 1-2 minutes after the infant begins sucking. Hindmilk is released from the breast alveoli into the ducts in response to oxytocin release. Colostrum is the milk that is present immediately after birth and until the mother's mature milk "comes in." Colostrum is a thick, yellow fluid with large amounts of immunoglobulin and protein and is relatively low in fat compared with mature milk.

28. A: A significant amount of blood loss can occur in the postpartum period before it becomes clinically apparent. As a result, the postpartum nurse needs to be aware of risk factors for postpartum hemorrhage and early signs of significant blood loss. Early postpartum hemorrhage (within 24 hours of delivery) may be caused by a combination of factors. Uterine atony (inappropriate relaxation of the uterine musculature) is a common cause of early postpartum hemorrhage. Risk factors for uterine atony include uterine distension (e.g., multiple gestation, macrosomic infant), preeclampsia, retained placental fragments, bladder distension, medication (e.g., magnesium sulfate), and instrumented delivery (e.g., forceps and vacuum extraction). Genital lacerations (e.g., perineum, cervix, vagina) can also cause significant postpartum blood loss. Risk factors for genital lacerations include instrumented delivery, macrosomic infant, nulliparous mother, and precipitous vaginal delivery. Retained placental fragments, vulvar or pelvic hematomas, and uterine inversion are additional causes of early postpartum hemorrhage.

29. B: Intrapartum fetal heart rate monitoring requires documentation and interpretation of five variables: baseline fetal heart rate, baseline heart rate variability, presence or absence of fetal heart rate accelerations, fetal heart rate decelerations, and changes in the fetal heart rate pattern as labor progresses. Interpretation of fetal heart rate monitoring can be complex and challenging but is an important component of intrapartum fetal monitoring. In general, when fetal heart rate monitoring demonstrates a normal baseline rate with accelerations, moderate variability, and no late or variable decelerations, the fetus is neither hypoxemic nor acidotic. Early decelerations with normal variability are associated with uterine contractions; fetal head compression, which occurs with the uterine contraction, leads to stimulation of the vagus nerve, leading to a decrease in fetal heart rate, which resolves as the contraction subsides. Early decelerations are not associated with fetal hypoxia and require no intervention.

30. A: Cephalohematoma may occur in up to 2% of births and is far more common in vertex vaginal delivery than cesarean births. Blood vessels between the cranial bone and the periosteal layer rupture, leading to the formation of a hematoma in the subperiosteal space, which is limited in its extension by cranial suture lines. Cephalohematoma typically becomes clinically apparent in the first 1-2 days after birth and may take weeks to months to resolve. This is in contrast to a caput succedaneum, a subcutaneous collection of edematous fluid, which crosses suture lines, is typically present at birth, and resolves within hours to days after birth.

31. C: Mastitis is an infection of the connective tissue of the breast that occurs almost exclusively in lactating women. Mastitis is unusual in the immediate postpartum period, and is typically seen beginning 2-3 weeks after delivery in the breastfeeding patient. Human milk is an excellent medium for bacterial (and fungal) growth and typically becomes infected when bacteria from the infant's mouth or maternal skin ascend through a traumatized nipple. Mastitis typically presents with focal, unilateral breast pain and may be accompanied by fever and flu-like symptoms. The affected breast region is typically warm, red, and tender. Treatment of mastitis includes continuance of usual breastfeeding routines, gently massaging the area of discomfort, ice packs, pain relievers, and antibiotics. Because nipple trauma and milk stasis are major contributing causes of mastitis, proper nipple care and breastfeeding technique can prevent many cases of mastitis. The postpartum patient who is breastfeeding her newborn should be instructed in proper infant latch, nipple care, and positioning techniques, which enhance complete emptying of both breasts.

32. B: Jaundice is common in the neonatal period, occurring in up to 50% of full-term newborns and 80% of preterm infants. Prenatally, fetal unconjugated bilirubin crosses the placenta to be conjugated and excreted. Postnatally, unconjugated bilirubin is converted in the liver to its water-soluble form and then excreted in the infant's urine and stool. The infant is physiologically vulnerable to hyperbilirubinemia in the first several weeks of life for several reasons: there are low levels of hepatic enzymes necessary to convert bilirubin to its water-soluble form; there is a large unconjugated bilirubin load as a result of an increased rate of red blood cell destruction (in the newborn), and there is an increased reabsorption of bilirubin from the immature gastrointestinal tract. Physiologic jaundice as a result of these expected factors does not become clinically apparent until after 24 hours of life. Jaundice that is present in the first 24 hours after birth is considered pathologic and may result from abnormal hemolysis (e.g., ABO incompatibility) or underlying liver disease.

33. B: Group B *Streptococcus* (GBS) remains a common cause of neonatal sepsis and may lead to early-onset illness (within 1 week of birth) or late-onset illness. Infants with early-onset GBS disease are seriously ill and may present with pneumonia, apnea, and shock. Meningitis is more common in late-onset GBS disease. Approximately 20-25% of pregnant woman are colonized by GBS in their lower gastrointestinal or urinary tracts and can transmit the infection to the infant during vaginal delivery. Intrapartum antibiotic administration in pregnant women with positive GBS cultures (or other risk factors) at least 4 hours before delivery significantly reduces the incidence of early-onset GBS disease in newborns. *Gardnerella vaginalis* is the etiologic agent in bacterial vaginosis and is not a cause of neonatal sepsis. *Neisseria gonorrhoeae* may cause neonatal conjunctivitis but is not a cause of neonatal sepsis.

34. C: Postpartum "blues" (or adjustment reaction with depressed mood) occurs in more than half of postpartum mothers and is characterized by mild depressive symptoms in addition to happier periods. Postpartum "blues" typically occurs within a few days of delivery and lasts approximately 1-2 weeks. The postpartum "blues" are thought to be caused by rapid swings in prolactin, estrogen, and progesterone levels after delivery. Typical features include frequent tearfulness, fatigue, anxiety, irritability, and feelings of being overwhelmed. Signs of major depression (e.g., suicidal ideation) or psychosis are not features of the postpartum "blues."

35. B: The newborn infant is equipped with multiple behavioral and sensory mechanisms for interacting with his or her environment. Orientation describes the newborn's ability to notice, follow, and fixate on appealing visual and auditory inputs. The infant's ability to orient in this way encourages parent-infant bonding as the infant responds to caregivers' faces and voices. The newborn's ability to decrease his or her response to a repetitive stimulus (e.g., ambient noise, flashing lights) is habituation. Self-quieting refers to the infant's ability to calm him- or herself (e.g., with hand-sucking) when distressed. The degree to which an infant can habituate or self-quiet is often a large component of parental perception of the infant's temperament.

36. C: Proper care of the umbilical cord is important to prevent infection. Hospitals and families differ in the specifics of umbilical cord care, depending on tradition and cultural beliefs. Some medical providers advocate daily use of alcohol or antibacterial ointments, although there is no definitive data supporting their use. In general, the umbilical cord stump should be kept dry and either exposed to air or covered loosely with clean dressings or clothing. The base of the cord stump and the skin around the umbilicus can be cleaned several times daily with water and a cotton swab. Baths involving submersion of the abdomen in water should be avoided until the stump has fallen off. Pulling the cord stump is not recommended.

37. A: Infants in breech presentation at the time of delivery have a markedly increased incidence of perinatal injury and death, regardless of whether delivery is vaginal or surgical. Breech presentation occurs in 3-4% of all deliveries and is more common with congenital fetal anomalies, preterm deliveries, uterine or placental malformations, and multiple gestation. Risks to the fetus or newborn with breech presentation include increased risk of umbilical cord prolapse, fetal asphyxia/nonreassuring fetal status, spinal cord/brachial plexus injuries, dystocia, and perinatal death. Most infants in breech presentation at the time of delivery are delivered by cesarean section.

38. A: Breast engorgement differs from the normal feeling of fullness that the breastfeeding mother experiences when milk first "comes in." Engorgement is characterized by firm, warm, and painful breasts. Engorged breasts often appear taut and shiny and may be accompanied by axillary swelling and low-grade fever. The infant often has difficulty latching onto the engorged breast. Treatment of breast engorgement in the breastfeeding mother includes more frequent feedings at least 10-15 minutes on each breast to allow adequate emptying of both breasts, warm (or cold) compress application to stimulate let-down and soften the breasts, and pain relievers as needed for further relief. Supportive nursing bras may help with discomfort between feedings. Antibiotics are only indicated in the case on infection, such as mastitis.

39. A: Postpartum patients vary a great deal in the timing of their return to sexual activity. Because pregnancy can occur with the first ovulation after pregnancy (before first menstruation occurs), contraception and family planning issues should be discussed with all postpartum patients before discharge. Women who are not breastfeeding generally have a faster return of ovulation and menstruation compared with women who are breastfeeding. Breastfeeding is a fairly effective contraceptive method in the postpartum period (lactational amenorrhea method) provided that the mother is fully breastfeeding (day and night), is amenorrhoeic, and less than 6 months postpartum. A decrease in breastfeeding leads to an increased likelihood of ovulation and, therefore, an increased risk of pregnancy. Therefore, it is possible to get pregnant while breastfeeding. Other forms of postpartum contraception include progestin-only oral contraceptives, combined estrogen/progestin oral contraceptive, intrauterine devices, sterilization, and barrier methods. Depending on whether the patient is breastfeeding, recommended timing for each method varies.

40. B: Cyanosis limited to the distal extremities and perioral regions is known as acrocyanosis and is a common and normal finding in newborn infants. Central cyanosis (lips and tongue in addition to the trunk and extremities) in the newborn infant is not a normal finding. Central cyanosis in the neonate that persists after appropriate immediate post-delivery resuscitation is usually a sign of serious pulmonary disease (e.g., persistent pulmonary hypertension, respiratory distress syndrome), congenital heart disease (e.g., transposition of the great vessels, total anomalous pulmonary venous return), and sepsis. Fever may be present in the infant with sepsis/neonatal infection, but is not a finding that is highly specific for congenital heart disease.

41. C: The full-term healthy newborn infant can be expected to lose 5-10% of birth weight in the first 5-7 days of life as a result of fluid shifts and adjustment to feeding. Infants who are exclusively breastfed generally lose more weight than formula-fed infants as a result of the wait for maternal milk production to begin. Preterm infants and infants who are large-for-gestational age may have increased weight loss after birth as well. If an infant is having difficulty with feedings or is losing more weight than would be expected, close monitoring is warranted with feeding evaluation and support and frequent weight checks. Most healthy infants should return to their birth weight by 2 weeks of age.

42. A: Care of the postpartum patient after a cesarean delivery involves the usual postpartum care, in addition to close attention to the conditions unique to the mother who has undergone abdominal surgery. Postsurgical patients have an increased need for analgesic medications and other pain-relieving techniques after delivery. Early contact with her infant and early breastfeeding help with mother-infant bonding. Patients should be encouraged to take deep breaths regularly after cesarean delivery to minimize the risk of pulmonary infections. Leg exercises and early ambulation after cesarean delivery decrease the risk of venous thrombosis and speed the return of normal gastrointestinal motility.

43. C: Preeclampsia is a disease unique to pregnancy and typically presents anytime from late pregnancy to the postpartum period. Preeclampsia is characterized clinically by new onset hypertension with or without proteinuria, and edema. Preeclampsia is more common in first pregnancies. Preeclampsia leads to decreased organ perfusion, including the uterus and placenta. A form of preeclampsia with severe features is known as the HELLP syndrome in which lab findings include: hemolysis (H), elevated liver enzymes (EL), and low platelets (LP). Eclampsia is characterized by the onset of seizures or coma in women with preeclampsia, assuming the absence of alternate etiologies of seizure or coma.

44. B: Estimation of gestational age in the stable newborn infant is an important component of newborn assessment. Complications in the neonatal period more commonly occur in association with gestational age rather than birth weight. In other words, a small-for-gestational-age infant born at 35 weeks' gestation has a less complicated newborn course than a large-for-gestational-age infant born at 31 weeks' gestation. There are multiple tools available for estimation of gestational age, all of which combine evaluation of both external physical characteristics and neuromuscular development. Preterm infants tend to have decreased muscle tone, resulting in a less flexed resting posture. Preterm infants also have more lanugo, thinner skin, fewer plantar foot creases, less developed ear cartilage, and less breast bud tissue than term infants. Tests for neuromuscular development include assessment of the angle of the wrist, assessment of the popliteal, hip, and ankle flexion, and observation of the infant's resting posture.

45. C: Chronic maternal narcotic use during pregnancy leads to neonatal withdrawal symptoms within 72 hours of birth. Symptoms of drug withdrawal include high-pitched cry, vomiting, irritability, seizures, diarrhea, and sneezing. Maternal alcohol use can lead to fetal alcohol syndrome, which is characterized by specific facial features, developmental disability and feeding or growth problems. Fetal exposure to cocaine may lead to abnormal brain development, behavioral disturbances, and an increased risk for sudden infant death syndrome. Heavy maternal marijuana use may be associated with mild neonatal withdrawal symptoms, but a link between isolated marijuana use and neonatal withdrawal symptoms has not been definitively established.

Heavy maternal caffeine ingestion may lead to symptomatic withdrawal in the exposed infant but is less likely to cause neonatal withdrawal syndrome.

46. A: Although circumcision rates in the United States have been dropping in recent years, at least half of newborn males are circumcised. There are multiple clamp devices used for neonatal circumcision, as well as the Plastibell. Home care of the penis recently circumcised with one of the clamp devices should involve gentle warm water cleaning with diaper changes, petroleum ointment application, and monitoring for bleeding or infection. A thin, yellow layer of granulation tissue is an expected finding on the recently circumcised penis and should not be removed. If a Plastibell is in place, no ointment should be applied until the Plastibell has fallen off (usually by 7 days after circumcision).

47. A: Periodic breathing is a normal respiratory pattern in the newborn infant and is observed more commonly in preterm infants. As opposed to true apnea, periodic breathing is not associated with any cardiorespiratory compromise and resolves without intervention or stimulation. A pause in respiration that is prolonged (>15-20 seconds) or of any duration with associated with signs of cardiorespiratory compromise is not consistent with periodic breathing. Periodic breathing most commonly occurs during sleep. Transient tachypnea of the newborn is due to retention of excess lung fluid during delivery and is characterized by 12-72 hours of tachypnea with variable degrees of hypoxia and respiratory distress. Central apnea is due to an abnormality in brain control of respiratory stimulation and effort.

48. A: The newborn infant's first bowel movement (meconium) is a sticky, greenish black substance made up of bile salts and intestinal debris. Meconium may be passed during birth as a response to perinatal stress and can lead to respiratory distress and meconium aspiration syndrome if inhaled before or during delivery. Most healthy infants pass their first meconium stool by 24 hours of life. Delayed passage of meconium beyond 48 hours of life can indicate underlying disease, such as cystic fibrosis or Hirschsprung disease. Once feeding has been established, the stools transition to normal breastfed or formula-fed stools typical in infants. Breastfed stools are mustardy yellow in color with a cottage cheese consistency, while formula fed stools are slightly darker orange/tan, and slightly thicker in consistency (similar to peanut butter).

49. A: There are several reflexes found in the healthy term newborn. The rooting reflex occurs when the infant's cheek is touched, causing the infant to turn the head toward the side of contact with their mouth (to "find" the site for feeding). The Moro reflex is demonstrated when the infant is startled by sudden noise or movement and consists of the infant extending the arms suddenly and then slowly pulling them back to the body, often accompanied by a brief cry. The tonic neck reflex ("fencing" reflex) describes the extension of the infant's arm or leg on the side toward which the head is turned with associated flexion of the contralateral extremities. Other normal newborn reflexes include the grasping, sucking, and stepping reflexes.

50. B: Sudden infant death syndrome (SIDS) is the leading cause of death in 1-12-month-old infants. Rates of SIDS have declined by more than 50% since the initiation of the Back to Sleep campaign, which educates parents about the risks of placing infants on their stomachs to sleep. Other important recommendations that decrease the risk of SIDS include placing the infant on a firm surface to sleep, minimizing or eliminating second-hand cigarette smoke exposure, and using a pacifier during sleep. Gastroesophageal reflux symptoms may be more prominent in the supine position. The incidence of bronchiolitis is not affected by the infant sleep position.

51. B: Characteristics of jitteriness include:

- Clonic jerking with both fast and slow elements
- Halted by gentle restraints
- Elicited by stimulation
- Lack of ocular deviation
- Absence of autonomic response (increased heart rate, respirations, blood pressure)

Jitteriness is tremors of the chin and extremities, and is common in infants within a few days and may persist for up to months. Jitteriness is a benign condition but may indicate drug withdrawal, hypoglycemia, hypocalcemia, and encephalopathy.

52. A: After using a breast pump, the woman should rinse the equipment in cold water and then wash it in warm soapy water. If this isn't possible (such as when a woman is away from home), the woman should at least rinse the removable parts and then place them in a plastic bag so they can be washed later. The removable parts should be boiled for 20 minutes to sterilize or run through a dishwashing cycle once every 24 hours.

53. C: The most common neonatal bacterial infection is Group B *Streptococcus* (GBS) because most woman are carriers but asymptomatic. For this reason, women should be screened at 37+0 to 37+6 weeks of gestation and those who are positive administered antibiotics during labor. The woman needs at least 4 hours of antibiotics to provide adequate protection of the neonate from infection. Signs of infection in the neonate usually occur about 24 hours after birth although some infants have delayed symptoms 10-14 days after birth.

54. B: The neonate usually passes meconium within 8-24 hours although it may be delayed as long as 48 hours. First meconium is thick, dark, and tarry. Transitional stools for the next few days are usually brown to green, after which the child should pass normal stools. Stools of breastfed babies are usually yellow-gold and mushy, while bottle-fed are pale yellow and pasty in color. Bowel sounds can usually be heard within 30-60 minutes of birth as air begins to move down the GI tract (first to the stomach) as the child breathes.

55. A: If a few weeks after delivery, a woman complains that she cannot sleep, has little appetite and has begun having anxiety attacks and fears that she cannot take adequate care of her neonate, the most likely cause is postpartum depression. Onset may occur within the first 6 months but is not usually present initially, unlike postpartum blues. Symptoms of postpartum psychosis are much more severe and may include paranoia, hallucinations, and disorientation.

56. C: If a neonate's hemoglobin is 19.3 g/dL at birth, a typical value at 7 days is 17.4 g/dL. Hemoglobin is high immediately after birth because the placental environment is relatively hypoxic, but the hemoglobin begins to fall after birth with exposure to the higher oxygen content of ambient air and with an increase in adult hemoglobin. By 3 months, the hemoglobin usually ranges from 9.3-13.3 g/dL

57. C: HELLP syndrome is characterized by (H) hemolysis, (EL) elevated liver enzymes, and (LP) low platelet count. HELLP syndrome is most common in multiparous women during weeks 27-37 but may occur within 24 hours after delivery. Pain in the right upper quadrant related to liver dysfunction may be misdiagnosed as gastrointestinal upset or gall bladder disease. Initial symptoms are often flu-like, including headache, nausea and vomiting and visual disturbances. Mortality rates are high without prompt diagnosis and treatment.

58. B: The vaccination that should be routinely administered to all newborns within 24 hours of birth is hepatitis B. The second dose should be given within the first to second month and the third dose between 6 and 18 months. If the neonate's mother is hepatitis B positive, then the neonate should receive the vaccination within 12 hours of birth and 0.5 mL of hepatitis B immune globulin (HBIG). If the mother's status is unknown, the neonate should also receive the vaccination within 12 hours of birth and the mother tested.

59. A: The Quad Screen includes: (1) Alpha-fetoprotein (AFP), (2) Human chorionic gonadotropin (hCG), (3) Estriol (uE^3), and (4) Inhibin A (INH-A).

Disorder	AFP	hCG	uE^3	INH-A
Neural tube defects	High	Normal	Normal	Normal
Trisomy 21	Low	High	Low	High
Trisomy 18	Low	Low	Low	Low
Multiple gestation	High	High	Normal	Normal

60. C: The infantile form of Tay-Sachs disease is classified as a metabolic defect. The infant lacks an enzyme necessary to metabolize fatty substances, so these build up in the body and damage the brain and nerve cells. Symptoms are usually evident by about 6 months, but there is currently no treatment. The child progressively loses control of muscles and becomes blind and paralyzed. Life expectancy ranges from 4-5 years.

61. A: The nutritional supplement given to women to prevent neural tube defects is folic acid. Folic acid deficiency causes megaloblastic anemia in which immature red blood cells enlarge rather than divide, so there are fewer red blood cells. However, because cells need to duplicate during pregnancy as the fetus grows, adequate folic acid is critical. Women should receive 0.4 mg folic acid daily and, for deficiency, 1mg folic acid and iron supplements (because folic acid deficiency is associated with iron deficiency anemia).

62. C: If a woman complains that she is exhausted because the neonate nurses so frequently during the night that the woman cannot get any sleep, the nurse should advise the woman to sleep when the baby sleeps, day and night. Over time, the baby will establish a more regular nursing schedule, but initially neonates often want to nurse very frequently, especially in the evening, and irregularly. Bottle-fed babies usually go longer between feedings than babies that are nursed.

63. A: The CARE principles applied to the care of a pregnant woman refer to

- (C) Communication: Sharing information through speaking, writing, signs, or other means. Exhibiting mutual understanding and sympathy
- (A) Advocate: Speaking for the person and the person's rights
- (R) Respect: Paying attention, showing consideration, and respecting another
- (E) Enable: Empowering the person through information, resources, and support

64. B: The recreational drug that most increases the risk of spontaneous abortion is methamphetamine (commonly referred to as "meth" or "crank"). Methamphetamine is a stimulant drug that can be snorted or smoked. Methamphetamine has been associated with increased placental abruption and premature delivery. Infants may go through a form of withdrawal and exhibit tremors and poor muscle tone at birth. They may also have congenital abnormalities and may develop neurobehavioral problems.

65. C: While infants vary, by about the sixth day after birth, over a 24-hour period, most infants urinate approximately 6-8 times, having increased steadily from one diaper on the first day and two on the second day. The neonate's output depends on the intake, so if urinary output is inadequate, the patient may not be getting enough milk. Urine should be pale yellow in color. If the baby is jaundiced, the infant may excrete dark urine.

66. B: The neural tube defect that is most likely to result in hydrocephalus is myelomeningocele, which is a condition in which there is an opening in the spine through which the meninges and spinal cord protrude, in an exterior sac. Myelomeningocele is also associated with weakness or paralysis of the lower extremities and poor or no control of bowels and bladder. Surgery is done to close the defect and prevent CSF infection. Some require a ventriculoatrial shunt.

67. A: The mnemonic BUBBLE-HE is used to remember the steps to a comprehensive postpartal assessment:

- B: breasts—inspect carefully for firmness, color, temperature, abnormalities.
- U: uterus—check fundal location and tone.
- B: bladder—determine time of last urination and palpate bladder.
- B: bowels—determine last BM and presence of flatus.
- L: lochia—assess color, amount, presence of clots, signs of bleeding (free flow of blood).
- E: episiotomy (incision)—use REEDA assessment.
- H: Homan's signs (legs)—check for pain, swelling, redness, warmth in calves and pulses and sensation in legs and feet.
- E: Emotions: Assess level of exhaustion/fatigue and affect.

68. B: Human milk can be kept frozen in the freezer section of a side-by-side (separate door) refrigerator-freezer for 3-4 months. If the freezer compartment is inside the refrigerator (at the top) the milk should not be kept for more than 2 weeks because the temperature varies as the refrigerator is opened and closed. Deep freezers with a temperature of 0° C/32° F maintain temperature the best, so human milk can be frozen and stored for up to 6 months. Human milk is safe to use for up to 4 hours if stored at room temperature and up to 7 days if refrigerated.

69. C: If a pregnant woman at 38-weeks of gestation complains of dizziness when lying flat, the most likely cause is supine hypotensive syndrome. This drop in blood pressure and associated dizziness results when the enlarged uterus and growing fetus cause pressure on the inferior vena cava, resulting in decreased cardiac output. Similar symptoms may occur with anemia, hypoglycemia, and dehydration, but if these are ruled out, the woman should be advised to lie on the side rather than flat and to take deep breaths and raise herself slowly from lying to sitting position.

70. B: If a woman's pregnancy classification is G4, T2, P1, A1, L3, the number of total pregnancies is 4. The woman has been pregnant 4 times with 2 pregnancies carried to term, 1 premature birth, 1 abortion, and 3 living children. This classification system is in general use do describe a woman's reproductive history:

- G: Gravida refers to the number of times that a woman has been pregnant
- T: Term pregnancies, the number of pregnancies carried to term
- P: Preterm delivery, the number of preterm deliveries
- A: Abortions, may be spontaneous or induced
- L: Living births, the number of infants born living

71. C: If the fundal height is halfway between the woman's symphysis pubis and umbilicus, the approximate weeks of gestation are 16. The fundal heights directly correlate to the weeks of gestation from week 22, but the weeks of gestation can be estimated by the fundal position:

- Symphysis pubis: 12 weeks
- Halfway between symphysis pubis and umbilicus: 16 weeks
- At umbilicus: 22 weeks
- One-third of distance between umbilicus and xyphoid process: 28-30
- Two-thirds of distance between umbilicus and xyphoid process: 32 weeks
- At xyphoid process: 36 weeks. Then begins to drop again at 38-40 weeks as the head engages

72. A: The cell free fetal DNA test assesses for chromosomal disorders. Testing typically covers 3 common chromosomal disorders: trisomy 21 (Down syndrome), trisomy 18 (Edwards syndrome), and trisomy 13 (Patau syndrome). The DNA testing may also test for other rarer disorders, especially if there is a family history indicating increased risk. The cell free fetal DNA test, which can be done during or following week 10 of gestation, is presently still considered a screening test and must be verified by further testing, such as chorionic villus sampling or amniocentesis.

73. B: During pregnancy, a woman with BMI of 22.0 (which is classified as a normal weight for the mother) is expected to gain 25-35 pounds. Weight gains are recommended according to the woman's BMI:

BMI	Classified	Recommended weight gain
<18.5	Underweight	28-40 pounds
18.5-24.9	Normal weight	25-35 pounds
25-29.9	Overweight	15-25 pounds
30+	Obese	11-20 pounds

Women pregnant with twins should generally gain about 15-25 pounds more than women with singletons.

74. C: The presence of bilirubin in amniotic fluid usually indicates Rh-sensitized pregnancy and fetal hemolytic syndrome. Bilirubin may be monitored routinely beginning at 25-weeks of gestation to evaluate the severity of the syndrome in the developing fetus. Rh incompatibility occurs if the mother is Rh- and the father is Rh+, putting their infant at risk for hemolytic disease of the newborn (HDN) or Rh disease, (erythroblastosis fetalis). Sensitization can occur during abortion, placental abruption, amniocentesis, cesarean section, chorionic villus sampling, cordocentesis, delivery, ectopic pregnancy, and toxemia.

75. A: Severe post-dural puncture (spinal) headache is best treated with an epidural blood patch, which seals the cerebrospinal leak that causes the headache. Caffeinated beverages or medication with caffeine may provide temporary relief of the headache, and hydration is important, but usually not adequate alone. With the woman lying prone, the physician takes 20-25 mL of venous blood from a vein and then slowly injects it into the epidural space. The patient may feel some initial pressure, but this should prevent further leakage and resolve the headache within a few hours.

76. C: If bottle feeding a neonate with cleft lip and cleft palate, the nipple should be longer than normal size so the milk is delivered to the back of the throat, past the open cleft. The neonate should be fed in upright position to prevent aspiration. The mother should be encouraged to breast feed the neonate as breastfeeding is often successful with cleft lip and cleft palate although the mother must be sure to keep the infant upright.

77. B: Ultrasonography can be used to estimate fetal age with crown-rump length (CRL) at approximately 7-12 weeks. The heart rate can be assessed at 6-7 weeks gestation. Other measurements used to estimate fetal age include gestational sac dimensions at about 8 weeks and biparietal diameter (BPD) and femur length after 12 weeks. Ultrasonography can be used throughout pregnancy to estimate gestational age, to confirm the viability of the fetus, to identify gender, and to identify fetal abnormalities.

78. A: When palpating the uterus after delivery, it is necessary support the lower uterine segment with one hand while palpating with the other. Applying pressure to the fundus without properly supporting the lower uterine segment may result in increased bleeding, hemorrhage, and/or uterine inversion. The lower segment is supported by placing one hand directly above the symphysis pubis firmly (but avoiding distal pressure) while placing the other hand at the umbilicus and pressing inward and downward until the fundus is palpated.

79. C: Asymmetric intrauterine growth restriction is caused by problems that occur during the third trimester and typically result from problems with the function of the uterus and placenta and/or nutritional deficiency. Usually, the brain and heart have normal development and the neonate has normal length but is in less than the 10th percentile for weight. The abdominal organs may be underdeveloped. The neonate will usually develop normally with adequate nutrition after birth.

80. A: If a woman in labor is receiving a benzodiazepine to relieve anxiety, nausea, and pain, the medication that should also be available on the unit is flumazenil. Flumazenil is an antagonist for benzodiazepines and may be necessary to reverse the effects if excessive sedation occurs. Benzodiazepines may result in some degree of amnesia, so some women may want to avoid their use. Naloxone should also be available for patients receiving narcotic analgesia. N-acetylcysteine is a reversal agent for acetaminophen overdoses.

81. B: A patient who experienced placenta previa is at increased risk of hemorrhage during the postpartal period because the area of implantation does not contract effectively. With placenta previa, the placenta implants very low in the uterus or over the cervical os. Additionally, the blood supply in the lower segment of the uterus is less than in the upper segment, so the placenta tends to grow to a larger size to compensate. This leaves a greater denuded area that can bleed after expulsion of the placenta.

82. A: Following spontaneous rupture of the membranes during labor, if the fetal heart rate becomes markedly bradycardic with variable decelerations, this likely indicates cord prolapse, which occurs when part of the cord is below the presenting part of the fetus, blocking blood flow. While prolapse may be occult and occur at any time during labor, it is most common after rupture of the membranes because the pressure literally washes the cord downward. Risk increases with an exceptionally long cord, mal-presentations, multiple gestations, hydramnios, and preterm birth.

83. C: During the process of lactation, the breasts usually being filling and feel firm and warm by the third day. The breasts are usually soft during the first two days but produce colostrum in small amounts, as the neonate's stomach capacity is very small immediately after birth. By the fourth day, the breasts will feel full before the neonate nurses and then should feel soft if the emptying of the breast was adequate. If the mother's breasts remain very firm and uncomfortable after nursing, a breastfeeding specialist should review breastfeeding techniques with the mother to ensure the neonate is latching and nursing effectively.

84. B: The most common cause of subinvolution is retained placental fragments and infection. Subinvolution is a restricting of the rate at which the uterus returns to nonpregnant size. Indications of subinvolution include prolonged lochia, pelvic pain or discomfort, intermittent bleeding or hemorrhage, backache, and lethargy and malaise. An unpleasant or foul vaginal odor is usually present with infection. Treatment requires identifying and treating the cause. Methylergonovine (Methergine®) is often given to promote contractions and antibiotics for infection.

85. A: If shoulder dystocia (difficult delivery of the shoulders) occurred during delivery, the newborn should be examined for fractured clavicle and Erb's palsy. The anterior or posterior (less common) shoulder becomes literally stuck behind the pubis. Shoulder dystocia poses risks to both the mother and fetus and may result in death of the fetus or severe impairment because the cord becomes compressed and the lungs cannot expand because the fetus is lodged in the birth canal. Risk factors for shoulder dystocia include macrosomia, diabetic mother, obese mother, abnormal anatomy of pelvis, prolonged pregnancy, older maternal age, and induced labor.

86. B: Labor and delivery is defined as precipitate if labor lasts less than three hours. Women who are multiparous are at greatest risk because of loss of muscle tone. They may experience dilation of 10 cm within an hour while nulliparous women may experience dilation of 5 cm an hour. In some cases, the mother may have experienced little pain prior to delivery. Precipitate labor may also occur with hypertonic uterine contractions. If there is inadequate relaxation of the uterine muscle between contractions, the fetus may suffer hypoxia.

87. C: Autonomy is the ethical principle that the individual has the right to make decisions about her own care, based on informed consent and understanding of risks and benefits. Beneficence is an ethical principle that involves performing actions that are for the purpose of benefitting another person. Nonmaleficence is an ethical principle that means healthcare workers should provide care in a manner that does not cause direct intentional harm to the patient.

88. C: If a woman complains of persistent constipation in the postpartal period, the best treatment approach is usually a stool softener, such as docusate sodium or Bisacodyl, both of which can be taken while the woman is breastfeeding. While the woman should be encouraged to drink ample fluids and to include fiber in the diet, constipation is common because hormonal changes decrease bowel motility. Also, if the woman had an episiotomy or tearing, the woman may avoid bearing down because of pain.

89. C: When conducting a review of the literature as part of evidence-based research, the level of evidence based on a quasi-experimental study, such as a matched case-control study, would be categorized as level III:

- Level I: Meta-analysis, randomized controlled studies
- Level II: One or more well-designed study, may or not be randomized
- Level III: As above
- Level IV: Comparative non-experimental studies
- Level V: Case reports and clinical examples but without empirical evidence

90. B: In the postpartal period, the uterine fundus should no longer be palpable after 10 days. Immediately after delivery, the fundus should be palpable at about the midline point between the umbilicus and the symphysis pubis, and it should continue to descend at about the rate of 1 cm per day. It's important that the woman urinate prior to assessment of the fundus because a full bladder may displace the fundus. The nurse should note the position of the fundus vertically as well as any lateral deviation.

91. A: The antibiotic agent that should be avoided for long-term use (>14 days) when a woman is breastfeeding is tetracyclines. While some studies indicate that short-term use may be acceptable, tetracycline is usually avoided because it may result in permanent tooth staining and enamel defects in the infant's developing teeth. Tetracycline should also be avoided during pregnancy because it may restrict skeletal growth in the fetus and cause the same dental problems. Cephalosporins and erythromycin are safe to use while breastfeeding.

92. C: If a nurse administers the wrong drug to a patient but the patient suffers no ill effects, the elements of malpractice that are missing are damages (because the patient suffered no ill effects) and causation (because there must be damages before there can be causation). The four elements necessary for malpractice are: duty to use care, breach of duty, damages, and causation. In order to prove malpractice, evidence must show that all 4 elements are present.

93. A: Necrotizing enterocolitis in a preterm infant is usually caused by ischemic bowel. If the neonate has episodes of hypoxia, oxygen is shunted to the heart and lungs and other organs, such as the intestines, may become hypoxic. If oxygenation is inadequate, areas of necrosis occur, and this interferes with peristalsis, so stool begins to build up. Sepsis may also occur, putting the neonate at grave risk.

94. B: If, on palpating the uterus in the postpartal period, the nurse finds the fundus is displaced superior to the umbilicus and to the right, the nurse should suspect that the cause is bladder distension. The nurse should ensure the bladder is empty prior to uterine palpation. Spontaneous urination usually occurs within 6-8 hours. The woman should urinate an average of 150 mL per hour to prevent bladder distension. The postpartal period is one of diuresis up to 3000 mL a day for the first few days, and the bladder can easily become distended because of decreased bladder tone.

95. A: Methylergonovine (Methergine®) may be administered to a woman after delivery in order to promote uterine contractions. Uterine atony or subinvolution may result in postpartal hemorrhage if not treated. Methylergonovine is usually administered at 200 mcg IV at 2- to 4-hour intervals after delivery or at 200-400 mcg PO every 6-12 hours for 2-7 days. Blood pressure must be carefully monitored, and methylergonovine should be used with care in hypertensive patients.

96. C: A woman who is breastfeeding and needs to take smoking cessation medication in order to stop smoking should avoid varenicline. Low dose nicotine patches (14-mg or 7-mg) decrease exposure to nicotine and other chemicals compared to smoking. Blood levels of nicotine vary considerably with nicotine gum, depending on how fast and frequently the gum is chewed, so women should be advised to avoid using the gum for 2-3 hours before breastfeeding.

97. B: A woman who has taken methadone during pregnancy and wants to breastfeed should continue the same dose of methadone. The danger to the infant is greater if the mother reduces the doses or stops the methadone and returns to substance abuse. However, the infant should be monitored for excessive drowsiness. The drug's peak occurs 4-5 hours after the woman takes an oral dose, so the mother should try to avoid breastfeeding at that time. When breastfeeding, the infant receives about 2-3% of the maternal dose.

98. A: If a neonate's skin is dry and peeling with no vernix and loss of subcutaneous fat, the likely gestational age is 42-44 weeks. Post-term infants may weigh >4000 g. Other indications include long and thin body, long fingernails (meconium staining may be evident), long hair, and hypothermia. The neonate may suffer from cold stress because of decreased brown fat, and may have hypoglycemia. Post-term infants are at increased risk of meconium aspiration and seizures resulting from hypoxia.

99. C: In the immediate postpartum period, a woman's gastric motility is generally decreased because of both hormonal effects and the lack of adequate abdominal muscle tone. Because of this, the postpartal woman often experiences abdominal distension from gas and constipation. Spontaneous bowel movements usually occur by the second or third day after delivery, but the woman may benefit from increased fluids and fiber and stool softeners, especially if the stool is hard and the woman must strain to defecate.

100. B: If a woman's white blood cell count was 20,000 after delivery and increased to 40,000 by the second day, this likely indicates an acute infection. The WBC count is commonly between 20,000 and 30,000 after delivery but it should start to fall and return to normal levels within 3-7 days. A sudden marked increase is always cause for concern and further tests and should be carried out to determine the cause of the increase.

101. C: If testing after birth shows that a neonate has inherited galactosemia, an inborn error of metabolism, the neonate should be fed soy-based formula. Because the child cannot metabolize galactose, which is derived from metabolism of lactose, the infant can never have any product that contains either, and this eliminates all milk products, including human milk. Failure to diagnose and treat can result in organ damage (liver, kidneys), intellectual disabilities, cataracts, and death.

102. A: If a breastfeeding woman shows a nonimmune rubella titer prior to discharge, the woman should be given and MMR vaccine and continue breastfeeding. The MMR vaccination should not be taken by the woman during pregnancy or the month prior to becoming pregnant because the live virus used in the vaccine poses a risk to the developing fetus. The varicella vaccination should also be avoided. Safe vaccinations include tetanus and diphtheria toxoids, hepatitis B, influenza, rabies, and meningococcal.

103. B: The breastfeeding position that is good to relive plugged milk ducts and engorged breasts is the football hold. The baby's legs are tucked under the arm on the side the child is nursing. This position is often used with twins if the woman wants to nurse both infants at the same time. The football hold is also a good position for women who have had a Cesarean and have abdominal tenderness.

104. A: When assisting with the lumbar puncture of a preterm neonate, the correct position for the neonate is lateral with the trunk flexed (being careful to avoid over-flexion). If the neonate is term, this position or sitting position with the head supported may be used. Following the procedure, the infant should be kept flat for at least 60 minutes and cardiorespiratory and oxygen saturation continuously monitored during that period. If the infant received narcotic sedation for the procedure, monitoring should continue for 4 hours and the infant should remain NPO for 2 hours.

105. C: When an infant latches only to the nipple, the nipple is not able to extend as deeply into the infant's mouth as required for effective breastfeeding. The nipple must extend into the infant's mouth to the soft palate because if it ends at the hard palate, the suckling movements will result in irritation and discomfort. If, when a new mother is trying to breastfeed, the neonate latches on to just the nipple, the nurse should advise the woman to insert a finger at the side of the infant's mouth to break the suction and to start over. Appropriate latching (to both the nipple and areola) typically does not cause discomfort or irritation.

106. A: If a neonate exhibits neck rigidity after birth, this may indicate injury to the sternocleidomastoid muscle. The neonate should be able to hold the head up slightly when lying prone, but the head lags because of weakness of the neck muscles when lifted from supine position. The sternocleidomastoid muscle, one of the largest in the neck, allows the head to turn from right to left and the neck to flex. Because the muscle originates in the clavicle and sternum, clavicular injuries can damage the muscle.

107. B: A demarcated unraised red-purple lesion caused by capillaries below the skin on a child's face is a nevus flammeus (port-wine stain). Nevus vasculosus (strawberry mark) is a capillary hemangioma and is a raised, demarcated dark red lesion. Erythema toxicum is a transient rash characterized by perifollicular lesions (1-3 mm), white or yellow with pustules, which appears suddenly over all of the body (except the palms and soles). The cause of erythema toxicum is not known.

108. B: If a woman with flat nipples has started using a nipple shield while breastfeeding but the infant is not gaining adequate weight, the nurse should advise the woman to use the nipple shield for only 1-2 minutes and then remove it for the rest of the nursing period as the nipple usually elongates enough for the infant to latch on within this time. The breast stimulation is inadequate with a nipple shield, and the infant must work harder to nurse.

109. A: If a nursing neonate has a 5:1 suck/swallow ratio, this indicates non-nutritive suckling. The normal suck/swallow ratio is 2:1 or 1:1, which indicates that an adequate volume of milk is being obtained. If the suck/swallow ratio is 5:1 or greater, the neonate is probably getting very little or no milk and may become exhausted from trying to suckle, and the milk supply will decrease because of inadequate stimulation of the breast. The woman may need assistance from a breastfeeding specialist.

110. C: If a woman asks about bottle feeding human milk so the infant's father can experience feeding the infant, she should be advised to wait for at least 4 weeks. The suckling effort the infant makes is different with a woman's nipple than with a rubber nipple, and starting bottle feeding too early may result in nipple confusion and make the child resistant to nursing. Some infants are more sensitive to nipple changes than others.

111. B: Until a neonate regains body weight, the neonate should be nursed at least every 3 hours. If the neonate is sleeping, the mother should awaken the neonate because small infants can easily become dehydrated. Additionally, if the child wants to nurse more often, the neonate should be allowed to do so. Neonates usually nurse every 1-3 hours, so pacifiers should not be used to extend the time between feedings. Each session of nursing usually takes 20-40 minutes, so the mother gets very little rest in the first few weeks.

112. A: A normal percentage of weight loss for a neonate in the first few days of life is 5%. A weight loss of greater than 7% is cause for concern and may mean that the infant is not nursing adequately. As the mother's milk production increases, the neonate's weight should stabilize and then begin to increase at the rate of about 0.5-1.0 ounce (15-30 g) daily for the next few months.

113. B: When expressing milk from the breast, a woman should start by grasping the breast with a C hold with the fingers about 2-3 centimeters from the areola and should move about the breast in a clockwise manner. If the hand stays in a fixed position, not all of the milk ducts will empty. Once the breast is grasped, the woman pushes back and then squeezes while moving the hand forward (milking motion).

114. A: Women may experience exacerbation of autoimmune disorders, such as lupus erythematosus, after labor and delivery because the woman's immune system is no longer suppressed. So that the mother's body does not reject the fetus as "foreign," the immune system remains suppressed during pregnancy. Because of this suppression, women with autoimmune disorders often experience reduction of symptoms or remission during pregnancy.

115. C: If, on the first post-partum day, the woman's fundus is firm and lochia appears normal but the woman complains of perineal discomfort and BP falls to 88/50 and pulse increases to 112, the nurse should suspect a hematoma. Hematomas occur with bleeding into the connective tissues and may occur in the vulvar, vaginal, and retroperitoneal areas. In the vulvar region, the discoloration and bulging are noticeable, but vaginal and retroperitoneal hematomas are hidden and harder to detect.

116. C: If a neonate's cardiac status appeared normal at birth but 48 hours later the neonate experiences a precipitous drop in circulation to the lower body, the likely congenital heart defect is coarctation of the aorta, which is a stricture of the aorta, proximal to the ductus arteriosus intersection. As the heart tries to pump the blood past the stricture, the blood pressure to the head and upper extremities increases decreasing blood pressure and circulation to the lower body and extremities. Symptoms may not occur until the ductus arteriosus closes, causing sudden loss of blood supply to the lower body.

117. A: Following delivery, if the fundus feels contracted and in the right position but free flow of bright red blood is evident vaginally, this is likely due to vaginal or cervical lacerations. Lochia is usually a darker red and dribbles more slowly. Anytime bleeding occurs with a contracted uterus, this is a warning sign that the patient should be examined for lacerations because the patient may experience significant loss of blood if the laceration is undetected and untreated.

118. C: The hormone that stimulates the alveoli to produce milk is prolactin. As the infant suckles, this stimulates the breast and causes the pituitary gland to release increased oxytocin, which in turn causes the muscles around the alveoli to contract and send the milk into the main lactiferous (milk) ducts (the "let down" reflex). If the breasts do not receive adequate and frequent stimulation, the level of prolactin begins to fall and eventually milk production stops.

119. B: If a woman reports that her neonate cries frantically when hungry, this likely means that the woman is missing signs of hunger because crying is usually a late sign. Signs of hunger include the infant making licking or sucking motions, rooting, and head bobbing. The infant may also hold the hands in fists or bring the hands to the mouth. If the woman strokes the infant's lips or cheek, the infant will turn the head and try to suck.

120. B: Following an unmedicated delivery, a neonate should ideally begin breastfeeding during the first 1-2 hours. During this time period, the neonate is usually most alert. The smell of the amniotic fluid remaining on the baby and the mother's smell are similar, and this smell helps to guide the infant to the breast and facilitate nursing. Therefore, the neonate should be offered the breast before the first bath.

121. A: A woman who develops postpartal DVT should be carefully monitored for signs of pulmonary embolus because small clots can easily dislodge and travel to the lungs. Signs and symptoms include dyspnea, tachycardia, pallor, cough, falling oxygen saturation level, and anxiety. Any woman with onset of these symptoms should immediately have head elevated to relieve dyspnea and be administered oxygen per facemask at 8-10 L/min and the physician notified.

122. C: Stages of milk production:

- Stage 1: Occurs during late pregnancy. Increased progesterone and estrogen levels to bring about changes in the breasts that prepare them for lactation.
- Stage 2: Occurs postpartum. Both progesterone and estrogen levels fall and prolactin levels increase in order to promote milk production.
- Stage 3: Occurs with weaning. Prolactin levels fall as the breasts have decreased stimulation.

123. B: In order to prevent post-dural puncture (spinal) headache, the woman should lie flat for several hours. When spinal anesthesia is administered, a small amount of cerebrospinal fluid may leak out, and if the fluid level in the brain is low, this can cause a headache, especially if the head is elevated, until the volume builds up again. Adequate hydration is also important, and caffeinated beverages may provide temporary relief.

124. A: During the *claiming* part of parent-neonate attachment, the parent usually first compares the child to other family members by looking for family traits and noticing how the neonate is similar: "She has her father's eyes." This is usually followed by the parent noticing differences: "His hair is darker than his brothers'." Last, the parent begins to notice those things that make the neonate unique: "Look at those long fingers!"

125. C: After delivery, a woman is likely to exhibit signs and symptoms of hypovolemic shock with blood loss greater than 1500 mL. The blood volume typically increases by about 1500 mL during pregnancy, so the woman usually tolerates considerable blood loss. Once the extra 1500 mL of blood is lost, every 500 mL of additional blood loss usually results in a 3% drop in hematocrit. Hypovolemic shock results in hypotension, tachycardia, pallor, cool skin (from vasoconstriction), anxiety, and confusion.

126. C: The phase of maternal role transition during which the woman begins to feel like a mother is letting go. Phases:

- Taking in (0-48 hours): Needs assistance of others and is focused on her personal needs, but may want to talk about labor and delivery and may exhibit excitement.
- Taking hold (2-10 days or weeks): Eager to learn and to take care of neonate but needs support and approval of others to gain confidence.
- Letting go: Gives up fantasies of "perfect baby," begins to see herself as a mother and part of a family, and resumes role with partner.

127. B: If a neonate's chest circumference is 34 cm, the head circumference would normally be about 36 cm. Normal measures:

Weight	2500-4000 g (average about 3400). Physiologic weight loss is 5-10% for full term and 15T for preterm.
Length	45-55 cm (average 50 cm).
Head circumference	32-38 cm (usually 2 cm greater than chest circumference)
Chest circumference	30-36 cm
Blood pressure	56-77/33-50 mm Hg
Pulse	120-120 bpm awake; 100 bpm asleep; 180 bmp crying
Respiration	30-60 per minute

128. A: An indication that the woman may not be bonding with her neonate is when the mother exhibits disgust when the infant urinates and refuses to change the diaper. Other indications include showing a lack of concern if the neonate cries; failing to try to talk to, touch, or interact with the neonate; ignoring the neonate completely; or expressing disappointment with the neonate's appearance or gender.

129. B: Paternal transition to parenting includes three stages:

- Commitment: The father accepts the responsibilities of parenthood and begins to make plans.
- Attachment: The father bonds with the infant through touch and interaction, such as singing to the neonate or holding and helping to care for the neonate.
- Preparation: The father adjusts his life to accommodate the needs of the infant.

130. B: If a woman admitted in labor plans to relinquish her infant for adoption, the nurse should acknowledge the adoption plans: "I understand the adoptive parents have been notified that you are in labor." Broaching the subject in a supportive manner allows the mother to express feelings about the adoption if she chooses to do so. It's unlikely that little else is on the woman's mind, so pretending otherwise only isolates the woman and her feelings.

131. C: To prevent contamination, reconstituted formula (or any opened formula) for bottle feeding should not be stored in the refrigerator for more than 24 hours. It's best to prepare one bottle at a time for use although women often prepare multiple bottles for use, such as during the night or while the woman is away from the infant and others are feeding the child, and liquid formula containers may hold enough to fill multiple bottles.

132. A: To facilitate bonding between the woman and her neonate if the woman chooses to bottle feed, the nurse should encourage the woman to maintain eye contact with the neonate during feedings. Maintaining skin-to-skin contact while feeding also helps to promote bonding. Holding the infant with the head higher than the body helps to prevent the child from aspirating and decreases risk of subsequent ear infections.

133. B: The neonate of a diabetic mother whose blood glucose levels were elevated above 145 mg/dL during labor is likely to experience hypoglycemia (<45 mg/dL) and hypocalcemia (<8 mg/dL). Hypoglycemia occurs because the mother's elevated glucose levels during pregnancy cause hyperplasia of insulin producing cells and increased insulin production. Hypocalcemia is common with neonates of diabetic mothers although the reason is not clear.

134. C: The primary risk factor for metritis (uterine infection) is Cesarean birth. The risk of infection is approximately 25 times higher with Cesarean birth than vaginal birth, a concern with the increased numbers of Cesarean births. For this reason, most women are administered single-dose antibiotic prophylaxis after delivery. Colonization of bacteria in the genital tract increases the risk of infection. Incidence tends to be highest in those of lower economic status although infection can occur in any woman.

135. B: A woman with gestational diabetes is at risk of delivering a neonate with macrosomia (birthweight > 4500 g). The maternal elevated glucose results in excess production of insulin in the fetus, and this causes excessive growth. These infants often exhibit extra fat deposits in the trunk and shoulder, and this increases the risk of shoulder dystocia. Macrosomia also increases the risk of Cesarean birth because of the size of the neonate.

136. A: If a woman with a history of bipolar disease develops marked hyperactivity about two weeks after delivery with signs of postpartum psychosis, including confusion and anger toward the infant, the first intervention should be to ensure the safety of the infant. The infant needs to be removed from the mother's care because of the risk of infanticide with postpartum psychosis. In some cases, especially if no other family member can care for the infant, child protective services may need to be notified.

137. C: If a neonate is born with gastroschisis (stomach and intestines herniating through an opening in the abdominal wall) the exposed organs should be immediately covered with moist gauze dressings and wrapped in plastic (around the neonate's body) to secure and prevent further fluid loss and hypothermia. The infant must be maintained in supine position to prevent intestinal ischemia. Surgery is usually done within 2-4 hours of delivery.

138. B: Following delivery, the best preventive measure to reduce the risk of developing deep vein thrombosis (DVT) is early ambulation. Whether Cesarean or vaginal birth, the woman should be assisted to ambulate within a few hours of delivery. Early ambulation also encourages urination and stimulates bowel motility, reducing the risk of constipation. The woman should be advised to avoid crossing the legs because doing so may decrease peripheral blood flow.

139. A: A first-line treatment for gestational hypertensive disorders is nifedipine, although hydralazine or labetalol may also be used. However, they are administered intravenously while nifedipine is administered orally. Adverse reactions include dizziness, headache, flushing, and palpitations. The woman should be advised to avoid grapefruit. Use of nifedipine to control blood pressure must be balanced against potential fetal risk. Diuretics are generally avoided during pregnancy because of the risk of compromised placental perfusion.

140. C: A woman should be encouraged to room-in with her neonate during hospitalization in order to facilitate bonding. However, the woman should be assured that she can call for assistance with infant care at any time and that nurses will monitor both the mother and the neonate frequently. If the woman prefers to place her infant in the nursery for part of the time, the woman should also be supported in this choice.

141. C: On the day of delivery, a diabetic woman who has been receiving insulin for type 1 diabetes will probably require a lower dosage of insulin (and sometimes no insulin). The glucose level often drops precipitously after delivery, so the woman may require treatment for hypoglycemia. Regular insulin should be administered rather than longer acting insulin until glucose levels stabilize.

142. A: If a neonate has a hematocrit of 67%, this likely indicates polycythemia. Polycythemia (hematocrit >65%) develops in utero in response to oxygen deprivation. The fetus produces additional red blood cells as a compensatory measure. Polycythemia may also occur in neonates who are small or large for gestational age if the cord is milked after delivery. Polycythemia increases the viscosity of the blood. An exchange transfusion may be done to reduce the hematocrit to prevent neurological deficits.

143. B: If a Haitian woman states that she does not want to name her baby girl, the nurse should assume that delayed naming is a cultural norm. In fact, Haitians usually wait until after the first month to give their neonates a name. Naming holds special importance in many cultures, and names may be chosen to reflect religion, such as names chosen from the Bible or the Koran. Some Africans believe that the name may affect the child's fate. In some cultures, such as traditional Chinese, the father decides on the name.

144. B: Postpartum blues typically begins a day or two after delivery, peaks at 5 days, and subsides by about 10 days. Postpartum blues is characterized by emotional lability during which the woman may have mood swings and feel depressed and anxious. The cause is not clear but is likely some combination of physical factors (hormonal and body changes), psychological factors (anxiety, fear of caring for the child), social factors (loss of support), and/or cultural factors (unhappiness with gender of child, cultural expectations).

145. A: X-linked disorders affect primarily male offspring. The female carries two X chromosomes—one from the father and one from the mother. Because one chromosome is normal, this chromosome can compensate for the defective chromosome. However, if the male offspring receives a defective X chromosome, the Y chromosome cannot compensate, and the male will exhibit the disorder.

146. C: If a woman expresses concern that her 3-year-old child does not seem to love the neonate, the nurse should advise the woman that young children develop affection over time. It is normal for a young child to feel some degree of jealousy when an infant is brought into the home, and since the infant interacts minimally in the first few weeks, the young child may show little interest, but this should change over time if parents remain attentive and supportive.

147. B: A woman who is nursing her neonate usually needs to increase fluid intake by about 1000 mL per day to compensate for the 23-27 ounces of milk produced each day for the neonate. She should also increase calories by about 500 per day. However, this may vary depending on the woman's usual caloric intake and weight. If a woman is overweight and trying to lose weight, the woman should avoid reducing calories for at least the first 6 weeks until milk production is well established.

148. C: An antidepressant that is generally considered reasonably safe to continue during pregnancy for women with a history of severe depression is citalopram (Celexa®) although some studies indicate it may slightly increase the risk of persistent pulmonary hypertension in the neonate. Other SSRIs that are often continued during pregnancy are sertraline and fluoxetine. The risks should be balanced against the risk of exacerbation of depression. Paroxetine (Paxil®) has been linked to heart defects, and MAO inhibitors, such as tranylcypromine (Parnate®), should be avoided during pregnancy.

149. B: A neonate exposed to or infected with herpes simplex is treated with acyclovir. The risk of transmission of maternal infection to the neonate is about 50% with primary infection and 1-2% with secondary outbreaks. Infected neonates usually exhibit symptoms by 10-12 days, including skin, eye, and mucous membrane blistering. HSV may spread to internal organs, including the brain. Women with active lesions should have Cesarean birth within 4 hours of membranes rupturing.

150. A: Conditions associated with oligohydramnios (<500 mL) include urinary tract anomalies. After week 20 of gestation, most amniotic fluid is produced by fetal urine, so if urine production is inadequate, the volume decreases. Oligohydramnios can lead to pressure deformities (such as club foot), pulmonary hypoplasia, and compression of the umbilical cord. Chromosomal abnormalities (trisomy 21, 18, and 13) and obstructional lesions of the GI tract are associated with polyhydramnios (>500 mL).

151. C: Laboratory findings associated with disseminated intravascular coagulation include:

- Prolonged prothrombin and partial prothrombin times.
- Decreased platelet counts and fragmented RBCs.
- Decreased fibrinogen.

DIC is a secondary disorder of pregnancy, triggered by various conditions, including placental abruption, hypovolemic shock, eclampsia, post-partal hemorrhage, and sepsis. Treatment includes replacement blood products, anticoagulants, cryoprecipitate, coagulation inhibitors, and coagulation factors.

152. B: When assisting a patient to take a sitz bath to relieve swelling and discomfort of hemorrhoids, the nurse should assure that the water temperature does not exceed 105° F (41° C). Patients should continue a sitz bath for approximately 20 minutes. Patients who will continue sitz baths at home should be taught that, at this temperature, the water feels comfortably warm when tested on the wrist but not hot.

153. A: If the normal speaking voice is 50-60 decibels, the noise levels in the nursery and NICU should be maintained at 45 decibels or lower because excessive noise can be very stressful to neonates, resulting in overstimulation. Women should be advised to avoid exposing their neonates to loud noises, such as radios and TVs at high volume. If the neonate becomes stressed, the neonate's oxygen requirements increase, and the neonate may experience increased episodes of apnea and bradycardia.

154. B: With kangaroo care, the neonate in minimal (or no) clothing is placed between the mother's bare breasts to provide warmth and skin-to-skin contact. This can be done immediately after birth, but provides benefits to both mother and infant if continued, especially for preterm neonates. Neonatal benefits include better regulation of vital signs, calming, decreased periods of apnea, increase in weight gain, fewer nosocomial infections, and enhanced bonding.

155. C: If a neonate has a patent ductus arteriosus, the usual initial treatment is indomethacin. If given within 10 days of birth, the medication closes about 80% of defects. Patent ductus arteriosus (PDA) occurs when the ductus arteriosus that connects the pulmonary artery and aorta fails to close after birth. This results in left to right shunting of blood from the aorta back to the pulmonary artery, increasing the blood flow to the lungs and causing an increase in pulmonary hypertension that can result in damage to the lung tissue.

156. B: In the neonate, the nurse should immediately report any periods of apnea that last more than 20 seconds. Periodic breathing with periods of apnea lasting for 5-15 seconds is common in the neonate, but prolonged apnea is abnormal and may indicate respiratory distress. The neonate should be carefully examined for changes in skin color and depressed heart rate during episodes.

Stimulating the infant may trigger respirations. Other indications of respiratory distress include grunting respirations and sternal and intercostal retraction.

157. A: The wet neonate's temperature falls rapidly after birth if not promptly dried and warmed because of evaporation when the wet skin is exposed to air currents. Temperature drops rapidly (skin temperature falls 0.3 °C/minute) after birth with exposure to ambient room temperature but should stabilize within 8-12 hours. Temperature is often measured by axillary method (for 3 minutes) and ranges from 36.3-37.0 °C. To avoid a temperature drop, the neonate should be examined under a warmer.

158. C: Following birth, damage to the neonate's upper brachial plexus (C5 to C7) is likely to result in Erb's palsy, which affects both the upper arm and the forearm. Movement is diminished or absent with the arm extended at the side and the forearm prone. Brachial plexus injury is associated with macrosomia, breech presentation, and shoulder dystocia. In most cases, recovery occurs within 3-6 months, but some infants may require surgical repair although prognosis is poor for surgical intervention. Pseudoparalysis (lack of movement because of fracture) may be misdiagnosed as brachial plexus injury.

159. A: The purpose of administering vitamin K to a neonate it to facilitate clotting. Neonates lack vitamin K at birth, and are, therefore, at risk of developing clots until vitamin K begins to be synthesized in the intestines when the neonate begins to feed. The neonate is administered an injection of vitamin K1 (AquaMEPHYTON) in a single dose of 0.5-1.0 mg to prevent episodes of bleeding in the first week of life.

160. A: Parents should be taught to place a neonate on the back when the neonate is sleeping and unattended at all times to decrease the risk of sudden infant death syndrome (SIDS). Ideally, the baby should sleep in the same room with a parent for the first year, but in a separate crib on a firm mattress with a fitted sheet but no blankets, toys, of other bedding. The slats of the crib must be no more than 6 cm apart to prevent the neonate from getting the head caught between the slats.

161. A: Starting immediately after hospital discharge, the neonate should have "tummy time" 2-3 times daily for 3-5 minutes each time. During this time, the neonate should be constantly attended. Tummy time helps to prevent flat areas of the head and helps to strengthen the neck and shoulder muscles as the child lifts the head. The frequency and duration of tummy time should increase as the neonate gets older.

162. B: The normal position for the neonate's ears is with the insertion point of the top of the ear parallel to the outer canthus of the eye. The ears should be proportionate to the head size, soft and pliable, and cartilage should be firm by term. Low set ears are associated with a number of different congenital disorders, including trisomy 13 (Patau syndrome), trisomy 18 (Edwards syndrome), and intellectual disabilities.

163. A: When placing a newborn in a safety car seat, the seat should be rear facing and reclined 30-45 degrees (about half-way back) as this prevents the neonate's head from falling forward in a crash and blocking the airway. If the seat is reclined too far, the infant may slide backward (toward the front of the car) during a crash, injuring the head. A safety car bed may be necessary for premature infants.

164. C: If a neonate must undergo a medical procedure, sucrose analgesia (SweetEase™) should be given to the infant 2 minutes before the procedure begins. A pacifier is dipped in sucrose analgesia (24% solution) and given to the neonate to suck. The pacifier can be redipped every 2 minutes up to 4 times. Sucrose solution may be used in addition to other analgesia to provide comfort.

Contraindications include less than 32 weeks of gestation, hyperglycemia, feeding problems, severe illness, opioid sedation, paralysis, and NPO status (unless okayed by physician).

165. C: Score of 10. Silverman-Anderson Index:

Characteristic	0	1	2
Chest/abdomen	Rise together with inspiration.	Abdomen rises but upper chest lags or sinks.	See-saw movement
Intercostals	No retraction	Minimal retraction	Pronounced retraction
Xiphoid process	No retraction	Minimal retraction	Pronounced retraction
Nasal flaring	None	Minimal	Pronounced
Grunt (expiratory)	None	Grunt heard with auscultation.	Audible grunt

166. B: The newborn hearing test that measures the integrity of the middle and inner ear and the outer hair cells of the cochlea is the otoacoustic emissions test. Otoacoustic emissions (OAE) are sounds generated by the cochlea, the inner ear structure. The audiologist conducts the OAE test by inserting a probe into the infant's external auditory canal, and stimulating the cochlea with several clicking noises. The audiologist uses a microphone to measure the evoked OAE sent off by the cochlea.

167. A: The eye prophylaxis for neonates that is generally the drug of choice is erythromycin to reduce the risk that the neonate will develop neonatal ophthalmia because of maternal infection with *Neisseria gonorrhoeae.* Erythromycin is effective against both gonococcal and chlamydial infections and is less irritating than silver nitrate. If the mother has had prenatal care and received a negative screening for sexually transmitted disease, the prophylaxis, although required by most states, can probably be refused with little risk to the neonate.

168. C: If air becomes trapped in the alveoli because of meconium aspiration during labor and delivery, the neonate is at risk for pneumothorax. Thick meconium staining of the amniotic fluid poses considerable risk that the fetus will aspirate and develop obstructions. During inspiration, the bronchioles dilate to accommodate air, and this usually allows air to enter the lungs, but the bronchioles contract on expiration, and this can result in air trapping. If the alveoli become too distended, they may rupture, resulting in the pneumothorax.

169. B: ABO incompatibility can occur if the mother is O and the fetus is B or A. In this case, the mother carries no antigens for A or B but has anti-A and anti-B antibodies. If the antibodies cross the placenta and enter the fetal circulation, they can cause fetal hemolysis. ABO incompatibility causes less severe problems than Rh incompatibility, but ABO incompatibility can cause problems during the first pregnancy because the anti-A and anti-b antibodies are already present.

170. C: If a neonate with Down syndrome has skin that appears mottled at times (pale in some areas and flushed in others), especially if the neonate is exposed to cool air, the most likely cause is cutis marmorata. With this disorder, the blood vessels contract and dilate at the same time. This condition is benign and resolves over time. Neonates with Down syndrome are prone to having cutis marmorata, so the parents should be advised about the condition to allay their fears.

171. A: In order for a child to be born with cystic fibrosis, an autosomal recessive disorder, both parents must carry the defective gene. When both parents carry the defective gene (carriers), then the risk that the fetus in each pregnancy will have the disease is 25% and the risk that the child will be a carrier is 50%. With most genetic disorders (but not all), carriers have no symptoms and must be detected through genetic testing.

172. C: If a neonate is born to an HIV infected mother, the neonate should begin antiretroviral medications within 6-12 hours. The neonate is tested (ELISA and rapid tests) within 24 hours of birth to determine if the neonate is positive with confirmatory testing carried out by DNA PCR. The neonate should take medications for the first 6 weeks, and the mother should avoid breastfeeding as there is a risk of 0.7% transmission for each month of breastfeeding.

173. C: In order to prevent intracranial hemorrhage, a neonate with thrombocytopenia requires a platelet count of at least 30,000. Thrombocytopenia in the neonate is rare but may be caused by increased rate of destruction or decreased production. Thrombocytopenia is common with neonatal infections, which increase the rate of platelet destruction. The need for platelet transfusion varies according to the condition of the neonate with stable neonates requiring transfusion at counts <25,000 and unstable <50,000.

174. B: If a neonate's mother was addicted to methamphetamine use during her pregnancy, the neonate in withdrawal will likely exhibit high-pitched crying, hyperreflexia, excessive lethargy and sleeping with abnormal sleep patterns, poor feeding, frantic fist sucking, fever, and tremors. Neonates of amphetamine-addicted mothers are usually small for gestational age and may have a small head circumference because of the vasoconstrictive effects on placental circulation and nutrition to the fetus.

175. A: Neonates who are bottle fed need to be burped every 2-3 ounces. Breastfed neonates should be burped after nursing on each breast. Bottle fed neonates swallow more air than breastfed neonates and need to be burped more frequently. Indications that the neonate is uncomfortable because of gas in the stomach include grimacing, squirming, regurgitating, and crying. The neonate may be burped while held on the shoulder or in sitting position.

Maternal Newborn Nurse Practice Test #2

To take this additional Maternal Newborn Nurse practice test, visit our bonus page: **mometrix.com/bonus948/matnewnurse**

SCAN HERE

How to Overcome Test Anxiety

Just the thought of taking a test is enough to make most people a little nervous. A test is an important event that can have a long-term impact on your future, so it's important to take it seriously and it's natural to feel anxious about performing well. But just because anxiety is normal, that doesn't mean that it's helpful in test taking, or that you should simply accept it as part of your life. Anxiety can have a variety of effects. These effects can be mild, like making you feel slightly nervous, or severe, like blocking your ability to focus or remember even a simple detail.

If you experience test anxiety—whether severe or mild—it's important to know how to beat it. To discover this, first you need to understand what causes test anxiety.

Causes of Test Anxiety

While we often think of anxiety as an uncontrollable emotional state, it can actually be caused by simple, practical things. One of the most common causes of test anxiety is that a person does not feel adequately prepared for their test. This feeling can be the result of many different issues such as poor study habits or lack of organization, but the most common culprit is time management. Starting to study too late, failing to organize your study time to cover all of the material, or being distracted while you study will mean that you're not well prepared for the test. This may lead to cramming the night before, which will cause you to be physically and mentally exhausted for the test. Poor time management also contributes to feelings of stress, fear, and hopelessness as you realize you are not well prepared but don't know what to do about it.

Other times, test anxiety is not related to your preparation for the test but comes from unresolved fear. This may be a past failure on a test, or poor performance on tests in general. It may come from comparing yourself to others who seem to be performing better or from the stress of living up to expectations. Anxiety may be driven by fears of the future—how failure on this test would affect your educational and career goals. These fears are often completely irrational, but they can still negatively impact your test performance.

Elements of Test Anxiety

As mentioned earlier, test anxiety is considered to be an emotional state, but it has physical and mental components as well. Sometimes you may not even realize that you are suffering from test anxiety until you notice the physical symptoms. These can include trembling hands, rapid heartbeat, sweating, nausea, and tense muscles. Extreme anxiety may lead to fainting or vomiting. Obviously, any of these symptoms can have a negative impact on testing. It is important to recognize them as soon as they begin to occur so that you can address the problem before it damages your performance.

The mental components of test anxiety include trouble focusing and inability to remember learned information. During a test, your mind is on high alert, which can help you recall information and stay focused for an extended period of time. However, anxiety interferes with your mind's natural processes, causing you to blank out, even on the questions you know well. The strain of testing during anxiety makes it difficult to stay focused, especially on a test that may take several hours. Extreme anxiety can take a huge mental toll, making it difficult not only to recall test information but even to understand the test questions or pull your thoughts together.

Effects of Test Anxiety

Test anxiety is like a disease—if left untreated, it will get progressively worse. Anxiety leads to poor performance, and this reinforces the feelings of fear and failure, which in turn lead to poor performances on subsequent tests. It can grow from a mild nervousness to a crippling condition. If allowed to progress, test anxiety can have a big impact on your schooling, and consequently on your future.

Test anxiety can spread to other parts of your life. Anxiety on tests can become anxiety in any stressful situation, and blanking on a test can turn into panicking in a job situation. But fortunately, you don't have to let anxiety rule your testing and determine your grades. There are a number of relatively simple steps you can take to move past anxiety and function normally on a test and in the rest of life.

Physical Steps for Beating Test Anxiety

While test anxiety is a serious problem, the good news is that it can be overcome. It doesn't have to control your ability to think and remember information. While it may take time, you can begin taking steps today to beat anxiety.

Just as your first hint that you may be struggling with anxiety comes from the physical symptoms, the first step to treating it is also physical. Rest is crucial for having a clear, strong mind. If you are tired, it is much easier to give in to anxiety. But if you establish good sleep habits, your body and mind will be ready to perform optimally, without the strain of exhaustion. Additionally, sleeping well helps you to retain information better, so you're more likely to recall the answers when you see the test questions.

Getting good sleep means more than going to bed on time. It's important to allow your brain time to relax. Take study breaks from time to time so it doesn't get overworked, and don't study right before bed. Take time to rest your mind before trying to rest your body, or you may find it difficult to fall asleep.

Along with sleep, other aspects of physical health are important in preparing for a test. Good nutrition is vital for good brain function. Sugary foods and drinks may give a burst of energy but this burst is followed by a crash, both physically and emotionally. Instead, fuel your body with protein and vitamin-rich foods.

Also, drink plenty of water. Dehydration can lead to headaches and exhaustion, especially if your brain is already under stress from the rigors of the test. Particularly if your test is a long one, drink water during the breaks. And if possible, take an energy-boosting snack to eat between sections.

Along with sleep and diet, a third important part of physical health is exercise. Maintaining a steady workout schedule is helpful, but even taking 5-minute study breaks to walk can help get your blood pumping faster and clear your head. Exercise also releases endorphins, which contribute to a positive feeling and can help combat test anxiety.

When you nurture your physical health, you are also contributing to your mental health. If your body is healthy, your mind is much more likely to be healthy as well. So take time to rest, nourish your body with healthy food and water, and get moving as much as possible. Taking these physical steps will make you stronger and more able to take the mental steps necessary to overcome test anxiety.

Mental Steps for Beating Test Anxiety

Working on the mental side of test anxiety can be more challenging, but as with the physical side, there are clear steps you can take to overcome it. As mentioned earlier, test anxiety often stems from lack of preparation, so the obvious solution is to prepare for the test. Effective studying may be the most important weapon you have for beating test anxiety, but you can and should employ several other mental tools to combat fear.

First, boost your confidence by reminding yourself of past success—tests or projects that you aced. If you're putting as much effort into preparing for this test as you did for those, there's no reason you should expect to fail here. Work hard to prepare; then trust your preparation.

Second, surround yourself with encouraging people. It can be helpful to find a study group, but be sure that the people you're around will encourage a positive attitude. If you spend time with others who are anxious or cynical, this will only contribute to your own anxiety. Look for others who are motivated to study hard from a desire to succeed, not from a fear of failure.

Third, reward yourself. A test is physically and mentally tiring, even without anxiety, and it can be helpful to have something to look forward to. Plan an activity following the test, regardless of the outcome, such as going to a movie or getting ice cream.

When you are taking the test, if you find yourself beginning to feel anxious, remind yourself that you know the material. Visualize successfully completing the test. Then take a few deep, relaxing breaths and return to it. Work through the questions carefully but with confidence, knowing that you are capable of succeeding.

Developing a healthy mental approach to test taking will also aid in other areas of life. Test anxiety affects more than just the actual test—it can be damaging to your mental health and even contribute to depression. It's important to beat test anxiety before it becomes a problem for more than testing.

Study Strategy

Being prepared for the test is necessary to combat anxiety, but what does being prepared look like? You may study for hours on end and still not feel prepared. What you need is a strategy for test prep. The next few pages outline our recommended steps to help you plan out and conquer the challenge of preparation.

Step 1: Scope Out the Test

Learn everything you can about the format (multiple choice, essay, etc.) and what will be on the test. Gather any study materials, course outlines, or sample exams that may be available. Not only will this help you to prepare, but knowing what to expect can help to alleviate test anxiety.

Step 2: Map Out the Material

Look through the textbook or study guide and make note of how many chapters or sections it has. Then divide these over the time you have. For example, if a book has 15 chapters and you have five days to study, you need to cover three chapters each day. Even better, if you have the time, leave an extra day at the end for overall review after you have gone through the material in depth.

If time is limited, you may need to prioritize the material. Look through it and make note of which sections you think you already have a good grasp on, and which need review. While you are studying, skim quickly through the familiar sections and take more time on the challenging parts.

Write out your plan so you don't get lost as you go. Having a written plan also helps you feel more in control of the study, so anxiety is less likely to arise from feeling overwhelmed at the amount to cover.

Step 3: Gather Your Tools

Decide what study method works best for you. Do you prefer to highlight in the book as you study and then go back over the highlighted portions? Or do you type out notes of the important information? Or is it helpful to make flashcards that you can carry with you? Assemble the pens, index cards, highlighters, post-it notes, and any other materials you may need so you won't be distracted by getting up to find things while you study.

If you're having a hard time retaining the information or organizing your notes, experiment with different methods. For example, try color-coding by subject with colored pens, highlighters, or post-it notes. If you learn better by hearing, try recording yourself reading your notes so you can listen while in the car, working out, or simply sitting at your desk. Ask a friend to quiz you from your flashcards, or try teaching someone the material to solidify it in your mind.

Step 4: Create Your Environment

It's important to avoid distractions while you study. This includes both the obvious distractions like visitors and the subtle distractions like an uncomfortable chair (or a too-comfortable couch that makes you want to fall asleep). Set up the best study environment possible: good lighting and a comfortable work area. If background music helps you focus, you may want to turn it on, but otherwise keep the room quiet. If you are using a computer to take notes, be sure you don't have any other windows open, especially applications like social media, games, or anything else that could distract you. Silence your phone and turn off notifications. Be sure to keep water close by so you stay hydrated while you study (but avoid unhealthy drinks and snacks).

Also, take into account the best time of day to study. Are you freshest first thing in the morning? Try to set aside some time then to work through the material. Is your mind clearer in the afternoon or evening? Schedule your study session then. Another method is to study at the same time of day that you will take the test, so that your brain gets used to working on the material at that time and will be ready to focus at test time.

Step 5: Study!

Once you have done all the study preparation, it's time to settle into the actual studying. Sit down, take a few moments to settle your mind so you can focus, and begin to follow your study plan. Don't give in to distractions or let yourself procrastinate. This is your time to prepare so you'll be ready to fearlessly approach the test. Make the most of the time and stay focused.

Of course, you don't want to burn out. If you study too long you may find that you're not retaining the information very well. Take regular study breaks. For example, taking five minutes out of every hour to walk briskly, breathing deeply and swinging your arms, can help your mind stay fresh.

As you get to the end of each chapter or section, it's a good idea to do a quick review. Remind yourself of what you learned and work on any difficult parts. When you feel that you've mastered the material, move on to the next part. At the end of your study session, briefly skim through your notes again.

But while review is helpful, cramming last minute is NOT. If at all possible, work ahead so that you won't need to fit all your study into the last day. Cramming overloads your brain with more information than it can process and retain, and your tired mind may struggle to recall even previously learned information when it is overwhelmed with last-minute study. Also, the urgent nature of cramming and the stress placed on your brain contribute to anxiety. You'll be more likely to go to the test feeling unprepared and having trouble thinking clearly.

So don't cram, and don't stay up late before the test, even just to review your notes at a leisurely pace. Your brain needs rest more than it needs to go over the information again. In fact, plan to finish your studies by noon or early afternoon the day before the test. Give your brain the rest of the day to relax or focus on other things, and get a good night's sleep. Then you will be fresh for the test and better able to recall what you've studied.

Step 6: Take a Practice Test

Many courses offer sample tests, either online or in the study materials. This is an excellent resource to check whether you have mastered the material, as well as to prepare for the test format and environment.

Check the test format ahead of time: the number of questions, the type (multiple choice, free response, etc.), and the time limit. Then create a plan for working through them. For example, if you have 30 minutes to take a 60-question test, your limit is 30 seconds per question. Spend less time on the questions you know well so that you can take more time on the difficult ones.

If you have time to take several practice tests, take the first one open book, with no time limit. Work through the questions at your own pace and make sure you fully understand them. Gradually work up to taking a test under test conditions: sit at a desk with all study materials put away and set a timer. Pace yourself to make sure you finish the test with time to spare and go back to check your answers if you have time.

After each test, check your answers. On the questions you missed, be sure you understand why you missed them. Did you misread the question (tests can use tricky wording)? Did you forget the information? Or was it something you hadn't learned? Go back and study any shaky areas that the practice tests reveal.

Taking these tests not only helps with your grade, but also aids in combating test anxiety. If you're already used to the test conditions, you're less likely to worry about it, and working through tests until you're scoring well gives you a confidence boost. Go through the practice tests until you feel comfortable, and then you can go into the test knowing that you're ready for it.

Test Tips

On test day, you should be confident, knowing that you've prepared well and are ready to answer the questions. But aside from preparation, there are several test day strategies you can employ to maximize your performance.

First, as stated before, get a good night's sleep the night before the test (and for several nights before that, if possible). Go into the test with a fresh, alert mind rather than staying up late to study.

Try not to change too much about your normal routine on the day of the test. It's important to eat a nutritious breakfast, but if you normally don't eat breakfast at all, consider eating just a protein bar. If you're a coffee drinker, go ahead and have your normal coffee. Just make sure you time it so that the caffeine doesn't wear off right in the middle of your test. Avoid sugary beverages, and drink enough water to stay hydrated but not so much that you need a restroom break 10 minutes into the test. If your test isn't first thing in the morning, consider going for a walk or doing a light workout before the test to get your blood flowing.

Allow yourself enough time to get ready, and leave for the test with plenty of time to spare so you won't have the anxiety of scrambling to arrive in time. Another reason to be early is to select a good seat. It's helpful to sit away from doors and windows, which can be distracting. Find a good seat, get out your supplies, and settle your mind before the test begins.

When the test begins, start by going over the instructions carefully, even if you already know what to expect. Make sure you avoid any careless mistakes by following the directions.

Then begin working through the questions, pacing yourself as you've practiced. If you're not sure on an answer, don't spend too much time on it, and don't let it shake your confidence. Either skip it and come back later, or eliminate as many wrong answers as possible and guess among the remaining ones. Don't dwell on these questions as you continue—put them out of your mind and focus on what lies ahead.

Be sure to read all of the answer choices, even if you're sure the first one is the right answer. Sometimes you'll find a better one if you keep reading. But don't second-guess yourself if you do immediately know the answer. Your gut instinct is usually right. Don't let test anxiety rob you of the information you know.

If you have time at the end of the test (and if the test format allows), go back and review your answers. Be cautious about changing any, since your first instinct tends to be correct, but make sure you didn't misread any of the questions or accidentally mark the wrong answer choice. Look over any you skipped and make an educated guess.

At the end, leave the test feeling confident. You've done your best, so don't waste time worrying about your performance or wishing you could change anything. Instead, celebrate the successful completion of this test. And finally, use this test to learn how to deal with anxiety even better next time.

Review Video: Test Anxiety
Visit mometrix.com/academy and enter code: 100340

Important Qualification

Not all anxiety is created equal. If your test anxiety is causing major issues in your life beyond the classroom or testing center, or if you are experiencing troubling physical symptoms related to your anxiety, it may be a sign of a serious physiological or psychological condition. If this sounds like your situation, we strongly encourage you to seek professional help.

Additional Bonus Material

Due to our efforts to try to keep this book to a manageable length, we've created a link that will give you access to all of your additional bonus material:

mometrix.com/bonus948/matnewnurse

www.ingramcontent.com/pod-product-compliance
Lightning Source LLC
LaVergne TN
LVHW062147200926
848484LV00007B/1871